Current Problems in Dermatology

Vol. 48

Series Editors

Peter Itin Basel
Gregor B.E. Jemec Roskilde

Tattooed Skin and Health

Volume Editors

Jørgen Serup Copenhagen
Nicolas Kluger Helsinki
Wolfgang Bäumler Regensburg

110 figures, 85 in color, and 25 tables, 2015

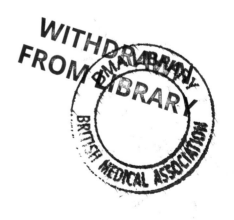

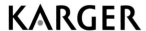

KARGER

Basel · Freiburg · Paris · London · New York · Chennai · New Delhi ·
Bangkok · Beijing · Shanghai · Tokyo · Kuala Lumpur · Singapore · Sydney

Current Problems in Dermatology

Prof. Jørgen Serup
Bispebjerg University Hospital
Department of Dermatology D
Copenhagen (Denmark)

Dr. Nicolas Kluger
Department of Skin and Allergic Diseases
Helsinki University Central Hospital
Helsinki (Finland)

Prof. Wolfgang Bäumler
Department of Dermatology
University of Regensburg
Regensburg (Germany)

Library of Congress Cataloging-in-Publication Data

Tattooed skin and health / volume editors, Jørgen Serup, Nicolas Kluger,
Wolfgang Bäumler.
    p. ; cm. -- (Current problems in dermatology, ISSN 1421-5721 ; vol.
48)
  Includes bibliographical references and indexes.
  ISBN 978-3-318-02776-1 (hard cover : alk. paper) -- ISBN 978-3-318-02777-8
(electronic version)
  I. Serup, Jørgen, editor. II. Kluger, Nicolas, editor. III. Bäumler,
Wolfgang, 1959- , editor. IV. Series: Current problems in dermatology ; v.
48. 1421-5721
  [DNLM: 1. Tattooing--adverse effects. 2. Coloring Agents. 3.
Epidermis--pathology. 4. Tattooing--legislation & jurisprudence. 5.
Tattooing--methods. W1 CU804L v.48 2015 / WR 140]
  GT2345
  391.6'5--dc23
                                    2015000919

Bibliographic Indices. This publication is listed in bibliographic services, including MEDLINE/Pubmed.

© Copyright 2015 by S. Karger AG, P.O. Box, CH-4009 Basel (Switzerland) and DOT/UETA (chapter by Schmidt)
www.karger.com
Printed in Germany on acid-free and non-aging paper (ISO 9706) by Kraft Druck, Ettlingen
ISSN 1421–5721
e-ISSN 1662–2944
ISBN 978–3–318–02776–1
e-ISBN 978–3–318–02777–8

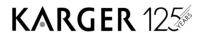

Contents

Preface

With some 100 million Europeans being tattooed, i.e. 10–20% of the adult population, it is timely to highlight tattooed skin and health.

Tattoos have been part of human history for thousands of years and have flourished due to people's emotions, aspirations and wishes to permanently express themselves as individuals. Today, as in the past, people hold the ownership of tattoos. Tattoos have a sunny side and a rebellious drive as well as a shadow. In modern society, tattoos are mainly decorative, used by both genders and span a broad range of social segments, age groups and ethnicities. The tattoo culture is global and serviced by a huge industry that operates across national borders and continents.

Unlike in the past, when soot and soil minerals were used for tattooing, tattoo colorants are now based on modern-pigment chemistry, which has allowed elaborate artwork on the skin. These pigments, however, entail a complex chemistry that is injected into the skin when getting a tattoo. Pigment particles are also sized in the nano-range. Modern scientific technologies that should be used to provide safer tattoo colorants and minimise the risk of the possible health concerns that come along with tattooing are now available. Tattooing can be considered the largest on-going human experiment on the injection of particles and chemicals into the human skin. However, this experiment has not been protocolled, has been off record, and has had no systematic surveillance. In contrast to the injection of medications based on one highly pure drug chemical, which passes astronomical regulatory requirements before being launched, the lack of regulation of tattooing is not logical.

The adverse events that we see in the clinic and know about have cast a shadow on tattooing and include allergic reactions from red tattoos, papulo-nodular reactions from black tattoos, scars and technical complications, psycho-social complications, and bacterial and viral infections, particularly those that may be life-threatening, such as acute blood infection and death, followed by slow-progressing viral infections and possible organ failure with a fatal outcome. The growing concern about multi-resistant bacteria, especially methicillin-resistant *Staphylococcus aureus*, as expressed in a warning by the World Health Organisation, is the number one future risk of tattooing. Therefore, the control of hygiene and sterility of inks is an urgent need. We *don't* see skin malignancies or malignancy of regional lymph nodes, which can be tattooed in cognito along with the skin. The potential carcinogenic risk of ink ingredients, such as polycyclic aromatic hydrocarbons, remains unconfirmed in the clinic, despite tattooed individuals being exposed to such a potential risk for a century. However, the research is scattered, and the potential risks to the body, internal organs and foetus are not excluded. The manufacturing of tattoo inks and chemical ingredients in inks cannot remain being not safeguarded.

Professional tattooists and recognised producers of tattoo inks are motivated and wish to contribute to the improvement of the safety of tattooing; however, amateurs, called 'scratchers', and producers of discount inks are significant players in the price-sensitive marketplace who are ready to occupy a larger volume if serious players are weakened under the weight of regulation. Regulation of the tattoo business is a very special challenge, and manufacturers face difficulties in their access to raw material pigments that are documented as safe. The 29 leading international pigment suppliers, under the Ecological and Toxicological Association of Dyes and Organic Pigments Manufacturers, will not run any corporate risk and will not sell their pigments for tattoo ink manufacturing. Therefore, the need for realism is obvious, and wisdom beyond technical insight and bureaucratic reference is necessary for the fulfilment of the ultimate goal, improvement of tattoo safety in real life.

The Council of Europe, with resolutions ResAp(2003)2 and ResAp(2008)1, initiated a development towards safer tattooing. In a very recent work documenting the safety assessment of tattoo inks, the Council experts have pointed out that dedicated animal experiments are necessary to assess tattoo inks. In 2014, the European Union committed the Directorate-General for Health and Consumers to prepare common European requirements for tattoo ink products to protect consumers. This was paralleled by the development of hygiene standards by the Comité Européen de Normalisation, with Deutsches Institut für Normung as the project leader. These important initiatives will mark a new era.

Improvement of the safety of tattooing is hampered by the massive deficit of academic insight into tattooing. The current research is truly premature and is covered by only a few hundred scientific publications in the world literature. Tattooing is a modality of its own; it is the multiple injection of ink particles across the skin barrier. Knowledge from other fields, such as cosmetics, laboratory research and traditional toxicology, cannot be uncritically applied to tattooing without proper validation.

The European Society of Tattoo and Pigment Research (ESTP) was founded on 13 November 2013 at the first European Congress on Tattoo and Pigment Research, ECTP2013, at Bisbebjerg University Hospital, Copenhagen, Denmark. The ESTP shall contribute to future research in the field. This book, which was edited by ESTP and inspired by the book 'Dermatologic Complications with Body Art', by ESTP board member, Dr. Christa de Cuyper in 2010, shall contribute to the future development of safe tattooing. This book is written for a broad range of people who are involved in tattooing, including clinicians who treat adverse events associated with tattooing.

This publication was only possible due to the generous contributions of the faculty of esteemed authors, each a specialist in their particular field. Karger Publishers did a marvellous job. This book was completed in only 10 months, from first inviting the authors to the final print and launch. Thank you!

European Society of Tattoo and Pigment Research (ESTP), April 2015

Jørgen Serup, MD, DMSc, Professor of Dermatology, Chairman of ESTP Bispebjerg University Hospital, the 'Tattoo Clinic' Copenhagen, Denmark

Nicolas Kluger, MD, Co-chairman of ESTP Helsinki University Hospital, Department of Dermatology, Helsinki, Finland

Wolfgang Bäumler, MSc, PhD, Professor, Treasurer of ESTP University of Regensburg, Department of Dermatology, Regensburg, Germany

Serup J, Kluger N, Bäumler W (eds): Tattooed Skin and Health.
Curr Probl Dermatol. Basel, Karger, 2015, vol 48, pp 1–5 (DOI: 10.1159/000369174)

The Cultural Heritage of Tattooing: A Brief History

Lars Krutak

Repatriation Office, National Museum of Natural History, Smithsonian Institution, Washington, D.C., USA

Abstract

For millennia, peoples around the world have tattooed human skin to communicate various ontological, psychosocial, and sociocultural concepts encompassing beauty, cultural identity, status and position, medicine, and supernatural protection. As a system of knowledge transmission, tattooing has been and continues to be a visual language of the skin whereby culture is inscribed, experienced, and preserved in a myriad of specific ways. If we are to fully comprehend the meanings that tattoos have carried across human history and into the present, then it would be useful to explore some of the ways tattoos, as instruments that transmit culture, have been deployed cross-culturally through time.   © 2015 S. Karger AG, Basel

Adornment

Across the indigenous world, tribal peoples rarely describe tattooing as an artistic or aesthetic practice because there are no terms for 'art' or 'artist' in the majority of indigenous languages. Instead, tattooing is integrated into the social fabric of community and religious life, and typically speaking, it is a cultural, clan, or family-mandated ritual that anchors societal values on the skin for all to see [1]. The tattooed dermis is a potent source of pride, precisely because it reenacts ancestral or mythological traditions. Wrapped in images of gods, ancestors, and spirits, tattoos have become venerated as symbols of protection, tribal unity, and genealogy.

However, it should be recognized that tattooing is sometimes used for beautification and is occasionally considered an artistic endeavor. Archaeological evidence indicates that the earliest tattoo, a 7,000-year-old tattooed mustache from South America, was cosmetic [2, 3]. Other anciently tattooed and mummified individuals from Nubia (ca. 2000 B.C.) and the Siberian Altai (3rd century B.C.) were adorned with ornamental tattoos that probably enhanced their sexuality and outward appearance [4]. In other locations, indigenous tattooists themselves have spoken about their indelible achievements. Alice Yaavgaghsiq, the last living Yupik tattooer of St. Lawrence Island, Alaska, approaches her tattooed creations the way a sculptor evaluates a piece of marble. When employing the timeworn technique of skin stitching, or needle and thread tattooing, Alice said: 'My designs came from my heart' [1].

Identity

Aesthetic considerations aside, the painful sensations and subsequent bloodletting associated with permanent body marking corresponds metaphorically to the process of being born, or rather, rebirth [5]. People gain new knowledge of themselves through painful stimuli like tattooing, and these sensate experiences model ways in which humans arrive at their ideas of existence and identity through imprinting new memories upon their consciousness and bodies [6].

In its traditional context, tattooing most often served to induct the recipient into indigenous society as a properly enculturated community member. As a rite of passage that belonged to the people, it also honored individual achievement and reinforced ancestral lineage ties through re-enacting traditional ritual practices. But, it was not the physical manifestation of the tattoo on the body that was most important because the intangible meanings embodied in its creation, form, function, and associated history were of paramount concern. For example, on the Northwest coast of North America, clan crest tattoos were a primary vehicle through which collectivities demarcated their identities in the social milieu [1]. The origins of crests were tied to supernatural and mythic events, and these emblems were believed to embody the spirits of ancestors, some of whom were creatures of the land, sea, and air. Each crest, whether it was carved into an object or tattooed upon human skin, also embodied an intangible property, such as associated names, stories, songs, or even geographical locations, that

belonged to the owner of the clan crest. The use of a clan crest set the group (clan) apart from others, while also defining its social position. Therefore, in Northwest Coast culture, the ownership of a crest, or the right to use the emblem, was more valuable than the possession of any physical object that might portray it, including a tattooed human body [1].

Status and Position

In many indigenous societies, tattoos were not applied by just anyone. The actual process was usually ritualized and performed by experts who were initiated and/or apprenticed into their position. Occasionally, the domain of tattooistry was reserved for priestesses, female aristocrats, healers, and shamans [1, 3, 7].

The intrinsic value of tattooing, however, was not simply confined to the technical or performative aspects of the tattooist. Rather, the power of the tattooist often arose from deities or helper and ancestral spirits who channeled their supernatural agency into the tattooist. In Samoa, tattooing experts (*tufuga tā tatau*) were always male, and they participated in lengthy apprenticeships to earn a place in the guild of tattooers. These priestly men were compelled to honor patron deities and follow traditional rules and prohibitions; otherwise, their tattoos lacked *mana*, or spiritual potency [8]. On the Great Plains of North America, only tribal priests who were the keepers of sacred tattoo bundles derived from primordial beings could create tattoos [1]. These religious leaders were initiated into their ceremonial position and were required to purchase and learn the requisite tattoo rituals in order to perform them. Their clients included men who had proven themselves in battle through the performance of a series of ritually mandated acts that varied between tribes and aristocratic women of high birth, whose bodies were tattooed to activate 'life-giving' powers [1]. The cultural tradition of warrior

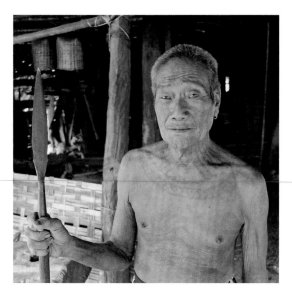

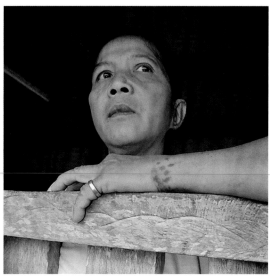

Fig. 1. Macham Naga tiger hunter U' Lum, 2014. © Lars Krutak.

Fig. 2. Kayan therapeutic tattoos of Wen Meriang, 2011. © Lars Krutak.

tattooing, where tattoos were earned and not freely given, was also widespread across Asia, Africa, Melanesia, South America, and Polynesia [3, 7]. Among the Yimchungru Naga of India and the Macham and Ponyo Naga of Myanmar, 'warrior tattoos' were also earned for killing tigers [9] (fig. 1).

Therapeutics

The medicinal aspects of tattooing have largely been underreported. The mummified, tattooed remains of a Neolithic 'Iceman' discovered in Europe in 1991 are the oldest known human evidence of curative tattooing, which was akin to acupuncture. More than fifty bluish-black tattoos were placed at major joint articulations, and radiographic analyses of the Iceman's corpse revealed considerable arthrosis in many of the same regions (e.g., lower back or lumbar spine, hip joints, knee joints, and ankle joints) [10]. The 2,500-year-old tattooed mummy of a tribal chieftain of the nomadic Pazyryk people of the Siberian steppes also displayed similar joint tattooing on his lower back and ankle joints [11]. In the historic period, the St. Lawrence Island Yupiit and Unangan (Aleut) of Alaska also practiced joint tattooing as a preventive against arthritic complaints and bodily pains [1, 3]. Today, the therapeutic tradition of joint tattooing continues among the Kayan of Sarawak and closely resembles that of the Iceman in placement and function [10] (fig. 2).

The efficacy of tattooing as a medical technology was great because the indigenous Ainu of Japan, the Yuki and Miwok of California, and the Chippewa, Menominee, and Meskwaki of the Great Lakes region of North America also tattooed to relieve rheumatism and joint sprains [10].

Utilizing carboniferous pigments, the tattooing was performed directly over the painful location. The Chippewa also tattooed to cure goiter, as did several peoples of the northern Philippines [10, 12]. Outside of these related cultural practices, tattooing was documented in Native North America as a treatment for a variety of other medical complaints, including heart disease (Deg Hit'an), lack of mother's milk (Chugach Eskimo, Canadian Inuit), consumption (Miwok), and toothache (Iroquois) [1].

Experimental biomedical research conducted in the 1950s and 1960s suggested that infants and young children who were unusually stressed through traumatic hardening practices (e.g., piercing, circumcision, scarification, inoculation, head modeling, etc.) displayed more rapid rates in growth and overall size at adulthood, perhaps due to the stimulation of hormones secreted from the pituitary gland [13, 14]. Belsky et al. [15] found that early childhood stress was also related to earlier onset of puberty. Studies in the 1990s concluded that individuals artificially stressed at the onset of puberty, which is another critical period in human development, also exhibited these and other biological benefits [16]. More recently, research has suggested that repetitive mild stress exposure has anti-aging effects and promotes longevity [17, 18]. All of this reminds me of the many historical statements made by indigenous peoples who recognized the biological benefits of tattooing in early youth and at puberty, specifically that these tattooing practices promoted health, fertility, and long life [1, 3, 19].

Apotropaism and Mimicry

Indigenous tattooists were often called upon by clients to apply preventive spiritual medicine upon their bodies via apotropaic tattoos. Spiritual possession and, even more so, being soul-less was greatly feared, and particular tattoo motifs were believed to repel the advances of malevolent spirits that infested the landscape [3, 7]. Sometimes, however, the dynamic power of the tattoo was instead related to the use of magical pigments and sacred tools that pierced the dermis [1, 3]. In other instances, the saliva of the tattooer was considered to embody supernatural power and was mixed with the tattooing pigment to neutralize or 'keep off evil spirits' from the tattooed client [1, 20, 21].

Many tribal peoples believed that spirits resided in communities, just like those of humans. They had camps and villages, they married and hunted, and they had their own habits and characteristics in the form of culture [22, 23]. Spirits could also take human or semi-human form, and I see no reason why they were not tattooed just like humans. Thus, when humans were provided with 'apotropaic' symbols on their bodies, perhaps this form of tattooing was not, strictly speaking, protective. Instead, this variety of tattooing may originally have been incorporative or created to mimic the symbols believed to be worn by spirits. In this way, tattooed spirits would see tattooed humans as fellow spirits and not as prey [1].

References

1 Krutak L: Tattoo Traditions of Native North America: Ancient and Contemporary Expressions of Identity. Arnhem, LM Publishers, 2014.

2 Allison JM: Early mummies from coastal Peru and Chile; in Spindler K, Wilfring H, Rastbichler-Zissernig E, Zur Nedden D, Nothdurfter H (eds): Human Mummies. A Global Survey of Their Status and the Techniques of Conservation 3. Vienna, Springer, 1996, pp 125–130.

3 Krutak L: The Tattooing Arts of Tribal Women. London, Bennett & Bloom, 2007.

4 Renaut L: Tattooing in antiquity; in Anne & Julien, Galliot S, Bagot P (eds): Tattoo. Paris, Musée du Quai Branly and Actes Sud, 2014, pp 22–26.

5 Gell A: Wrapping in Images: Tattooing in Polynesia. Oxford, Clarendon, 1993.

6 Jablonski NG: Skin: A Natural History. Berkeley, University of California Press, 2006.

7 Krutak L: Magical Tattoos and Scarification: Spiritual Skin. Aschaffenburg, Edition Reuss, 2012.

8 Galliot S: Samoan tattoos leave indelible global imprint. Voices 2011;27:10–11.

9 Krutak L: Tattooed tiger men of India and Myanmar. Total Tattoo 2013;106: 34–38.

10 Krutak L: The power to cure: a brief history of therapeutic tattooing; in Della Casa P, Witt C (eds): Tattoos and Body Modifications in Antiquity. Zurich Studies in Archaeology 9. Zurich, Chronos Verlag, 2013, pp 27–34.

11 Krutak L: St. Lawrence Island joint-tattooing: spiritual/medicinal functions and inter-continental possibilities. Etud Inuit 1999;23:229–252.

12 Krutak L: Kalinga Tattoo: Ancient and Modern Expressions of the Tribal. Aschaffenburg, Edition Reuss, 2010.

13 Landauer TK, Whiting JWM: Infantile stimulation and adult stature of human males. Am Anthropol 1964;66:1007–1028.

14 Levine SJ: Stimulation in infancy. Sci Am 1960;202:80–86.

15 Belsky J, Steinberg L, Draper P: Childhood experience, interpersonal development, and reproductive strategy: an evolutionary theory of socialization. Child Dev 1991;62:647–670.

16 Ludvico LR, Kurland JA: Symbolic or not-so-symbolic wounds: the behavioral ecology of human scarification. Ethol Sociobiol 1995;16:155–172.

17 Gems D, Partridge L: Stress-response hormesis and aging: that which does not kill us makes us stronger. Cell Metab 2008;7:200–203.

18 Rattan SIS: Hormesis in aging. Ageing Res Rev 2008;7:63–78.

19 Dias J, Dias M: Os Macondes de Moçambique. Lisboa, Centro de Estudios de Antropologia Cultural, 1964.

20 Karsten R: Civilization of the South American Indians: With Special Reference to Magic and Religion. London, Kegan Paul, 1926.

21 Searight S: The Use and Function of Tattooing on Moroccan Women. 3 vols. New Haven, Human Relations Area Files, 1984.

22 Bogoras W: The Chukchee. Publications of the Jesup North Pacific Expedition 7; Memoirs of the American Museum of Natural History 11. New York, G.E. Stechert, 1904–1909.

23 Viveiros de Castro E: Cosmological deixis and Amerindian perspectivism. J R Anthropol Inst 1998;4:469–488.

Lars Krutak
Repatriation Office, National Museum of Natural History, Smithsonian Institution
10th & Constitution Avenue NW, MRC 138, PO Box 37012
Washington, DC 20560 (USA)
E-Mail larskrutak@gmail.com

Serup J, Kluger N, Bäumler W (eds): Tattooed Skin and Health.
Curr Probl Dermatol. Basel, Karger, 2015, vol 48, pp 6–20 (DOI: 10.1159/000369175)

Epidemiology of Tattoos in Industrialized Countries

Nicolas Kluger

University of Helsinki and Helsinki University Central Hospital, Dermatology, Helsinki, Finland

Abstract

In 1974, the first professional French tattooist C. Bruno wrote a book, entitled 'Tatoués, qui êtes-vous?', depicting his experience as a tattooist in the picturesque Pigalle tourist district of Paris. However, we have come a long way since then. Tattooing has gained tremendous visibility, notoriety and popularity in Western countries. In Germany, 8.5% of the population (aged between 14 and 90 years) has a tattoo. Similar trends have been found in France, Finland and Australia, where approximately 10% of the populations have at least one tattoo. However, the overall tattoo prevalences overseas and in Europe are even higher, especially among the youth, for whom it is up to 15–25% according to the country. Much has been written about the tattooed and tattooists. However, who are they currently? What motivates them to get tattooed and give tattoos? How do they see themselves? Why do some individuals remove their tattoos? Is there a 'profile' of the tattooed? Are they really 'risk takers'? And how do the nontattooed perceive them? Through a critical review of the literature, we will reconsider tattooing from an epidemiological aspect, challenge current beliefs and explore new insights into the motivations and fears of tattoo artists and their clients.   © 2015 S. Karger AG, Basel

For the past 20 years, body art, mainly tattooing and piercing, has gained tremendous popularity and visibility in Western countries. Until quite recently, we had only limited data on the absolute prevalence of tattooing and piercing practices [1]. Recently, these practices have become the center of interest, and publications have flourished. This interest has included not only the prevalence of but also motivations for getting tattooed and the perceptions of tattooed individuals by other nontattooed subjects in addition to their self-perceptions. We review here the epidemiology of tattooed individuals in Western countries.

Tattooing as a Trademark of the X and Millennial Generations

Whether studies have been performed in the USA, in Europe or in Australia, the overall prevalence of tattooing is around 10–20% [2–12]. Results have varied according to the studied population, the country of origin and the time when the studies were performed. Currently, the 'elder' generations, known as the 'Boomers' and the 'Silent' Generation (especially individuals over 45 and 65 years of age), are clearly less tattooed than the young [5]. This observation is explained by the fact that getting tattooed in the 1950s–1960s was far from being mainstream and was definitely not accepted by the middle classes in the USA and in Europe [13]. Tattoos were then associated with sailors, the military, criminals, prostitutes and other marginal groups [13]. It is not surprising that in 2006, Stirn et al. reported 'only' an 8.5% prevalence of tattooed individuals in Germany in a study including individuals up to 90 years of age [8]. In their national survey in 2004, Laumann et al. clearly showed that the current tattooed generation was born at the end of the 1970s – beginning of the 1980s [2]. The prevalence was the highest among individuals between 18 and 29 years of age [2]. Interestingly, 8 years later, in 2012, the Harris Poll Interactive confirmed that the very same group (now aged 30–39) was still the predominant tattooed group in the USA [6].

The prevalence of tattooing in the general population is rising. The Harris Polls, which were performed successively in 2003, 2008 [4] and 2012 [6], reported an overall increase in tattooing from 2003 to 2012 for the general population, and for the men and women, prevalences increased by 16%, 16 and 15–21%, 19 and 23%, respectively [6].

Tattooing definitely belongs to Generation X and is a part of the Millennial Generation, mainly those born at the beginning of the 1980s [5]. It is still too early to know whether the next generation and the youngest group of the Millennial Generation will follow the tattooing trend as eagerly as the previous one. One could expect a decrease as a form of defiance and rejection against such trends belonging to the previous generation.

Are There More Tattooed Women than Men?

Traditionally, tattooing has been more prevalent among men, or at least it has been more accepted for a male to be tattooed than a female, as we will see below. Consequently, the numbers of women with tattoos used to be fewer than those of tattooed men (table 1). As illustrated in Australia,

tattooing is more common among older age groups, particularly in men over 40 years of age [12]. However, over the past 20 years, this trend has progressively changed. In the beginning of the 1990s, half of all tattoos were already being performed on women from every social class [14]. The incidence of tattoos among women has quadrupled, and today, the figures for the two genders approach equality [5]. In some studies, the trend has even inverted. In the USA, the prevalence of tattooed women has surpassed that of tattooed men (23 vs. 19%) [6]. In Australia, men are significantly more likely to be tattooed than women (15.4 vs. 13.6%) [12]. However, among individuals 20–29 years of age, tattooed women clearly predominate in Australia (29.4 vs. 22.3%) [12].

The choice of a tattoo is also guided somewhat by gender [1, 15]. Men often have multiple tattoos located mainly on the arms and upper back and on an exposed area. In contrast, women tend to choose more discrete, less visible, smaller and unique tattoos [1, 15]. However, the visibility of tattoos is variable. According to the Pew Research Center [5], over 70% of interviewed individuals reported that their tattoos were not usually visible. Visibility may, however, depend on the clothing worn [5].

Cosmetic tattoos (or permanent make-up) are usually performed on the faces of women (eyelids, eyebrows, and lips) for various reasons. It is not clear whether those tattoos are always included in studies or not, but they are an additional explanation of the increased prevalence of tattooing among women, both young and old [16].

The impact of peer influence is quite important. Indeed, 75% of young tattooed individuals have at least one close friend who is tattooed, and 29% have at least one immediate family member with tattoos [17]. Moreover, the number of tattoos is significantly related to the number of friends with tattoos, supporting the role of the friendship network [18]. Family influence is rather limited and at most weak. A correlation between the number of tattoos and the number of

Table 1. Prevalence of tattoos among adults in several industrial countries

Country/population	Year	N	Age, years	%	Men, %	Women, %
North America						
USA	2004	500	18–50	24	26	22
Random phone interview [2]			**18–29**	**36**		
			30–40	24		
			41–50	15		
USA	2008	452	Total	–	–	–
Internet survey [3]			18–49	–	18	29
			50–69	–	16	7
USA	2008	2,302	Total	14	15	13
National representative on-line poll			18–24	9		
(Harris Poll) [4]			**25–29**	**32**		
			30–39	25		
			40–49	12		
			50–64	8		
			65–	9		
USA						
National representative on-line poll	2012	2,016	Total	21	19	23
(Harris Poll) [6]			18–24	22		
			25–29	30		
			30–39	**38**		
			40–49	27		
Europe						
France	2010	958	Total	10	11	9
Nationally representative			18–24	8	–	–
phone interview [7]			**25–34**	**20**	–	–
			35–49	12	–	–
			50–64	5	–	–
			65–	1	–	–
France	2012	1,965	Total (mean	17	11.5	24
Random youth leaving a bar on			age: 20–22			
Saturday night [50]			years)			
Germany	–	2,043	Total	8.5	–	–
Face-to-face interview at home [8]			14–44	15	–	–
			25–34	–	22	–
Finland	2009	1,898	Total (15–29)	13	–	–
Youth barometer [9]			15–19	9		
			20–24	12		
			25–29	**19**		
Australia						
Random sample survey [10]	1998	10,030	>14	10	–	–
Random phone interviews [11]	2001–2002	19,000	16–59	12.6	14.5	10.6
Random phone interview [12]	2004–2005	8,656	Total	14.5	15.4	13.6

Bold values indicate the age group where the prevalence of tattooed individuals is the highest.

family members with tattoos has been noted [17]. Among family members, sisters have the highest influence [18].

According to Laumann et al., 65% of tattooed individuals got their first one before the age of 24 years [2], and in Germany, Stirn et al. found that 77% of individuals were tattooed before the age of 35 years [8]. In approximately 90% of cases, tattoos are performed in a professional tattoo shop [2]. In a rather limited number of cases (2.7–3.2%), they are performed at 'home' (home tattooing) [12, 19].

In 2009, a nation-wide internet-based survey was performed on German-speaking individuals that recruited 3,411 tattooed participants [19]. This study gave a fairly interesting snapshot of the 'typical' west European tattooed individual at the end of the first decade of the 2000s [19]. Overall, the mean age of the tattooed subjects was 30 years. They possessed professional tattoos (96%), usually one to 3 tattoos (73%), and many were of a single color (63%), typically black (59% of cases). These tattoos covered more than 300 cm^2 of the surface of the skin in 61% of the cases. The first tattoo was typically acquired during early adulthood, between the ages of 18 and 35 years (77%) was rarely acquired as a minor (17.6% were minors when they were first tattooed). Women tended to have tattoos on the trunk (54%), and men had more on the arms (48%). However, these results may be overestimates of the true values because this study selected tattooed aficionados who were more willing to participate and were more likely into tattoos. Tattooing was rarely performed at home (2.7%).

It's not possible to construct a general 'profile' of tattooed individuals because everyone is unique. However, several groups of subjects with tattoos sharing similar characteristics have been reported. Latreille et al. succeeded in defining 4 profiles of tattooed individuals based on a series of 151 consecutive French subjects asking for tattoo removal [15]. Of course, it is pointless and meaningless to try at all costs to put every tattooed individual into one of these groups. How-

ever, these data are of interest in terms of information campaigns about tattooing and tattoo removal to avoid unwanted tattoos, disappointment and unnecessary removal procedures. They are also useful in terms of creating more homogeneity with homogenous groups of tattooed subjects for further epidemiological studies. The four groups are summarized in figure 1.

Tattooing among Adolescents

Adolescents, e.g. high-school students under 18 years of age and college students, are undoubtedly the most studied group of interest (table 2). Studies have focused on subjects over 18 years of age [18] and under 18 years of age [20], disclosing different results. Tattooed adolescents see themselves as 'risk takers' [21]. They do not always seek advice nor inform their parents that they are getting a tattoo [22]. They may undergo tattooing despite not being allowed to by their parents [23]. According to a recent study in Naples, Italy, 73% of high-school students had body art that had been performed in unauthorized facilities [24]. There is a lack of perception of the possible risks related to body art, which indicates the need for proper information on body art-related health risks among adolescents [22, 24–26].

According to several North American studies [20, 27–30], body art, including tattooing, is associated with various risk-taking behaviours, such as substance use (cannabis, alcohol, and antidepressants) [27, 30], sexual activity, violent behaviour and school problems in adolescent populations aged 12–18 [20], 12–22 [28], and 11–21 [29]. Laumann et al. also have noted that a first tattoo acquired before the age of 18 years is associated with a time in jail of more than 3 days and the use of recreational drugs [2]. The age of acquisition of body art is related to a higher risk of the use of getaway drugs [28], as well as the receipt of amateur tattoos [28]. Nevertheless, other factors, such as the receipt of parental consent before

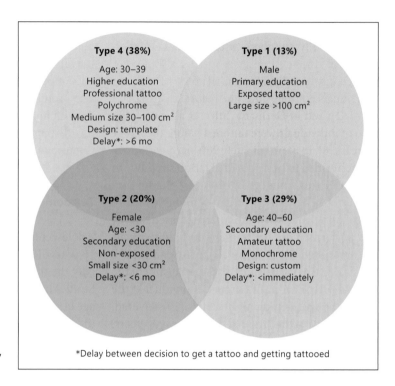

Type 4 (38%)

Age: 30–39
Higher education
Professional tattoo
Polychrome
Medium size 30–100 cm²
Design: template
Delay*: >6 mo

Type 1 (13%)

Male
Primary education
Exposed tattoo
Large size >100 cm²

Type 2 (20%)

Female
Age: <30
Secondary education
Non-exposed
Small size <30 cm²
Delay*: <6 mo

Type 3 (29%)

Age: 40–60
Secondary education
Amateur tattoo
Monochrome
Design: custom
Delay*: <immediately

*Delay between decision to get a tattoo and getting tattooed

Fig. 1. Tattooed individuals' characteristics grouped into 4 types, according to Latreille et al. [15].

obtaining a tattoo, a tattoo's meaning, and its location may come into account. Tattooing among high-school students and adolescents under the age of 18 years may be used as an indicator of risk behaviours.

Other Populations

Other populations have been studied regarding tattoos. Because they have been highly selected, results cannot be interpreted in any light other than the context in which they have been applied. Naturally, the same logic applies to the possible psychopathological implications of tattooing [31].

Although tattooing is illegal in most prisons throughout the world, it has completely integrated into the lifestyles of inmates. Tattoos may have been applied before imprisonment [32]. Of note, if tattoos are acquired in the community, a backyard tattooist or friend is rather frequently used [33]. Tattoos are more often applied during imprisonment for various reasons, including prison culture, protection, signs of strength and aggressiveness, remembrance, passing time/boredom, particular personality types or just because the prisoner liked tattoos [31, 33]. The prevalence of tattooed inmates is variable according to previous studies. It has been estimated that almost 40% of inmates get tattooed while in prison [32]. Results have differed according to the country. In Marseilles, France, 8.9% of inmates reported having been tattooed during the first 3 months of imprisonments [34]. In Chicago, Illinois, 66% of inmates have tattoos, but only 16% received them during incarceration [33]. In Victoria, Australia, 70% of prisoners have been tattooed, and 41% of them have been tattooed while in prison [32]. The main risk of prison tattooing is the transmission of blood-borne diseases, mainly hepatitis C, due to a lack of hygiene and asepsis [32–34], implying that

Table 2. Prevalence of tattooing among adolescents in several industrial countries

Country/population	Year	N	Age range (years) or mean age	%	Boys (%)	Girls (%)
North America USA Military beneficiaries attending an adolescent clinic [28]	2000–2001	552	12–22	13.2	8.1	16.6
USA School-based national representative sample [29]	1995–1996	5,837	11–21	4.6	4.8	4.2
Canada High schools, Quebec, Canada [20]	2002	2,145	12–18 12–13 14–15 16–18	8	5.8 4 4.9 8.5	9.8 3.5 7.6 18.1
Europe Questionnaire administered at high schools, Naples, Italy [24]	2008–2009	9,322	Mean age 16.1	11.3	11.7	10.9
Questionnaire administered at a university in the province of Naples [24]	2008–2009	3,610	Mean age 21.6	24	15.1	20.7
Questionnaire administered at public secondary schools, Veneto, Italy [25]	–	4,277	14–22	6	–	–
Anonymous written questionnaire self-administered to freshmen, University of Bari, Italy [22]	2009–2010	1,598	20.1	9.6	9	9.8
Other Brazil Examination of 18-year-old military recruiters (male) [23]	2010	1,968	18	10.8		–

prison administrations should take action to promote safe tattooing in prisons [35].

The military has been long reported as a subgroup for which tattoos are more frequently encountered. Tattoos may be performed by professional tattooists from the countries of origin of soldiers, abroad or more rarely, during deployment [36]. They are less frequently self-administered or performed by a friend [37]. They are usually performed in the context of peer group pressure [37]. The prevalence of tattoos ranges from 10% [23] to 44% [37–39]. The most common tattoo is a person's name [36]. However, in everyday practice, numerous French military individuals have been encountered with tattoos depicting their army corps. Currently, tattooing may be seen as a means of self-expression [36].

The body images of modern elite athletes have recently become important. An athlete's image reflects his or her identity and social, cultural and/or ethnic backgrounds. Most athletes follow current trends. Therefore, body art has gained increased popularity among athletes. Limited data are available on the true prevalence and incidence of body art among athletes. Benjamins et al. have reported a prevalence of 8.6%

for minority high-school athletes with tattoos [40]. Broadcasting and advertisements clearly show elite athletes harboring tattoos who participate in various sports, such as football, rugby and swimming.

The possible association between tattoos (and piercing) and eating disorders (anorexia nervosa, bulimia, or binge-eating disorders) has been raised by Carroll et al. [28]. However, thus far, this link appears to be at most low/modest [28, 41] and has not been confirmed [42]. Moreover, tattooing in this peculiar population could be seen as a sign of self-care and body image improvement rather than self-harm [42].

Background and Risk Factors among Tattooed Individuals

The question of whether tattoos could be a sign of deviance or of 'risk behaviours' always raises tension among tattooed individuals. This reaction is often the consequence of misunderstandings of the frame and extent of the interpretation of studies. Moreover, in our experience, it is not rare that media report only fragments of select data or that they are misinterpreted before being published to an inexperienced public. Any study has to be read and interpreted carefully. The reader always must consider the following: who, where, how many and how? Indeed, the reader must consider the specificity of each population (ethnicity, teenager versus adult, prisoner, military, etc.) and also the methodology of the study (face-to-face interview vs. self-reported anonymous survey, internet survey, etc.), the number of individuals included and whether the conclusions are adequate. There are always numerous factors and biases, such as studies among teenagers (usually way more frequent) versus a more general and adult population, the inclusion of other pieces of body art (piercings, microdermals, transdermal piercings, etc.), the number of tattoos, their sizes, their locations and even tattoo designs. Overall, the results of cohort studies are not applicable to a given tattooed individual, and association does not mean causality.

Education and Occupation

There is no doubt that the current prevalence of tattooing has increased in all social groups [2, 14]. However, tattooing remains more common among those of low socioeconomic and educational statuses [2, 12, 15, 23, 43–46]. The highest levels of education are associated with a diminished likelihood of being tattooed, especially in individuals who have completed secondary education [12]. In France, a difference in the working class is also notable. Up to 19% of workmen are tattooed, while only up to 7% of executives and 14% of middle managers are tattooed [7]. Stirn et al. have also reported that unemployment occurs significantly more often among tattooed individuals compared to controls [8].

Marital Status and Sexuality

Expressing sexual affectations or emphasizing sexuality through body art, tattooing or piercing, is a common motivation [13]. Clearly, piercing and tattoos can increase one's sexual attractiveness and sexual sensations. Popular beliefs have long related body art and piercing especially to male sexual orientation, sadomasochism or fetishism [45].

Individuals with tattoos are most often in a committed relationship, either living with a partner or being married or engaged similar to the general nontattooed population [2, 12, 47]. In Australia, tattooed women more often have a regular partner but do not live with them [12].

The sexual identity of either men or women is not associated with having tattoos [12, 45]. In Australia, men and women with more lifetime sexual partners are more likely to have a tattoo [12].

Having a tattoo is associated with being sexually active for both men and women [48] and early sexual initiation (e.g. a younger age at initiating sex) [45, 48]. Nowosielski et al. performed a study specifically focused on the sexual behaviours of young tattooed and/or pierced adults in Poland [45]. A younger age at first sexual intercourse and a higher number of lifetime sexual partners were observed among the tattooed participants. They may have more liberal attitudes towards sexuality, but importantly, tattooed adults do not engage in risky sexual behaviours. There was no statistical significance observed for the associations of tattoos with sexual preference, orientation, engaging in risky sexual behaviours, the frequency of masturbation or history of sexual abuse [45]. Recently, Swami corroborated that tattooed individuals are more likely to engage in sexual relations in the absence of commitment [49]. However, she also showed that this difference existed prior to obtaining a tattoo and therefore, this behaviour was not the result of tattoo procurement [49]. There is no difference in terms of sexually transmitted diseases between tattooed and nontattooed subjects [12]. Persons with tattoos should not be considered as belonging to a sexually transmitted infection risk group [45]. Of note, Stirn et al. [44] found among a group of 432 subjects with body art (piercings and tattoos) that 9% had reported to have been a victim of sexual abuse during childhood (7.4%) or adulthood (1.4%). These results were not found by Nowosielski et al. [45]. However, it is possible to regain a feeling of control over one's own body through body modifications [44].

Behaviours: Smoking, Alcohol and Drug Use

Tattooed individuals (men and women) more often disclose smoking habits compared to nontattooed individuals, as demonstrated by various studies in different countries [3, 12, 23, 43, 46, 50]. Not only smoking but also early smoking [50] and a higher level of daily cigarette consumption [50, 51] have been reported among youth. Having both piercings and tattoos is associated with an increase in smoking behaviours compared with having only tattoos [50].

The association of tattoos with alcohol consumption is far less clear-cut. It does not seem to be particularly increased among tattooed individuals in Australia [12]. According to Laumann et al., there are fewer 'never drinkers' among individuals with tattoos compared to those without them, and more tattooed individuals have a presumed drinking problem [2]. This same study reported a higher alcohol intake among tattooed individuals [2]. However, another self-reported study has reported that tattooed individuals are more frequently 'told to cut back alcohol,' although this finding was not statistically significant [3]. Tattooed adolescents report more binge drinking episodes than nontattooed adolescents [29]. Guégen has also observed that young French men and women with piercings and tattoos have higher levels of alcohol consumption on Saturday nights. However, adolescents with only tattoo(s) do not have higher levels than those who are nontattooed and nonpierced, which is suggestive of an association of cumulative body art with recreational alcohol consumption [52].

Recreational drug use (mainly cannabis use) has been reported to be more frequent among those with tattoos [2, 12]. This behaviour has been found in both adults and adolescents [28, 29].

Motivations to Get a Tattoo [13, 44]

The motivations that drive individuals to get one or more tattoos are plentiful. They have evolved from their primal uses for therapeutic purposes, as religious or subcultural group affiliation signs, as social status markers and as signs of strength [13] to simple fashion accessories. Understanding the motivations underlying the acquisition of tattoos is important to gain insights into the reasons why individuals modify their bodies and to contribute

Table 3. Motivational categories according to Wohlrab et al. [13]

Beauty, art and fashion   – Body embellishment
Individuality   – Self-identity, distinction from others, and control of one's own appearance
Personal narratives   – Expression of personal catharsis and personal values and reclamation of one's own body
Physical endurance   – Testing one's own pain threshold during the procedure and it's limits
Group affiliations and commitments   – Subcultural memberships
Resistance   – Resistance to society or to parents
Spirituality and cultural traditions
Addictions   – Physical addiction (endorphin release due to the pain experienced during the procedure) and psychological addiction ('tattoo collectors')
Sexual motivations
No specific reasons   – Impulsive decision, sometimes under the influence of drugs or alcohol

to the elimination of the negative stigmatization of body modification [13]. Wolhrab et al. divided motivations for tattooing (and piercing) into ten categories, as summarized in table 3. It appears that several motivations may be combined for any given individual, and they may change over time according to the tattoo and the evolution of the individual and their environment. The embellishment of one's body and the search for individuality seem to be the main driving forces for obtaining a tattoo. Due to the permanence of tattoos, the time needed to plan them, painful tattooing session(s) and after-care, it is reductive to consider tattooing *only* as a fashion accessory. Tattoos contain deeper personal meanings [13]. More recently, the results of a study of 432 subjects have confirmed that overall, individuals acquire tattoos and/or piercings mainly to express individuality and self-consciousness and to demonstrate autonomy and bodily control. Rarely, individuals

acquire tattoos to represent their belonging to a group or to be fashionable [44]. As Stirn et al. have stressed, currently, individuals want to be integrated into social environments and do not want to shock others. The Pew Research Center indirectly confirmed this point in their study, in which most adults (72%) acknowledged that they did not want to display their tattoos in public [5]. However, Stirn et al. observed that individuals with a higher number of body art modifications (tattoos and piercings) would be looking to shock others, provoke rejection, experience pain and feel that they are doing what they want with their body [44]. These very same individuals with high numbers of body modifications have also reported an addiction to body art and a desire to acquire more [44]. Moreover, some individuals who have reported past sexual abuse may see and use body art as an attempt to overcome their experience and reclaim their body. However, the efficacy of body art in this regard is debatable, as illustrated by those individuals who continually accumulate additional modifications [44].

How Do Tattooed Individuals See Themselves?

Among those with tattoos, 30% feel sexier. Twenty-five percent find that tattoos make them feel more rebellious, 21% more attractive or strong, 16% more spiritual and 9% healthier [6]. Only a limited number of tattooed individuals had opposite feelings about being tattooed (approximately 3%) [6]. However, the feelings of being sexier, more rebellious and more attractive were diminished when these findings were compared to the results from the same poll performed in 2003 [6]. The fact that less tattooed individuals currently feel more rebellious can be explained by the increased popularity of tattooing. The self-assessment of attractiveness has been confirmed in other studies [53]. Tattooed individuals are usually more extraverted, more experience seeking, and more often have a need to be unique [47, 49, 54]. Not surprisingly, they also have more positive attitudes towards tattoos than nontattooed individuals [47]. Even though tattooed individuals rate themselves as more rebellious, recent studies have pointed out that there are no significant differences between tattooed and nontattooed individuals' attitudes towards authority [49]. This result is in opposition with the old belief that tattooing is an act of rebellion/gang affiliation or truancy. This discrepancy may be explained by differences in methodologies between self-reported behaviours and the use of specific scales [49].

Tattoo Regrets and Reasons for Removal

Tattooing is permanent by definition; however, the human mind is versatile. Regardless of the origin of and reason for getting tattooed, some individuals will ultimately decide to have one of their tattoos removed. With the progression of removal techniques, the tattoo removal market has boomed within the past years.

However, the rate of regret may vary according to studied groups in terms of individuals' ages and interests (the general population, selected tattooed individuals, the military, etc.) and countries of origin, in addition to the time when the study was performed. Thus, in 2012, the Harris Poll reported that 14% of individuals regret getting a tattoo [6]. This proportion declined compared to the poll results from 2003 (17%) [6]. Similarly, according to Laumann et al., 17% have considered such a procedure (but had not yet received it at the time of the interview) [2]. One-third of British soldiers have acknowledged regretting their tattoos [37], while few have reported this regret in a very recent study of US military service members [36]. However, in studies performed on select groups of tattooed individuals, the rates of regret are lower. Indeed, Klügl et al. found that only 4.9% of tattooed individuals in a German-speaking country were not satisfied with their tattoos and were considering tattoo removal [19].

The reasons for tattoo removal are variable. The major reasons include never having been pleased with a tattoo, embarrassment or shame, and professional reasons [15]. Other motivations include the enhancement of self-esteem, social (change of lifestyle) and personal reasons (the tattoo feels incompatible with a patient's age or with their present attitudes/values), family pressure or a change of partner [55, 56]. According to Latreille et al., almost 25% of subjects who attended their laser clinic where not immediately satisfied with their tattoo upon acquisition [15]. Among a collegiate tattooed population, 13% did not like their first tattoo, 18% found that the artist did not meet their expectations and 22% were not happy with one or more of their tattoos [18]. These results stress the importance of carefully planning a first tattoo and of choosing a professional tattooist with artistic qualities.

How Do Nontattooed Individuals See the Tattooed?

Despite an obvious shift among the bearers of tattoos from marginal groups to the mainstream with tattooed individuals now being found in every social group, tattoos and tattooing are still associated with negative perceptions and connotations. According to the recent Harris Poll in 2012 [6], those without tattoos see people with tattoos as more rebellious (50%), less attractive (45%), less sexy (39%), less intelligent (27%), less healthy and less spiritual (25%) [6]. Moreover, retrospective analysis of the same poll administered previously in 2003 and 2008 showed a lack of variation. A recent study performed in the 10 largest US cities confirmed these results [57]. Twenty-four percent still considered that tattooed individuals were more likely to have deviant behaviours [6]. Women pay the highest price for being tattooed [14]. In a study of British soldiers, 67% of those without tattoos found that tattoos on girls were 'not attractive' [37]. Women with visible tattoos are rated more negatively [58, 59], and the size of a tattoo appears to be a predictor of the attitudes of individuals without tattoos [59]. Swami et al. have shown that tattooed women are perceived as less physically attractive, more sexually promiscuous and heavy drinkers. The more tattoos present, the higher the negative rankings were [60]. It seems that the participants of these studies held conservative attitudes with regard to gender, believing that women with tattoos, e.g. women with liberal gender attitudes, were not acceptable and rating them negatively. Interestingly, Swami et al. have observed that ratings are more negative if a woman is blonde compared to brunette (!), showing the impact of physical stereotypes on the ratings of individuals [60]. Guéguen has also confirmed that men perceive women with a tattoo on the lower back as more easily engaging in sexual intercourse on a first date [61]. However, some studies have shown different results. For undergraduate students, only the credibilities of tattooed men and women are affected but not their levels of attractiveness [62]. In other studies, students have reported a positive or supportive image of tattooed people [18, 63].

Unfortunately, the overall negative stereotypes are not only harmful to individuals in terms of their self-esteem and relationships with others, they may also impact their professional activities. The attitudes of employers toward prospective employees may be influenced by visible tattoos [64]. Several studies have been conducted on health care service employees in the USA. Stuppy et al. were the first to report the overall negative ratings of tattooed individuals by physicians and nurses [65]. Women respondents viewed tattooed people less favorably and yet again, they rated tattooed professional women more negatively than their male counterparts. Overall, these negative stereotypes may negatively affect the management and care of tattooed patients. We have observed that female anesthesiologists more often have a negative opinion about tattoos compared to their male colleagues and tend to more frequently refuse epidural analgesia in parturients with lumbar tattoos [66]. If tattooed patients are perceived negatively by health care providers, then some patients are also likely to perceive tattooed health care personnel more negatively. Thus, the nurse with the most body art (piercings and visible tattoos) would be perceived as the least caring, skilled and knowledgeable [67]. Again, tattooed female nurses are perceived as less professional than males with similar tattoos [68].

Tattooists

Interestingly, specific data regarding tattooists are lacking. There is currently no formation or training that qualifies someone to become a 'tattooist'. As such, a 'tattooist' is not considered thus far as belonging to a specific profession. Traditionally, tattooing is learned by years of apprenticeship in a

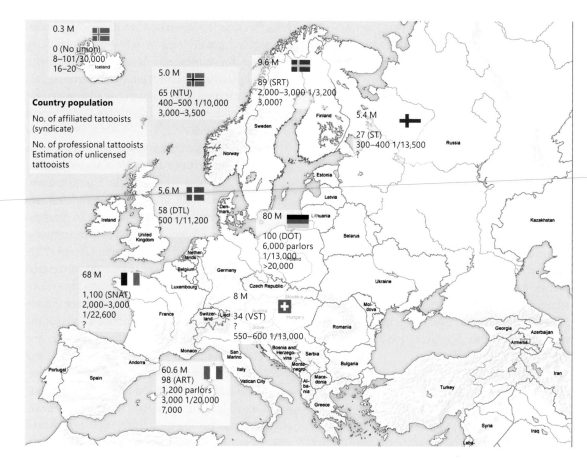

Fig. 2. Estimations of the numbers of tattooists in some European countries, including those belonging to a tattoo union, licensed tattooists and the estimated numbers of tattooists (including unlicensed ones) in 2013. Of note, the overall number of backyard/unlicensed tattooists is a self-estimation provided by tattoo unions upon request.

tattoo parlor in contact with experienced tattooist(s). Thus, tattooists are often 'self-educated'. Naturally, a tattooist needs to be gifted in the field of fine arts or plastic arts, although there are currently no schools that provide a 'tattooist' qualification. Virtually anyone can become a tattooist by buying tattooing materials and opening a tattoo shop as long the local legislation is respected. Such obligations vary according to the country. Because tattooists are often 'self-educated', it is important to insure for the safety of the customers and the tattooists themselves by providing them with a proper education and formation. In Western countries, despite the lack of legislation regarding the status of 'tattooist', tattooists have organized into unions/syndicates to promote tattooing and defend their rights as a specific profession. Meanwhile, national laws and legislation are starting to appear in an attempt to regulate this activity, ensure for the safety of customers and promote the proper functioning of the tattoo industry. For instance, in France, since 2009, tattooists have been obligated to be registered and to undergo training with regard to sepsis and hygiene. However, the tattoo industry has to face the rise of amateur or home tattooists (also called 'backyard tattooists' or 'scratchers'). The development of this market has been facilitated by the internet, which allows anyone to buy tattoo kits and inks. The tattoo industry considers them to be unfair competitors because unlicensed tattooists do not pay taxes or expenses related to parlor management. They usually can be found on the internet, providing inexpensive tattoos at home. In addition, home tattooing increases the risk of low-quality tattoos, which may lead to an increased number of tattoo removal procedures and an increased risk of infections because the sessions are not performed under adequate conditions of asepsis [69]. The real impact of this market is difficult to assess in terms of public health. Lastly, the proportion of allergic tattoo reactions that could be attributed to nonprofessional tattooing and the use of unauthorized inks is unknown. In figure 2, we summarize the number of 'official' tattooists in some European countries as well as an estimation of backyard tattooists, as determined by the tattoo syndicates.

Conclusions

Tattooing has grown in popularity and definitely belongs to the realm of generational conformity. Young adults and adults mainly see tattooing as a form of body art and not as a deviant behaviour [18]. Caution is necessary when it comes to attributing psychopathology to tattooed adults [70]. However, for adolescents, tattoos could be a sign of risk behaviours. Unfortunately, tattooing remains associated with negative stereotypes that may impact the personal and professional lives of tattooed individuals.

The tattooed generation is now aged between 20 and 40 years (born from 1975 to 1990). The youth may not always perceive the risks of tattooing. The proper education of young customers and also of tattooists is mandatory to prevent complications. Moreover, this very same population will grow old and age with their tattoos. Physicians may expect to see more tattoo-related complications, whether they are related to tattooing or are just coincidental. The long-term issues related to tattoo inks are unknown. Lastly, some tattooed individuals will attempt to remove one of their tattoos. The long-term safety of lasers used for tattoo removal and the effects of the dispersion of tattoo ink by-products after laser treatment are unknown. The increase in tattoo removal procedures has led to an unregulated market of tattoo removal by cosmetologists, tattooists, nurses and nonspecialized physicians as well as of 'do-it-yourself' tattoo removal procedures [71].

References

1 Laumann AE: History and epidemiology of tattoos and piercings. Legislations in the United States; in De Cuyper C, Pérez-Cotapos ML (eds): Dermatologic Complications with Body Art. Berlin/Heidelberg, Springer Verlag, 2010, pp 1–11.
2 Laumann AE, Derick AJ: Tattoos and body piercings in the United States: a national data set. J Am Acad Dermatol 2006;55:413–421.
3 Karagas MR, Wasson JH: A world wide web-based survey of nonmedical tattooing in the United States. J Am Acad Dermatol 2012;66:e13–e14.

4 Corso RA: Three in Ten Americans with a Tattoo Say Having One Makes Them Feel Sexier. Rochester, NY, Harris Poll, 2008. http://www.harrisinteractive.com/vault/Harris-Interactive-Poll-Research-Three-in-Ten-Americans-with-a-Tattoo-Say-Having-One-Makes-Them-Feel-Sexier-2008-02.pdf (accessed September 8, 2014).
5 Taylor P, Keeter S: Millennials: A Portrait of Generation Next: Confident. Connected. Open to Change. Washington, D.C., Pew Research Center, 2010. http://pewsocialtrends.org/files/2010/10/millennials-confident-connected-open-to-change.pdf (accessed September 8, 2014).

6 Braverman S: One in Five U.S. Adults Now Has a Tattoo. New York, NY, Harris Polls, 2012. http://www.harrisinteractive.com/NewsRoom/HarrisPolls/tabid/447/mid/1508/articleId/970/ctl/ReadCustom%20Default/Default.aspx (accessed September 8, 2014).
7 Fourquet J: Les Francais et les Tatouages. IFOP, 2010. http://www.ifop.com/?option=com_publication&type=poll&id=1220 (accessed September 8, 2014).

8   Stirn A, Hinz A, Brähler E: Prevalence of tattooing and body piercing in Germany and perception of health, mental disorders, and sensation seeking among tattooed and body-pierced individuals. J Psychosom Res 2006;60:531–534.

9   Myllyniemi S: Taidekohtia: Nuoriso-barometri 2009. Helsinki, Opetusministeriö, Nuorisotutki-musverkosto, Nuorisoasiain Neuvottelu-kunta, 2009. http://www.minedu.fi/OPM/Nuoriso/nuorisoasiain_neuvotte lukunta/julkaisut/barometrit/liitteet/Nuorisobarometri_2009.pdf (accessed September 8, 2014).

10 Makkai T, McAllister I: Prevalence of tattooing and body piercing in the Australian community. Commun Dis Intell Q Rep 2001;25:67–72.

11 Grulich AE, de Visser RO, Smith AM, Rissel CE, Richters J: Sex in Australia: injecting and sexual risk behaviour in a representative sample of adults. Aust N Z J Public Health 2003;27:242–250.

12 Heywood W, Patrick K, Smith AM, Simpson JM, Pitts MK, Richters J, Shelley JM: Who gets tattoos? Demographic and behavioral correlates of ever being tattooed in a representative sample of men and women. Ann Epidemiol 2012;22:51–56.

13 Wohlrab S, Stahl J, Kappeler PM: Modifying the body: motivations for getting tattooed and pierced. Body Image 2007; 4:87–95.

14 Armstrong ML: Career-oriented women with tattoos. Image J Nurs Sch 1991;23: 215–220.

15 Latreille J, Levy JL, Guinot C: Decorative tattoos and reasons for their removal: a prospective study in 151 adults living in South of France. J Eur Acad Dermatol Venereol 2011;25:181–187.

16 Armstrong ML, Saunders JC, Roberts AE: Older women and cosmetic tattooing experiences. J Women Aging 2009; 21:186–197.

17 Roberts AE, Koch JR, Armstrong ML, Owen DC: Correlates of tattoos and reference groups. Psychol Rep 2006;99: 933–934.

18 Armstrong ML, Owen DC, Roberts AE, Koch JR: College students and tattoos. Influence of image, identity, family, and friends. J Psychosoc Nurs Ment Health Serv 2002;40:20–29.

19 Klügl I, Hiller KA, Landthaler M, Bäumler W: Incidence of health problems associated with tattooed skin: a nationwide survey in German-speaking countries. Dermatology 2010;221:43–50.

20 Deschesnes M, Finès P, Demers S: Are tattooing and body piercing indicators of risk-taking behaviours among high school students? J Adolesc 2006;29:379–393.

21 Armstrong ML, McConnell C: Tattooing in adolescents: more common than you think–the phenomenon and risks. J Sch Nurs 1994;10:26–33.

22 Quaranta A, Napoli C, Fasano F, Montagna C, Caggiano G, Montagna MT: Body piercing and tattoos: a survey on young adults' knowledge of the risks and practices in body art. BMC Public Health 2011;11:774.

23 Bicca JF, Duquia RP, Breunig Jde A, de Souza PR, de Almeida HL Jr: Tattoos on 18-year-old male adolescents – characteristics and associated factors. An Bras Dermatol 2013;88:925–928.

24 Gallè F, Mancusi C, Di Onofrio V, Visciano A, Alfano V, Mastronuzzi R, Guida M, Liguori G: Awareness of health risks related to body art practices among youth in Naples, Italy: a descriptive convenience sample study. BMC Public Health 2011;11:625.

25 Cegolon L, Miatto E, Bortolotto M, Benetton M, Mazzoleni F, Mastrangelo G; VAHP Working Group: Body piercing and tattoo: awareness of health related risks among 4,277 Italian secondary school adolescents. BMC Public Health 2010;10:73.

26 Majori S, Capretta F, Baldovin T, Busana M, Baldo V; Collaborative Group: Piercing and tattooing in high school students of Veneto region: prevalence and perception of infectious related risk. J Prev Med Hyg 2013;54:17–23.

27 Braithwaite R, Robillard A, Woodring T, Stephens T, Arriola KJ: Tattooing and body piercing among adolescent detainees: relationship to alcohol and other drug use. J Subst Abuse 2001;13:5–16.

28 Carroll ST, Riffenburgh RH, Roberts TA, Myhre EB: Tattoos and body piercings as indicators of adolescent risk-taking behaviors. Pediatrics 2002;109:1021–1027.

29 Roberts TA, Ryan SA: Tattooing and high-risk behavior in adolescents. Pediatrics 2002;110:1058–1063.

30 Brooks TL, Woods ER, Knight JR, Shrier LA: Body modification and substance use in adolescents: is there a link? J Adolesc Health 2003;32:44–49.

31 Manuel L, Retzlaff PD: Psychopathology and tattooing among prisoners. Int J Offender Ther Comp Criminol 2002;46: 522–531.

32 Hellard ME, Aitken CK, Hocking JS: Tattooing in prisons – not such a pretty picture. Am J Infect Control 2007;35: 477–480.

33 Abiona TC, Balogun JA, Adefuye AS, Sloan PE: Body art practices among inmates: implications for transmission of bloodborne infections. Am J Infect Control 2010;38:121–129.

34 Rotily M, Delorme C, Obadia Y, Escaffre N, Galinier-Pujol A: Survey of French prison found that injecting drug use and tattooing occurred. BMJ 1998;316:777.

35 Gagnon H, Godin G, Alary M, Lambert G, Lambert LD, Landry S: Prison inmates' intention to demand that bleach be used for cleaning tattooing and piercing equipment. Can J Public Health 2007;98:297–300.

36 Lande RG, Bahroo BA, Soumoff A: United States military service members and their tattoos: a descriptive study. Mil Med 2013;178:921–925.

37 Gadd MC: A survey of soldiers' attitudes to tattooing. J R Army Med Corps 1992; 138:73–76.

38 Armstrong ML, Murphy KP, Sallee A, Watson MG: Tattooed Army soldiers: examining the incidence, behavior, and risk. Mil Med 2000;165:135–141.

39 Stephens MB: Behavioral risks associated with tattooing. Fam Med 2003;35: 52–54.

40 Benjamins LJ, Risser WL, Cromwell PF, Feldmann J, Bortot AT, Eissa MA, Nguyen AB: Body art among minority high school athletes: prevalence, interest and satisfaction; parental knowledge and consent. J Adolesc Health 2006;39: 933–935.

41 Preti A, Pinna C, Nocco S, Mulliri E, Pilia S, Petretto DR, Masala C: Body of evidence: tattoos, body piercing, and eating disorder symptoms among adolescents. J Psychosom Res 2006;61:561–566.

42 Iannaccone M, Cella S, Manzi SA, Visconti L, Manzi F, Cotrufo P: My body and me: self-injurious behaviors and body modifications in eating disorders – preliminary results. Eat Disord 2013;21: 130–139.

43 Rooks JK, Roberts DJ, Scheltema K: Tattoos: their relationship to trauma, psychopathology, and other myths. Minn Med 2000;83:24–27.

44 Stirn A, Oddo S, Peregrinova L, Philipp S, Hinz A: Motivations for body piercings and tattoos – the role of sexual abuse and the frequency of body modifications. Psychiatry Res 2011;190:359–363.

45 Nowosielski K, Sipiński A, Kuczerawy I, Kozłowska-Rup D, Skrzypulec-Plinta V: Tattoos, piercing, and sexual behaviors in young adults. J Sex Med 2012;9:2307–2314.

46 Kertzman S, Kagan A, Vainder M, Lapidus R, Weizman A: Interactions between risky decisions, impulsiveness and smoking in young tattooed women. BMC Psychiatry 2013;13:278.

47 Swami V, Pietschnig J, Bertl B, Nader IW, Stieger S, Voracek M: Personality differences between tattooed and non-tattooed individuals. Psychol Rep 2012; 111:97–106.

48 Koch JR, Roberts AE, Armstrong ML, Owen DC: College students, tattoos, and sexual activity. Psychol Rep 2005;97: 887–890.

49 Swami V: Written on the body? Individual differences between British adults who do and do not obtain a first tattoo. Scand J Psychol 2012;53:407–412.

50 Guéguen N: Tattoo, piercing, and adolescent tobacco consumption. Int J Adolesc Med Health 2013;25:87–89.

51 Drews DR, Allison CK, Probst JR: Behavioral and self-concept differences in tattooed and nontattooed college students. Psychol Rep 2000;86:475–481.

52 Guéguen N: Tattoos, piercings, and alcohol consumption. Alcohol Clin Exp Res 2012;36:1253–1256.

53 Kozieł S, Sitek A: Self-assessment of attractiveness of persons with body decoration. Homo 2013;64:317–325.

54 Tiggemann M, Hopkins LA: Tattoos and piercings: bodily expressions of uniqueness? Body Image 2011;8:245–250.

55 Varma S, Lanigan SW: Reasons for requesting laser removal of unwanted tattoos. Br J Dermatol 1999;140:483–485.

56 Armstrong ML, Roberts AE, Koch JR, Saunders JC, Owen DC, Anderson RR: Motivation for contemporary tattoo removal: a shift in identity. Arch Dermatol 2008;144:879–884.

57 Shannon-Missal L: Los Angeles is America's 'Most Inked Market'. New York, NY, Harris Poll, 2014. http://www.harrisinteractive.com/vault/Harris%20 Poll%2032%20-%20MMQ%20Tattoos_ 4.8.2014.pdf (accessed September 8, 2014).

58 Degelman D, Price ND: Tattoos and ratings of personal characteristics. Psychol Rep 2002;90:507–514.

59 Hawkes D, Senn CY, Thorn C: Factors that influence attitudes toward women with tattoos. Sex Roles 2004;50:593–604.

60 Swami V, Furnham A: Unattractive, promiscuous and heavy drinkers: perceptions of women with tattoos. Body Image 2007;4:343–352.

61 Guéguen N: Effects of a tattoo on men's behavior and attitudes towards women: an experimental field study. Arch Sex Behav 2013;42:1517–1524.

62 Seiter JS, Hatch S: Effect of tattoos on perceptions of credibility and attractiveness. Psychol Rep 2005;96:1113–1120.

63 Wiseman DB: Perceptions of a tattooed college instructor. Psychol Rep 2010; 106:845–850.

64 Bekhor PS, Bekhor L, Gandrabur M: Employer attitudes toward persons with visible tattoos. Australas J Dermatol 1995;36:75–77.

65 Stuppy DJ, Armstrong ML, Casals-Ariet C: Attitudes of health care providers and students towards tattooed people. J Adv Nurs 1998;27:1165–1170.

66 Kluger N, Sleth JC: Perception of tattoos among physicians: the example of anesthesiologists, tattoos and epidural analgesia (poster 13). 1st European Congress on Tattoo and Pigment Research ECTP, Copenhagen, Nov 13–14, 2013.

67 Thomas CM, Ehret A, Ellis B, Colon-Shoop S, Linton J, Metz S: Perception of nurse caring, skills, and knowledge based on appearance. J Nurs Adm 2010; 40:489–497.

68 Westerfield HV, Stafford AB, Speroni KG, Daniel MG: Patients' perceptions of patient care providers with tattoos and/ or body piercings. J Nurs Adm 2012;42: 160–164.

69 Kluger N, Saarinen K: Aspergillus fumigatus infection on a home-made tattoo. Br J Dermatol 2014;170:1373–1375.

70 Tate JC, Shelton BL: Personality correlates of tattooing and body piercing in a college sample: The kids are alright. Pers Individ Dif 2008;45:281–285.

71 Kluger N: The risks of do-it-yourself and over-the-counter devices for tattoo removal. Int J Dermatol 2015;54:13–18.

Nicolas Kluger
Departments of Dermatology, Allergology and Venereology, Institute of Clinical Medicine
University of Helsinki, Skin and Allergies Hospital, Helsinki University Central Hospital
Meilahdentie 2, PO Box 160
FIN–00029 HUS Helsinki (Finland)
E-Mail nicolaskluger@yahoo.fr

Serup J, Kluger N, Bäumler W (eds): Tattooed Skin and Health.
Curr Probl Dermatol. Basel, Karger, 2015, vol 48, pp 21–30 (DOI: 10.1159/000369177)

Tattoo Machines, Needles and Utilities

Frank Rosenkilde

Bel Air Tattoo, Copenhagen, Denmark

Abstract

Starting out as a professional tattooist back in 1977 in Copenhagen, Denmark, Frank Rosenkilde has personally experienced the remarkable development of tattoo machines, needles and utilities: all the way from home-made equipment to industrial products of substantially improved quality. Machines can be constructed like the traditional dual-coil and single-coil machines or can be e-coil, rotary and hybrid machines, with the more convenient and precise rotary machines being the recent trend. This development has resulted in disposable needles and utilities. Newer machines are more easily kept clean and protected with foil to prevent crosscontaminations and infections. The machines and the tattooists' knowledge and awareness about prevention of infection have developed hand-in-hand. For decades, Frank Rosenkilde has been collecting tattoo machines. Part of his collection is presented here, supplemented by his personal notes.

Electrical Tattooing

Before tattoo machines came into use, various types of handheld needles and other tools were used for tattooing, and I can only imagine that it must have been a good sales technique to be able to advertise electrical tattooing around 1890, when the electrical tattooing machines were developed. In this period, several persons applied for patents. The American Sam O'Reilly based his patent on Thomas Edison's electrical pen principle, which is a type of rotary machine. London-based Thomas Riley applied for a patent on a single-coil machine, and Alfred Charles South, who was also a Londoner, applied for a patent on a twin-coil machine. Technically, the modern machines are based on these principles, but they have, of course, been refined. Part of the author's collection of tattoo machines and equipment is presented in figs. 1–17, supplemented with detailed information in the legends.

Numerous types of machines that could be used for line, colour or shading functions have been developed over the years; some electrical, some even air powered, including dual-coil machines, single-coil machines, e-coil machines, rotary machines, hybrid machines. We could devote a whole book to the technical variations of all of these machines. Until recently, the dual-coil machine has been the most common in the world, but the refined technique behind the new rotary machines allows for adjustments that have been lacking in the old types.

The dual-coil machine is based on the same principle as the electrical doorbell. Its two coils cre-

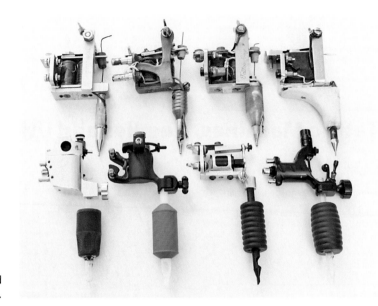

Fig. 1. This photo shows two types of tattoo machines. Old coil machines with fixed tubes and needles are shown in the upper row. This type is still used widely today. The bottom row shows different types of rotary machines with disposable grips. The main difference lies in the weight, materials and possibility of changing tubes and needles, a need that former times did not recognise.

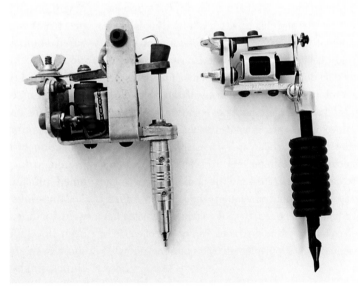

Fig. 2. The machine on the left is an old coil machine from around 1980, one of the first homemade machines I ever used. It has a non-disposable grip. A small, very light rotary machine from 2012 is shown next to it for comparison. It has a disposable plastic grip. Compared to the almost soundless and vibration-free rotary machine, the old machine is very noisy and vibrates violently. This is something that can be felt in the fingers after many years of working as a tattoo artist. The old machines weighed up to 400 g; the rotary machine on the right weighs 80 g.

ate an electromagnetic circuit, which makes the needle move up and down. The size of the coil and the number of copper wire wraps determine the strength of the machine. A liner can have eight-wrap coils, and a colour/shader may have 10–12 wrap coils.

A dual-coil machine consists of several components: the frame, which can be made of, for instance, brass, iron or aluminium, two copper-wire coils, a front and a back switch screw, a top adjustment screw, front and back springs, screws and washers, and a locking mechanism for the

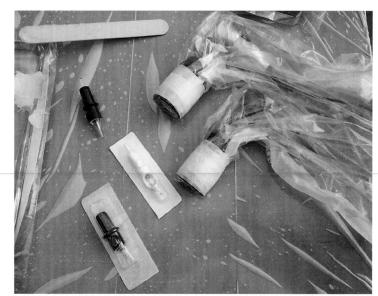

Fig. 3. This is a picture of a workstation covered in plastic. The special rotary machine, with its disposable needles, is ready to be assembled. The partially unpacked needle is of a type in which the tip is clicked into the tube. This system has become increasingly popular as price and availability have improved.

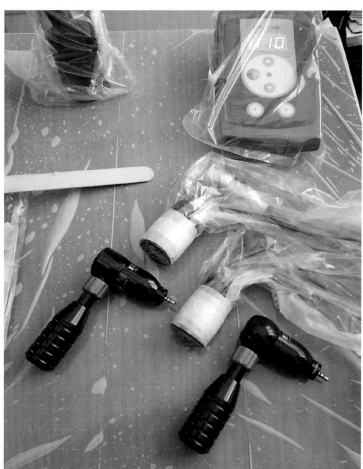

Fig. 4. Workstation with a special rotary machine for click-system needles. Two machines are covered in plastic, as are the wire, the bottle and the power supply; the two machines in front are uncovered.

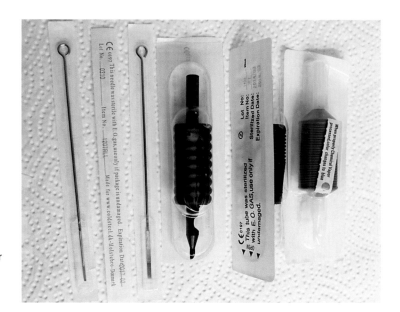

Fig. 5. Disposable needles and tubes. They come in sterile packaging and are mostly manufactured in China. They are usually of good quality, but in order to be 100% certain of quality and sterilisation, it is important to buy from a trustworthy supplier.

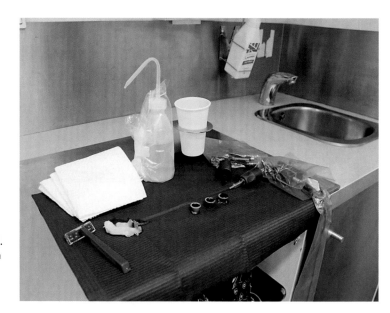

Fig. 6. A workstation on which all contact surfaces have been covered. Machines, wire, bottle (covered by a bag), machines with disposable grips and needles, disposable razor, jar, ink cups, ink and other objects.

grip, which forms an integrated part of the machine.

The combination of springs, hard/soft and short/long, and the distance to the top switch, with its adjustment screw, determine the impact of the needle. A liner machine, for instance, may have short, hard springs and a short distance to the top switch, which makes it run fast and consistently compared to a colour/shader machine, with its long, soft springs, which may run fast, but has a softer impact.

An adjustable power supply is used to set the speed; a liner machine with 8-wrap coils needed for a thin, three-needle line may run at 5–7 volts,

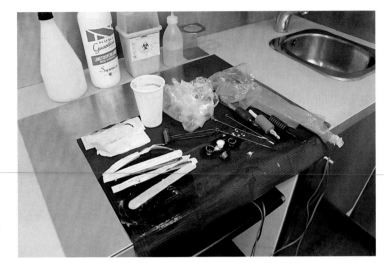

Fig. 7. A workstation after completion of a job. All material used for covering as well as the ink, excess Vaseline, razor, jar and needles will be disposed of. In the back, the container for used needles and various cleaning agents are shown.

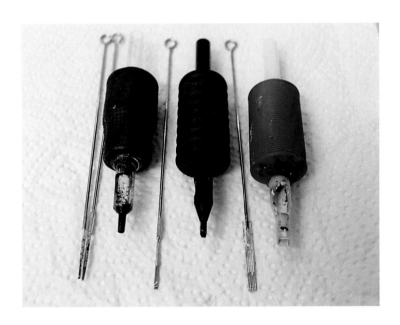

Fig. 8. Used disposable tubes and needles.

whereas a colour/shader machine with up to 15 needles may run at 7–10 volts.

Rotary machines have undergone a remarkable development over the last 10 years, but they are still powered by a small electrical engine. However, the old-fashioned direct drive with a shaft that forces the needle to go up and down usually has no adjustment possibilities, except for speed control, and an inexperienced tattoo artist may damage the customer's skin if he is unfamiliar with the machine.

There are many types of rotary machines being manufactured today: direct drive, hybrid, swash-drive, etc. Some are fitted with adjustment

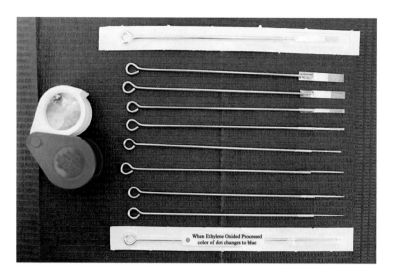

Fig. 9. Disposable needles are shown inside and outside their packaging. In the lower part of the figure, line needles and colour needles are shown; in the upper part of the figure, magnums, colour and shading needles. The thickness, length and point of a needle are all essential for the type of tattoo that is wanted. What we call a needle actually consists of several needles that are soldered together in various ways. A 'round' needle that is tightly soldered into a pointed shape may hold up to fifteen needles. This is used for outlining a tattoo. A soldering of up to fifteen needles will be used for colouring and shading. Magnums/flatshaders are soldered in layers. The larger the tattoo (for instance, a back tattoo with background), the larger the number of needles.

Fig. 10. With the use of a magnifying glass, it is possible to see if a needle is faulty or damaged. If you hit a sharp edge with the needle while working on a tattoo, the point may get flattened. The quality of needles from good suppliers is generally high, but if a customer bleeds excessively, it is important to check the needle to make sure that it is not causing the bleeding. A star pattern at the tip end of the needle means that it is faulty and must be disposed of.

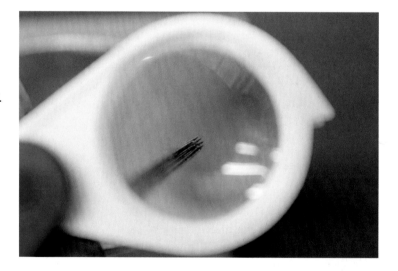

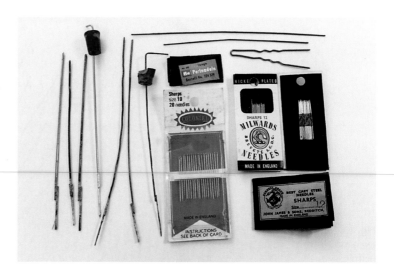

Fig. 11. Before the tattoo business developed into the industry that it is today, all tattoo artists made their own needles. This photo shows a selection of such needles. It took many hours to solder the needles into various combinations using jigs, soldering water, tin, metal sticks, etc. People had their own little tricks and, for lack of a better alternative, used ordinary sewing needles. But, over the years, we were able to get hold of better needles that mostly were manufactured in England.

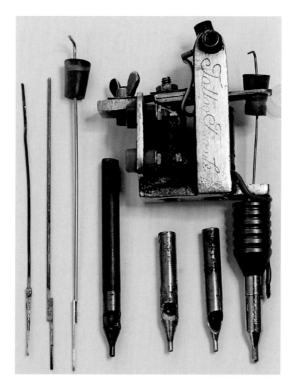

Fig. 12. This is a typical Danish finger-switch machine with a fixed grip and tube from the late 1970s that I have used myself. Some of these were still in use by the late 1980s, and their needles would often be left in for months – we didn't know any better! The used needles are lying next to the machine, and the tube still shows remnants of dried colour both inside and out. They were difficult to clean.

options and/or a spring dimmer that will cushion the impact of the needle. What they share is their sound. A coil machine can be very noisy, while rotary machines only make a humming sound – an advantage for nervous customers. Other advantages include their almost total lack of vibration and their low weight (some weigh below 50 g). This is beneficial to those tattoo artists who have wrist problems because the very old coil machines not only made a lot of noise,

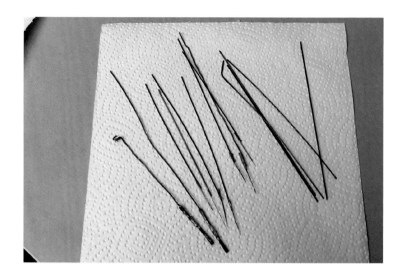

Fig. 13. Needles from the 1970s were mounted on spokes and hairpins.

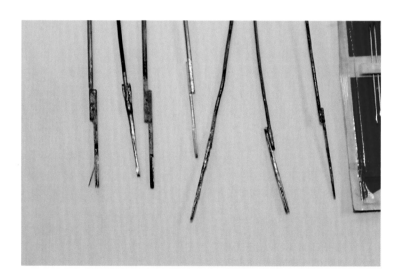

Fig. 14. These are the tip ends of used needles from the 1970s. They were often ordinary iron needles that could rust. Not such a good thing for a tattoo.

but also vibrated heavily and weighed up to 400 g.

Originally, the grips, with their tubes into which the needles were fitted, were fixed to the machine and were difficult to be replaced. At some point in the late 1960s, the American authorities demanded that tubes and needles be replaceable to facilitate mandatory sterilisation. The machines were developed accordingly, and needles and mounting methods were standardised. In Denmark, it was not until the late 1980s that we tattoo artists – at our own initiative – started working with sterilised, replaceable tubes and needles.

The grips consist of the grip itself and an inner tube that is made of steel, brass or aluminium. Some Danish and European tattoo artists fitted a wooden handle to a fixed grip, but since the late 1980s, most professional tattoo artists have been using stainless steel grips and tubes, which are cleaned and sterilised along with the needles in an

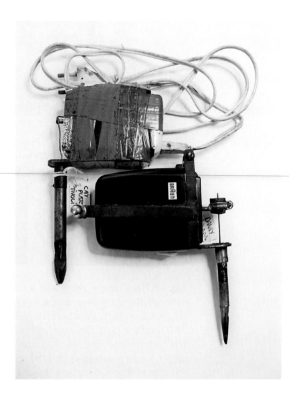

Fig. 15. These electrical razors have been rebuilt into tattoo machines and were often used in prisons. A prisoner with a bit of technical skill would easily be able to do this.

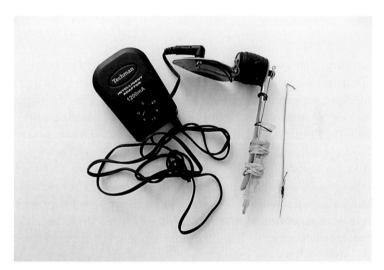

Fig. 16. This is a more recent prison machine. The engine is probably from a cassette player, and if you add to it a bit of scotch tape, a bent spoon, a ball-point pen and a sewing needle, you've got yourself a tattoo machine.

autoclave. This is now on the way out, as a wide variety of affordable, disposable plastic tubes are being marketed.

For many years, we exclusively used needles that were soldered in a round formation. Three needles for lines and seven needles for colour were the most common, and when lacking anything better, ordinary sewing needles could be used. But buying quality needles became easier over the years; particularly, British factories began manu-

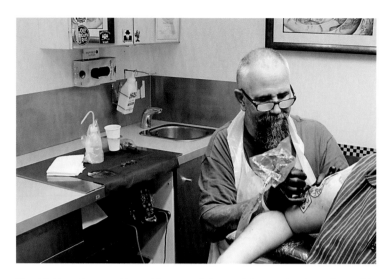

Fig. 17. Here, I am working with some of the machines and various disposable materials that have been described above. Working with modern machines and disposable materials is a big change from when I embarked upon my career in 1977, and the rapid development within my line of work has not stopped yet. The good thing is that we no longer have to do everything ourselves, for example, solder the needles, mix the colours, and build the machines. But, a lot of the charm that surrounded the old-fashioned tattoo parlours has definitely disappeared. I guess that is the price you have to pay for becoming popular and going mainstream; it still has been fantastic to be a part of it all.

facturing high-quality needles. Today, all needles are stainless steel. In the USA, magnums, rows of needles positioned in a slightly spread-out position on top of each other, have begun to be used and after a while we adopted this technique as well. For large tattoos and for fine shading, these needles can be very efficient. There are numerous types of needles, either long tapers or short tapers that indicate the point of the needle; #12/035 mm is most commonly used, and #10/030 mm is a type that mainly is used for lines, but there are many different contraptions round liner, round shader, flat shader, magnum, curved magnum.

Afterword

The development and popularity of the tattooing business since the year 2000 have been incredible. When I started out as a tattoo artist in the late 1970s, we were trying to refine the old sailor motifs. Today's tattoos can be veritable works of art. The business that was once quite small is now an industry, and machines, colours and techniques have been developed beyond belief. It has been fantastic to follow the development of tattooing and still be a part of it today. I am thankful for having been allowed to contribute to this book.

Frank Rosenkilde
Bel Air Tattoo
Aboulevard 31
DK–1960 Frederiksberg C (Denmark)
E-Mail belairtattoo@live.dk

Serup J, Kluger N, Bäumler W (eds): Tattooed Skin and Health.
Curr Probl Dermatol. Basel, Karger, 2015, vol 48, pp 31–36 (DOI: 10.1159/000369176)

The Technique and Craftsmanship of Tattooing in the Professional Tattoo Parlour

Lars Kristensen

DTL – Danish Tattooist Assoc., Sorø, Denmark

Abstract

This chapter will briefly explain the tools and techniques behind a good tattoo. Beside the fact that the professional tattoo artist needs to have talent for composing and drawing motives – the artistic part of his or her profession – the technical side of the process must also be mastered to make great tattoos. The craftsmanship behind the art. © 2015 S. Karger AG, Basel

Condition

The kind of tattooing described in this chapter is done with an electric tattoo machine.

This kind of tattooing has, in many ways, been unchanged since its patenting on the 8th of December 1891. The tattoo is coloured by getting under the skin of the customer, the same today as it was in 1891.

Since then, many technical improvements to other equipment that the tattoo artist uses, such as needles, colours, aftercare products, and the shop room, as well as improvements in the understanding of good hygiene, personal as well as for the shop room in which the tattoos are made, have been made.

Initial Customer Contact

The work process of a modern professional tattoo artist today starts at first contact with the customer. This could be over the phone, internet or in person.

From the beginning, it's important to make it clear to the customer that you, as a professional tattoo artist, take the customer's wishes and concerns seriously.

The professional tattoo artist takes time to guide and inform the customer about the known risks of using colour in a tattoo. Likewise, he or she informs the customer about aftercare of the tattoo: what you should do and what you shouldn't, and which products should be used, over the short- and long-term, when you take care of your tattoo.

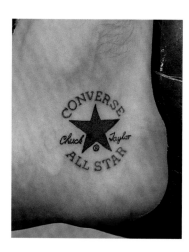

Fig. 1. Craftsmanship is not only about big tattoos. Sometimes, it's the detail that counts.

It's also very important to advise the customer regarding design, location, size, etc. (fig. 1). It's also a part of the work to say 'no' to tattoos that can't be made professional and satisfying, for example, tattoos on fingers.

A serious tattoo artist should also express his or her own subjective evaluation of a tattoo project. If the project is so controversial that the customer would get reactions that he or she did not expect from others, the tattoo artist should speak up. Then, the customer, based on the feedback from the tattoo artist, could decide whether he or she still wants the tattoo.

In the Shop

When a customer shows up in a shop to get a tattoo, the person – if he has chosen a professional tattoo artist, will enter a shop that is adapted to its purpose – the making of tattoos.

You will see many examples of shops that sell, for example, clothing or equipment. If this is the case, it's very important that the areas are clearly separated, so there is no doubt about where the tattoos are made. Also, this section should be ar-

ranged so the cleaning can be done in a proper and responsible manner.

You'll see that many tattoo artists have a tendency to collect souvenirs from their numerous trips around the world to tattoo conventions. Here, the same policy applies: the area where the tattoos are made should be easy to clean.

It must be clearly defined where the tattooing is done and where the waiting customers or accompanying friends should be seated.

Getting Started with the Tattoo

In the following, it is assumed that the professional tattoo artist follows the guidelines for good hygiene, which is described in one of the other chapters of this book.

The placing of the motive on the customer's body can be done in different ways. The most common ways are stencil or freehand drawing with skin markers – or a combination of both (fig. 2).

When the customer and the tattoo artist agree about the final design and placement of the tattoo, the actual work with the tattoo begins (fig. 3).

Nowadays, the tattoo artist can use different kinds of machines and needles, which is described in another chapter of this book.

It is important to use the right products in this process. Quality products. It does matter whether you work with a professional machine for USD 600 or a Chinese copy for USD 10. There is a difference. The expensive machine will transfer the ink with accuracy and uniformity into the customer's skin, whereas the Chinese copy typically works with irregularity and damages the skin.

The same applies for the needles. More expensive needles, purchased through a recognised dealer, work better and safer than the cheaper Chinese-copy products. You, as a tattoo artist, can directly import from the manufacturer.

You might be lucky to find one in a hundred cheap needles that work. However, the quality

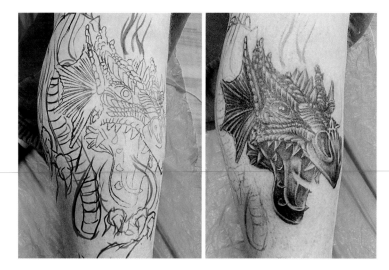

Fig. 2. Example of a combination of stencil and freehand drawing using a skin marker.

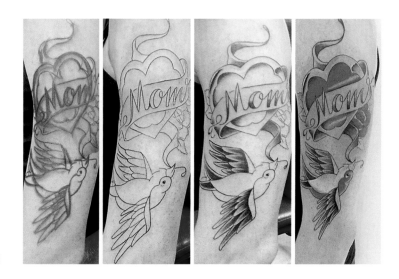

Fig. 3. Example of the process, from start to finish. First freehand drawing using a skin marker pen – then outlining – black and shading – and finally colours: Voila!

varies too much for you, as a tattoo artist, to consistently create quality work from time to time.

The same applies for the choice of colours. It's very important that you, as a professional tattoo artist, buy your colours at a dealer that you have knowledge about and trust. The market is filled with poor copies.

All of the major, recognised colour manufacturers find that their products are being illegally copied in countries such as China or Brazil. You can, as a user of the products, not tell the copies from the original. The only way you can be sure of what colours to use is to buy from a dealer approved by the manufacturer or to buy directly from the manufacturer.

The problems with the copy colours are, first of all, the manufacturer's product-sheets, which, of course, does not apply to the product you have purchased. So, you know nothing about what you are putting into your customer's skin. However, the analysis of the Chinese colours clearly shows that the manufacturer doesn't care at all. Several

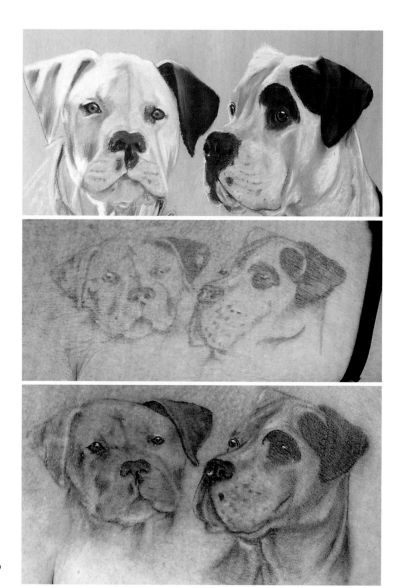

Fig. 4. Example of a poorly done tattoo – and the professional tattoo artist's fairly successful saving.

examples of contamination/bacteria in colours and on needles from dubious manufacturers have been found, and these products were sold as sterile.

Working on the Tattoo

While working on the tattoo, there are some basics you should be aware of. It's important to work at the correct depth of the skin. If you work too deep, you risk the colour flowing into the skin, giving a blurry, unclear outlining of the tattoo. However, if you don't work deep enough, the colour will disappear, and the customer will be left with a bad result, where parts of the tattoo will disappear as soon as the healing process is over. In the same way, it's important to work with a sufficient amount of colour in the needle tube so that the colour constantly flows evenly into the skin.

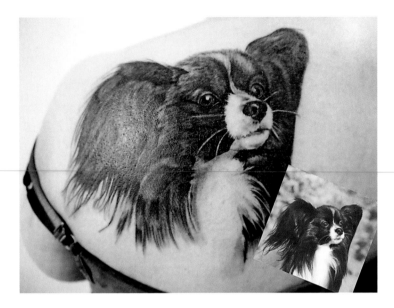

Fig. 5. Portrait of a Papillon – done by a professional.

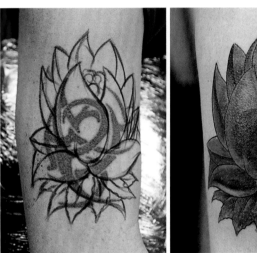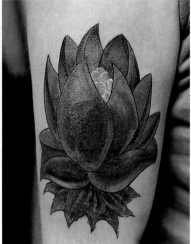

Fig. 6. Cover-up of an old black tribal-tattoo. Today, modern colours can, with some success, cover old black tattoos.

If you don't ensure this, you will to work too long on a single spot to fully colour the tattoo, with the skin being exposed to undue stress, and this will cause a prolonged healing process.

Especially, when you are doing a cover-up of an old tattoo, you must be aware of these things. First, the skin is already influenced by the old tattoo and therefore is more sensitive to the stress it's being exposed to by the new tattoo. In addition, you generally have to work harder and longer with the nee-dle to cover up the old tattoo, so the total impact on the skin is on average larger on cover-ups than on new tattoos made on untouched skin (fig. 4–6).

Aftercare

When the tattoo is done, the professional tattoo artist will make sure to advise the customer about taking care of the new tattoo. The new tattoo should

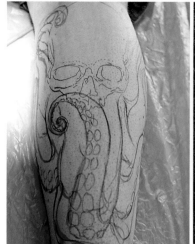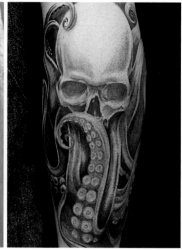

Fig. 7. From something that looks like random lines on a leg – to the final result: Art!

be kept clean with a sensitive, antiseptic and neutral soap. The tattoo needs to be lubricated 3–4 times daily with a product specifically for this purpose – typically an ointment containing panthenol. The customer should lubricate the tattoo until it has healed. In most cases, this will take about a week. Many studios hand out patient guidelines to the customer, where everything is described. Here, you can inform the customer on how to behave if any complications show up regarding the tattoo as well as give contact information for the studio.

Art and Craftsmanship in Union

Many of the professional tattoo artists you meet today make great art when they are working. However, the art is the finished tattoo (fig. 7), and the process behind it is good, old-fashioned craftsmanship.

The professional tattoo artist is a good craftsman who perfectly knows his equipment and materials and therefore becomes a person who makes art.

Lars Kristensen
Danish Professional Tattoist Association – Dansk Tatovoer Laug
Ringstedvej 39
DK–4180 Sorø (Denmark)
E-Mail formand@dansktatovoerlaug.dk

Serup J, Kluger N, Bäumler W (eds): Tattooed Skin and Health.
Curr Probl Dermatol. Basel, Karger, 2015, vol 48, pp 37–40 (DOI: 10.1159/000369180)

Tattoo as Art, the Drivers Behind the Fascination and the Decision to Become Tattooed

Liz Kierstein[a] · Kari C. Kjelskau[b]

[a]Independent Tattoo Artists, Copenhagen, Denmark; [b]Norwegian Tattoo Union, Oslo, Norway

Abstract

For many people, getting a tattoo is like purchasing art, and many professional and famous tattooists are artists who are acknowledged by colleagues and authorities. The history of tattooing goes back for thousands of years, and the reasons for getting tattooed are many. These permanent markings are always personal, they can be plain or elaborate, and they serve as amulets, healing and status symbols, declarations of love, signs of religion, adornments and even forms of punishment. Drivers behind the fascination of acquiring a tattoo may fall into four main groups, namely healing, affiliation, art and fashion.

© 2015 S. Karger AG, Basel

Introduction

We usually remember past history and associate tattoos with bikers, sailors and criminals, but today, tattoos can also be considered as fashion, aesthetics and art. A general acceptance of tattoos is on the rise in western countries, although in some communities, it is still seen as a negative practice. Females have in recent years become more visible in the industry, and more women are tattooed. It can be estimated that 15% of women are tattooed in contrast with 13% of men. As a result, the industry is more open and not as 'dangerous' as it once was.

In today's society, individuals can build their own status and identity because they are no longer born into a social status. In the pursuit of finding their identity, a lot of young people choose to get a tattoo. People from all parts of society are tattooed, including lawyers, doctors, priests, and nurses. Some consider that tattoos are for those who live on the edge, but they are so much more than risky behaviour and social stigma. They still involve identity and communication but also can represent art and fashion.

The reasons for getting tattooed are many. A tattoo can be a symbol of both individuality and group affiliation. From a psychological point of view, the reasons for getting a tattoo are complex. The industry is constantly being analysed by social anthropologists, psychologists, media scholars and art historians, and the results of these analyses can be as individual as the reasons why people get tattooed. However, tattoos are mainly acquired simply for the sake of vanity. Every individual has his or her own reason for getting tattooed. Two people can choose the same design

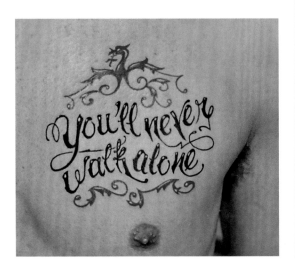

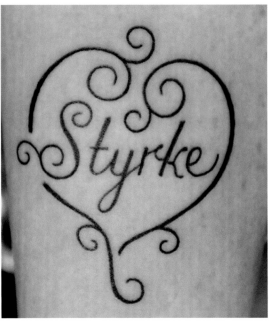

Fig. 1. Liverpool football fan. Photo: Ingwar Einebrandt, Art & Tattoo Studio Z.

Fig. 2. The text says 'Strength'. Photo: Kari Kjelskau, Memento Tattoo.

and have totally different reasons as to why they want to have that particular design. Tattoos show us that today's society is free, diverse and constantly changing. We have attempted to divide tattoos into 4 main groups as follows: healing, affiliation, art and fashion.

Healing

For some, having a tattoo is a form of healing. These individuals want to have control over pain caused to their bodies, physically or psychologically. It may be a form of controlled self-injury in which they can talk to an outsider (the tattooist) and at the same time feel controlled pain. The design often involves symbolism for strength or change, a life motto, or a memory. For these individuals, being tattooed is all about owning their own body and making their own choices, which can weigh up to the traumatic experiences from the past.

Affiliation and Sense of Belonging

Some people have tattoos involving symbolism and a sense of belonging. These tattoos can be a symbol of belonging to a particular group, such as a football team, a music logo, a family, a religion, or a criminal gang, especially for young individuals who are trying to find their identity. In today's society, identity is of high importance and is shown off. Often, individuals want to feel unique and special and at the same time, they want to have a sense of belonging (fig. 1, 2).

Art

For others, tattoos are art, similar to a piece of jewellery for others to admire. People allow themselves to get tattooed simply because it's beautiful. They choose a tattoo artist based on his or her ability to create art both on canvas and on the

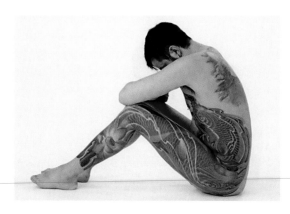

Fig. 3. Photo: Øygarden.

body and may travel far and pay a lot to get a tattoo from a specific tattoo artist. Some 'collect' this art and choose to be tattooed by various artists to amass a collection of tattoos on their body, while others stick to one tattoo artist who can decorate their entire body (fig. 3).

Younger people, professional artists and especially women are now seeking to be in the tattoo profession. They are often educated in the arts and can hold separate art exhibitions in addition to their actual tattooing practice. For the artists, this is an opportunity to make a living from their art, when paintings often can be difficult to sell. To 'use the body as canvas' is an expression that is used even by galleries. The difference is that tattoos on the skin are not appraised because they are not sellable and are only valuable to the wearer. They cannot be sold like paintings and sculptures at an international art auction.

Previously, tattooing at galleries was mainly considered performance art in the form of live tattooing, but recently, tattoos such as graffiti have gone from cult to art status and have been adopted by the art industry, especially in areas where art and fashion meet. The Musée du Quai Branly in Paris has welcomed this and hosted an exhibition in May 2014, the 'Tatoueurs, Tatoués', or 'Tattooists, Tattooed', to explore tattoos as an artistic medium. This exhibition had tattoos specifically designed for the exhibition by internationally known tattoo artists.

Fashion

In the last decade, tattoos have become increasingly visible in popular culture via television (TV) shows, such as Miami Ink, and LA Ink. In addition, idols, for example, those involved in sports and music, have presented tattoos as being fashionable. The fashion industry has picked up this trend by making clothes and perfumes that are tattoo-related, such as Ed Hardy, Diesel, and Gaultier. Trends spread quickly via social media. Those who choose tattoos based on fashion are often those who regret and want to cover up or remove them with lasers.

Idols are important as drivers. The tattoo world has always had tattoo artists who were idolised and admired. From early on, they called themselves professor, for example, Professor George Burchett, by whom sailors travelled from afar to get tattooed. Even the King of Denmark travelled to receive a tattoo from him. In the 1960s–1970s, Lyle Tuttle from San Francisco, CA, USA, was a prominent tattooist. He has tattooed famous people, including Janis Joplin, Chuck Norris, Cher and Peter Sellers and has been on the cover of Rolling Stones Magazine. He even ended up in Times Magazine, swimming from Alcatraz along with the Danish photographer, Bjoern Andersen. In recent years, TV shows have helped to popularise tattoo artists in the media, such as Kat von D, Ami James, and Lois Malloy. TV shows have greatly impacted those individuals who want a tattoo, and the designs shown on TV quickly become trendy.

People may choose a tattoo artist that they idolise or admire. Clients who really study the business often choose a tattoo artist based on what they want. Tattoo artists specialise in work styles more often than before. Some only do black/grey realism, while others only do old school, new school or Japanese. Based on talent, clients select a special tattoo artist in the same way one would choose an architect or an artist. The preparation and planning that these clients do in advance is impressive. They often travel around to conventions to see different pieces and search the Internet and Instagram to find the right tattoo artist. With the Internet, access to the best artists and the best quality has had a huge impact on the tattoo business.

Fashion also includes history and inspiration from the past. Tattoos have a long and interesting history, and many individuals want a tattoo performed in the traditional way, by hand with thorns, bone, or bamboo or sewn into the skin. Designs are often symbols from the old days that are of historical significance, and old designs from the South Pacific Islands have been well documented due to Captain Cook's voyages of discovery. Old wood carving designs are also

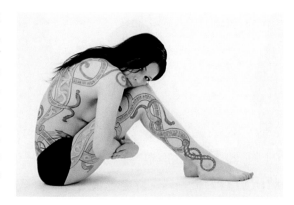

Fig. 4. Norwegian design inspired by the Urnes Stave church and the runes of the Håvamål. Photo: Øygarden.

turned into tattoos (fig. 4). Sailor tattoos remain popular. These designs are getting new lives in peoples' quests for original tattoos. Today, hipsters look to the 1950s to find inspiration for their designs.

Liz Kierstein
Independent Tattoo Artists
27, Fiolstraede
DK–1171 Copenhagen K (Denmark)
E-Mail tattoliz@gmail.com

Serup J, Kluger N, Bäumler W (eds): Tattooed Skin and Health.
Curr Probl Dermatol. Basel, Karger, 2015, vol 48, pp 41–44 (DOI: 10.1159/000369182)

Personal Records from My Tattoo Parlour: Deep Emotions Drawn as Life-Long Pictures on the Skin's Canvas

Liz Kierstein

Independent Tattoo Artists, Copenhagen, Denmark

Abstract

The author, who has been a professional tattooist for years, reports four individuals whose tragic life events led to decisions to be tattooed with illustrations of their life stories. The authors' personal experiences with tattooist-client interactions and clients' expectations and demands are reviewed. During the last decade, tattooing has moved in the direction of becoming more individualized and is often very personal. The working process and the intimacy between the client and tattooist create a comfort zone of trust and loyalty.

© 2015 S. Karger AG, Basel

Introduction

To introduce myself, I have been a Danish professional tattooist for 25 years. I have always been fascinated by the art of tattooing and have aimed to achieve and practice high professional standards. For periods, I also have worked in the USA and Spain. In this chapter, I shall report my personal experiences as a type of testimonial, starting with case reports from my parlour that have been printed in this book with permission.

Case Reports

Case 1: MP, 21-Year-Old Man

Tattoo: Memory tattoo on left side of chest (fig. 1a, b).

Design: Text in Danish: 'Et påtvunget ansvar, der ikke var ønsket – Livet. Så hvorfor ikke få det bedste ud af det?' English translation: 'An imposed, not wanted responsibility – Life. So, why not make the best out of it?'

Reason for Tattoo: His little brother committed suicide at the age of 19 years in January 2014 after 2 previous attempts.

Knowing that the youngest child of 3 would most likely succeed in committing suicide, the family tried to help him in any way they could. The boy suffered from depression and schizophrenic attacks after his parents divorced. He was frequently in fights, had a bad temper and found no reason to live. He left behind a family in grief, especially his older brother, MP, who wanted the life and tragedy of his little brother to be remembered. MP opted for text carved into his skin because the loss of his brother will be forever on his mind.

Encouraged by his cousin, who is a client at my studio, MP and his cousin showed up at my parlour one day and told their story. As a professional, I guided the young client with regard to the correct size of the

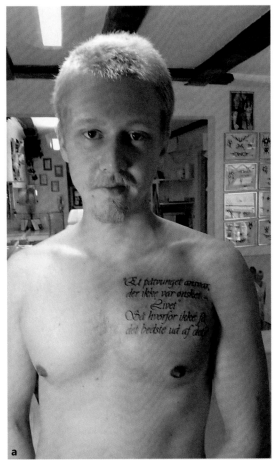

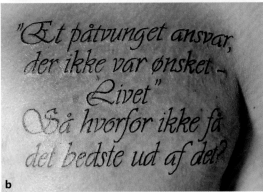

Fig. 1. a, b Memory tattoo. Tattoo and photo by author.

lettering in the tattoo and the correct placement of the tattoo on his chest over his heart. After a few days, MP returned and showed his preferred type of lettering, and he had chosen a decent size. We fitted the sentences, and the tattoo was performed. The redness of the surrounding skin in the photos is transient and due to tattoo needle trauma.

Case 2: KP, 48-Year-Old Male

Tattoo: Black and grey wash on right upper arm (fig. 2).

Design: Woman's face, pocket watch and devil.

Reason for Tattoo: His wife, who was only 63 years of age, recently died from Alzheimer's disease. The face symbolized the beauty of his wife, the pocket watch showed that time was running out, and the devil's face symbolized the terrible nature of the disease.

The client had never received a tattoo before and was trying to find comfort and some sort of acknowledgment of the fact that time really was running out. He wanted to mark his body during this terrible time, while waiting for his wife to pass away at a special care home.

Case 3: BNA, 40-Year-Old Woman

Tattoo: Colorful and on the left ankle (fig. 3).

Design: Tiger cub.

After a lot of homemade tattoos, this client finally came to me and got her 'first' professional tattoo. BNA's boyfriend and pals doubted that this was a real tattoo! The client was very, very happy and probably found comfort with this little innocent cub, which was helpless and fragile like BNA herself. She had been on drugs for years.

Case 4: JM, 53-Year-Old Male, Teacher and Guitar Builder

Tattoo: Left forearm – his 'music arm' (fig. 4).

Design: A graphic photo of Jimi Hendrix.

JM was divorced from his wife in 2013 and had an urge to turn the divorce into a positive situation. Because he had been a music lover for many years and was also a professional teacher who had been educated as carpenter and had his own shop as a guitar builder, he wanted to make a tattoo to honor one of his idols, the famous Jimi Hendrix, who was a left-handed guitar player like JM himself. Not wanting a realistic photo but rather a graphic tattoo, we designed this piece of art, and he was very happy with it.

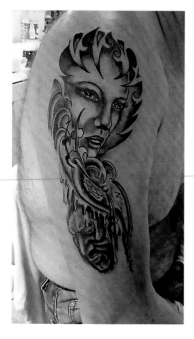 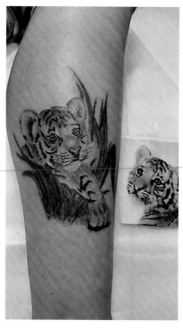 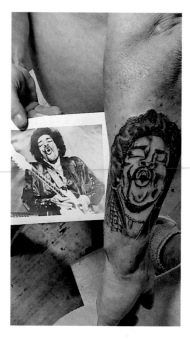

Fig. 2. Grief and eternal love. Tattoo and photo by author.

Fig. 3. Fragile soul. Tattoo and photo by author.

Fig. 4. Graphic style music legend. Tattoo and photo by author.

Comments

When I started getting tattoos in 1981, they were only for bikers, sailors, 'birds' in the streets (prostitutes) and guys down at the bar. When tribal art (black tattoos with intricate swirls and beautiful shapes) entered the tattoo scene in Denmark at the end of the 1980s and the beginning of the 1990s, other types of clients started to want tattoos. Tattoo designs don't necessarily need to have a specific look. This beautiful adornment of the body is drawn straight onto the skin with a pen following the anatomic shapes, resulting in a beautiful piece of art belonging only to the recipient. The very rigid and old-fashioned tattoo style of 'getting a tattoo from the wall' has changed, and individual artists' skills and talents are now challenged to create and draw according to their clients' recommendations.

It is very common that we are asked to help design artistic 'statements', or symbols with a certain meaning rather than just actual lettering, for example, the 'living in the moment desire' to tattoo a unique design to mark a special occasion, whether it is sad or joyful. The real tattoo artist does not necessarily want to hear the story, but most people are anxious to tell the reason for their tattoo and their decision to become tattooed.

People have many reasons for wanting a tattoo. Currently, tattoos are everywhere, including in ads, in the news, and on actors, musicians, soccer players, disc jockeys and artists. Because it is possible to be exposed to many more tattoos compared with just a decade ago, people have become fascinated by the beautiful artwork that we are able to do, and tattoos have become more and more realistic, colorful, larger and more personal.

The decision to become tattooed greatly differs depending on the situation. There are the young and impatient clients who just want to become decorated right there and then. Their parents may come to professional studios begging for tattoos for their minors because they know that the young kids will go to any extent to get tattooed, even using at-home scratchers.

Others might have wanted a tattoo for many years. For middle-aged individuals, a life-changing situation may have occurred, such as having grandchildren, a divorce, death or separation. In the 1980s, it was very common for young men to celebrate the completion of military training by getting a tattoo.

During my time as a tattoo artist in Spain, where I tattooed mostly navy personnel from the 6th US fleet, tattooing symbolized being away, longing for home and at times, the loss of friends in combat.

Tattoo artists are very lucky because our clients are very loyal. In the earlier days before the internet, word of mouth was very important to tattoo artists. The recommendation of one particular artist by one satisfied client to another individual led to more clients wanting to get tattooed by that artist. At that time (1989), I felt that a lot of people thought that if the tattooist (the tattoo artist) was female, she would be gentler, and the tattoo hurt less. However, this is not true. The professional tattooist knows how to let the machine do the 'dancing' on the skin.

It has always struck me how deeply involved clients are with every little detail of their design. This is what makes the job so interesting and challenging, to capture a client's desire and wishes and bring the first drawing to life and then to do the actual tattoo. Once the design is finished and approved, the most important part of the process awaits, the actual tattooing session. It is kind of a build up to complete satisfaction, seeing the tattoo on the skin for the first time.

While tattooing, it seems that the intimacy between the tattoo artist and client creates a comfort zone, and clients usually feel free to tell their story. The acts of touching the skin and tattooing create an invisible bond, and it becomes a mutual task to make a beautiful piece of art.

Clients are always offered a second visit for a check-up, and they often bring family or friends along. Once at the tattoo studio, non-tattooed people get inspiration from looking at all of the books and magazines, photos and tattoo paraphernalia that always decorate an 'old school tattoo studio'. Currently, a new type of tattoo studio has been introduced to the tattoo scene. Chains of shops with very little or no decor and charm but often with very skilled artists represent the new trend in our trade.

Liz Kierstein
Independent Tattoo Artists
27, Fiolstraede
DK–1171 Copenhagen K (Denmark)
E-Mail tattoliz@gmail.com

Serup J, Kluger N, Bäumler W (eds): Tattooed Skin and Health.
Curr Probl Dermatol. Basel, Karger, 2015, vol 48, pp 45–47 (DOI: 10.1159/000369184)

Tattooist-Customer Relationships in a Diversified Environment of Professional Tattooists and 'Scratchers'

Mads Wedel Kristensen

Institute of Sociology, University of Copenhagen, Copenhagen, Denmark

Abstract

The world of tattooing and body art has never been like it is today. This chapter seeks to investigate this situation through the lens of tattooing. One of the areas in which tattooing has changed is the relationship between the tattoo artist and his or her clients. Whereas being a tattoo artist used to be impersonal and very much just a job like any other, it has transformed tremendously today. The cause of this and, even more so, what exactly has changed are what this chapter will seek to shed light on. First of all, the format of the shops and how the art is done have changed, which allows for much greater flexibility from the perspective of the artist. Second, from the perspective of the client/customer, a transformation has also occurred, in some part thanks to developments such as the internet and other social/communication media, which give the client much more room and opportunity to discover and research tattoos. However, most importantly, this chapter seeks to map out a change in discourse when it comes to the relationship between the client and the tattoo artist and to explain how it has changed into a relationship based on mutual and reciprocated communication as well as focussed on making a product/piece of art that both can be satisfied with.

Before the Session

Even before the session, a lot has changed within the tattoo world and its mechanics. One of the key elements in the transformation of this process is social media, and particularly the internet [1, pp 97–100; 2, pp 3–6]. The focus here is not on how social media, such as TV shows, movies, and the internet, have helped in spreading the idea of tattoos in modern society as well as making them more commonly accepted; the focus is on how social media has served to help both clients and tattoo artists when it comes to research and preparation [3]. On the part of tattoo artists, the internet has helped them to research more of their craft, to get familiarised with different styles, and perhaps even to improve their own art. However, more importantly for clients, the internet has meant a great deal in terms of how to find the right artist, find the right motif for their tattoo, and find inspiration for their tattoo and has indeed helped to improve the whole experience on many accounts [2, p 3]. This means that both clients and tattoo artists expect a lot more from the planning part of the process. Clients research a lot about styles and different artists, making sure that they find the right guy to help them to achieve their dream tattoo. However, this also means that artists have started to expect a bit more preparation from their clients, or at least the ones who want a 'custom piece', and not just some 'fashion ink'. The end result of all of this planning often becomes a much more unique tattoo, and the planning will also result in the client reflecting a lot more on the motif that he or she wants for the tattoo and how he or she identifies with it [3]. There has also been a huge proliferation of (social) media that can help the client with this research. There are more and more so-called tattoo self-help books, which explain both the different genres of tattoos and their iconography. Most of them also have a chapter on 'how to find the perfect tattoo artist for your tattoo' and so on. This, along with tons of magazines and such, showing off artwork from all over the world, and the internet make sure that people can find an artist from anywhere in the world [1, pp 32–34]. This has made the tattoo artist-customer relationship one that focusses much more on reflection and art from the perspective of both parties [3, p 16]. There is even a much higher level of integrity today, as the tattoo artist may say no to a design if he or she earns enough to decline work and may rather recommend another artist, who might be better suited to meet the client's needs. Thus, there is more of a common goal and trust from the start. Additionally, the artist's reputation is much more at stake than it was in the past, as clients can now research the subject with great ease, including the quality of the work done. This means that if an artist short-changes a client or tricks him or her in another way, the artist's reputation will be ruined, so both parties need to respect each other [3, pp 29–30].

During the Process

When it comes to the process and how the relationship has changed in this regard, much can be said about how the process differs from tattoo to tattoo, especially since some smaller pieces will take a very short time, or perhaps only a few hours or less than one. However, regardless of this, as my previous research has shown [3], there is a much more relaxed and friendly atmosphere during the tattooing process than there was in the past. This, of course, cannot be said for all shops, but for the majority of what one may call 'modern tattoo shops', this holds true. This atmosphere makes the trust already established much stronger, and often, the aim is mutual satisfaction with the work being done. Because of that, the artist will often be very focussed on doing his or her best during the process. Especially because of how diversified the tattoo world is, communication between client and artist becomes paramount, as both want to be able to see themselves in the work being done [3, pp 24–25]; the client wants a unique piece that speaks to and about him or her, and the artist wants to put his or her artistic brand into the tattoo, such as a certain style of lines or colouring. This means that often, when a client finds a tattoo artist with the same artistic visions as the client has, the artist will be much more friendly and keen during the project than if the client came in and just asked to have a simple star made of black outlining done. However, all in all, during the process, the relationship between client and artist has transformed into that of comradery. This is not to say that an artist will befriend every client that he or she meets, but there is a lot more openness from the artist's side, which has played a large part in removing a lot of the stigmas surrounding tattoo shops and the like [1, pp 138–140]. The shop and artist are no longer seen as dangerous and deviant or as things to keep certain wariness about. Instead, the shop is seen as a place where one can come and pour out one's artistic ideas in a forum where they belong.

The Past and Now

It has already been briefly discussed above, but I would now like to discuss how the relationship between the artist and his or her clients has changed in a bit more of a general and academic sense. Most importantly, the whole societal context around tattoos has changed; they are no longer condemned to subcultural status or to be markers of deviants or villains. Instead, they have become culturally transcendent; individual; and, as the title of this chapter hints, diversified to a great extent. In line with the theories of Paul Sweetman, the tattoo has become the anchor of the self in late modern society [4]. This is, of course, inspired by the theories of sociologists such as Bauman [5] and Giddens [6], who all see the world as one of constant flux in our late modern society. Nothing is constant or certain like it was back in the time of tradition. Our identities are especially prone to change and transformation throughout our lives. What Sweetman tries to say is that tattoos and similar body art almost serve as a defragmentation of our identity because of how they make us reflect more carefully on ourselves and our identity. It has been discussed whether tattoos provide much individuality, something that artists doubt to an extent [3, pp 25–26]. However, there is great consensus among both clients and artists that what they are doing becomes a part of the wearer's and the artist's identities, as it is a piece of the artist's skills and the history of the artist's art as well as permanently positioned on another human being's skin (less so with piercings,

yet they can still have a similar effect). Whether a tattooed individual likes it or not, others will view him or her in light of the tattoos whenever the individual carries them visibly. This judgement does not necessarily have to be negative, but it should be considered. Because of this, tattoo artists, and especially the ones with at least some success, often take it upon themselves to be guides for their clients, counselling them on whether they are ready or able to carry the design that they have in mind or whether certain changes should be made for it to work [4, 7]. All in all, the relationship between artists and clients has, for the reasons listed in this chapter, become one of communication and dialogue. It is what marks the relationship more than anything in the modern tattoo/body-art culture. Without dialogue, a tattoo will often not end up as well done or thought out as it could have been, and that will lead to people regretting the tattoo and the artist not really being happy about the work [3, pp 29–30].

Thus, as already said, the paramount element in the modern artist-customer relationship between tattoo artists and their clients is communication/dialogue, with the mutual goal of creating something that will satisfy both parties; however, the focus is usually on the customer.

References

1 DeMello M: Bodies of Inscription: A Cultural History of the Tattoo Community. London, Duke University Press, 2000.
2 The Editors at Tattoofinder.com: Tattoo Sourcebook: Pick and Choose from Thousands of the Hottest Tattoo Designs. London, Harper Collins Publishers, 2008.
3 Kristensen MW: 'I am Not a Tattooist I am an Artist who Tattoos': A Sociological Analysis of the Professional Practice and Cultural Expression of Contemporary Tattooing. University of Portsmouth, School of Social, Historical and Literary Studies, Portsmouth, 2013.
4 Sweetman P: Anchoring the (postmodern) self? Body modification, fashion and identity. Body Society 1999;5:51–76.
5 Bauman Z: Liquid Life. Cambridge, Polity Press, 2005.
6 Giddens A: Modernitet og Selvidentitet: Selvet og Samfund under Sen-Moderniteten [Modernity and Self-Identity: Self and Society in the Late Modern Age]. Copenhagen, Hans Reitzel Forlag, 1996.
7 Ferreira VS: Becoming a Heavily Tattooed Young Body: From a Bodily Experience to a Body Project. Youth Society 2014;46:303–337.

Mads Wedel Kristensen, Stud. Cand. Scient. Soc.
Institute of Sociology, University of Copenhagen
Charlotte Muncks Vej 31, st th.
DK–2400 Copenhagen NV (Denmark)
E-Mail mads.k@hotmail.dk

Serup J, Kluger N, Bäumler W (eds): Tattooed Skin and Health.
Curr Probl Dermatol. Basel, Karger, 2015, vol 48, pp 48–60 (DOI: 10.1159/000369645)

Tattoo Complaints and Complications: Diagnosis and Clinical Spectrum

Jørgen Serup · Katrina Hutton Carlsen · Mitra Sepehri

Department of Dermatology, 'Tattoo Clinic', Bispebjerg University Hospital, Copenhagen, Denmark

Abstract

Tattoos cause a broad range of clinical problems. Mild complaints, especially sensitivity to sun, are very common and seen in 1/5 of cases. Medical complications are dominated by allergy to tattoo pigment haptens or haptens generated in the skin, especially in red tattoos but also in blue and green tattoos. Symptoms are major and can be compared to cumbersome pruritic skin diseases. Tattoo allergies and local reactions show distinct clinical manifestations, with plaque-like, excessive hyperkeratotic, ulcero-necrotic, lymphopathic, neuro-sensory, and scar patterns. Reactions in black tattoos are papulo-nodular and non-allergic and associated with the agglomeration of nanoparticulate carbon black. Tattoo complications include effects on general health conditions and complications in the psycho-social sphere. Tattoo infections with bacteria, especially staphylococci, which may be resistant to multiple antibiotics, may be prominent and may progress into life-threatening sepsis. Contaminated tattoo ink is an open-window risk vector that can lead to epidemic tattoo infections across national borders due to contaminated bulk production. Hepatitis B and C and human immunodeficiency virus (HIV) transferred by tattooing remain a significant risk needing active prevention. It is noteworthy that cancer arising in tattoos, in regional lymph nodes, and in other organs due to tattoo pigments and ingredients has not been detected or noted as a significant clinical problem hitherto, despite millions of people being tattooed for decennia. Clinical observation and epidemiology disagree with register data, which indicate an increased risk of cancer due to chemical carcinogens present in some inks. Registers rely on chronic dosaging of cell lines and animals. However, tattooing in humans is essentially a single-dose exposure, which might explain the observed discrepancy.

© 2015 S. Karger AG, Basel

Introduction

Tattooing of skin via deposition of pigment particles and ink ingredients in the dermis changes normal skin into abnormal skin. Fortunately, this often causes no harm and no disease, although with important exceptions. The tattooed individual may risk disablement, and death may even occur under exceptional circumstances.

In the medical literature, case reports and reviews have outlined the wide spectrum of adverse events related to tattooing [1–9]. Reports should always be read in the context of the development of tattoo inks and the tattoo business at the time of the report. Inorganic pigments such as mercury and cadmium salts are now being replaced by organic pigments. The tattoo ink products of today remain composite, with unknown ingredients and a range of chemical contaminants. The bacterial contamination and uncertain sterility of inks are even challenges today [10, 11].

Tattoo inks contain soluble ingredients, which supposedly are distributed, metabolised, and excreted within a few days, and the pigment. Tattooing is a single-dose injection of a large local dose, depending on the size of the tattoo. However, robust pigment particles remain permanently in the skin and make up the desired colouring. Pigments in the skin slowly vanish over time, along with a slow release of minute amounts of chemicals and metabolites, which may actually cause harm, such as allergy. The release is triggered by enzymatic and cellular processes in the tissues that are very different from harsh chemical degradation, with the formation of chemical cleavage products, in the laboratory, which is an artificial and unrealistic scenario. Pigments instilled into the tattoo partly escape via the lymph and become deposited in the regional lymph nodes. The nodes are invisibly dyed along with the skin. However, unknown amounts of pigment nanoparticles might reach the blood stream and theoretically cause harm somewhere in the body.

It has been documented that many tattoo inks, as referenced to register data, contain carcinogenic, mutagenic, and reprotoxic substances. However, concerns about tattoos' induction of skin cancer, including malignant melanoma, have *not* been confirmed in the medical literature and remain hypothetical [12]. A systematic review of the world literature only detected 50 reports of skin cancers situated in tattoos, which was concluded to be a coincidence since spontaneous skin malignancy related to sun exposure is very common and may affect tattooed skin independent of the pigment [12]. The literature, including the cited reviews, has not indicated a risk of distant organ cancer or foetal hazards, although such risks have not been excluded. Bispebjerg University Hospital, Department of Dermatology includes a centre for cutaneous oncology. Neither 'Oncology' nor the 'Tattoo Clinic' noted cases in which the origin of skin cancer was attributed to a tattoo and its pigment. Clinical observation and epidemiology disagree with register data, which indicate an increased risk of cancer due to chemical carcinogens present in inks. Registers rely on chronic dosaging of cell lines and animals, however, tattooing in humans is essentially a single-dose exposure, which might explain the observed discrepancy.

Since 2008, the 'Tattoo Clinic' of Bispebjerg University Hospital has collected some 400 medical cases of tattoo complications and has additionally researched other groups of tattooed individuals not admitted to the clinic as referenced below. This chapter provides a brief outline of our clinical experience and introduces a descriptive and observational approach, based on clinical pattern recognition, for the diagnosis of medical tattoo reactions. This approach is not a simple translation of diagnosis by histology of tattoo reactions into clinical skin conditions, as is often practised by clinicians. We rely on patient history and clinical signs and symptoms and use histology as a valuable tool for supplementary information and grading of severity prior to treatment. In our clinic, this treatment is preferably surgery by dermatome shaving, with effective removal of the culprit tattoo pigment in the outer dermis, where it is concentrated. The chapter will not address healing or the phases of recovery following a tattoo, problems, or the issue of aftercare other than what is mentioned in the context of infections.

Definitions of Tattoo Complaints and Complications

Tattoo *complaints* concern mild subjectively or objectively abnormal experiences or observations acquired along with and caused by a tattoo. Complaints may address local problems with the tattoo or may be general. Complaints may be acute or subacute and taper out as the tattoo heals. Complaints may also be chronic or chronically intermittent. The tattooed individual in general does not seek medical advice for the complaint.

Tattoo *complications* are more serious adverse reactions or events after tattooing that manifest as objective abnormalities or pathologies associated with clinical and subjective symptoms of a severity that is considered as a disease or disablement. The tattooed individual with complication in general requests professional medical advice and treatment.

Complaints Associated with Tattoos

In 2010, Klügl et al. [13] reported health problems associated with tattooed skin based on 3,411 spontaneous reports collected over the internet in German-speaking countries after an open public invitation. In total, 67% of respondents reported skin problems, and 7% reported general reactions, which had primarily occurred a few weeks after tattooing. Thus, several hundred complaints were counted. However, the study design did not allow conclusions about the pre-cise incidence or prevalence of complaints and complications.

A Danish study performed in a group of 154 younger persons attending a clinic for sexually transmitted diseases reported tattoo-related complaints of any kind and at any time in 27%, with 58% of complaints, related to sun exposure [14]. The predominant symptoms were itching/stinging/pain and elevation/inflammation.

Another study, the 'beach study', was conducted at summertime along the coastline of Denmark. Among 144 sunbathers with 146 tattoos, 42 reported complaints of any kind, with 52% of complaints, related to sun exposure [15].

The studies show that tattoo complaints dominated by itching and swelling are remarkably common and affect approximately 1/3 of tattooed individuals, with 1/5 of tattooed individuals having sun-related problems. Complaints were often reported in dark tattoos, which absorb more light. Skin reactions differed and could be instantaneous, appearing within seconds or minutes after sun exposure, or delayed, appearing within hours and lasting for days. Complaints that were independent of light could last for several weeks and could be constant or intermittent.

Non-Infectious Complications and Adverse Events

Non-infectious complications can be characterised according to clinical signs and symptoms and according to pathophysiology. Allergic reactions are frequent.

The diagnosis of allergy due to tattoos is performed in the absence of a valid test reference and based on the following clinical criteria:
– Allergic reactions are monomorphic, i.e. uniformly manifested in one particular colour and at all sites where that particular colour is applied in the tattoo
– There is latency of primary sensitisation lasting weeks, months, or years since the

tattoo was obtained until the reaction appears
- Once elicited and full blown, the reaction is constant, chronic, cumbersome and refractory to topical corticoid therapy
- A definite criterion for allergy is induction of alike reaction(s) in a hitherto-tolerated tattoo of the same colour located in another anatomical region, i.e. a manifestation of allergic cross-reactivity

In a series of 90 patients with chronic tattoo reactions, an allergy patch test with common allergens, dispersed textile dyes, a battery of risky tattoo inks, and identified culprit inks from individual cases demonstrated that patch test reactions cannot be elicited by application of the potential allergens mentioned [16]. Thus, allergic reactions are not elicited by an allergen directly present in the tattoo ink stock product but rather due to a hapten formed inside the skin over a longer period of time, i.e. months or years. Standard test methods used for cutaneous allergy are consequently not useful in the diagnostic evaluation of suspected allergic reactions. Similarly, in the evaluation of the potential allergy risk of new or known tattoo ink products and ink ingredients, methods such as the Buehler test, the guinea pig maximisation test, and the lymph node assay are inappropriate in rationale and design and are not applicable. These tests are bound to show false-negative results.

The term 'lichenoid', dating back centuries, to early French dermatology, is sometimes used to describe tattoo reactions with inflammation of the outer skin and epidermal thickening observed by histology. However, the term is imprecise and is used for a broad range of very different skin conditions. The traditional microscopic findings, with lichenoid, granulomatous, and pseudolymphomatous tattoo reactions, does not have a distinct clinical correlate and should not be used to label tattoo reactions as they appear in the clinic. The histologic patterns are not specific and may overlap in the same biopsy.

On clinical and morphologic grounds, reactions and complications can be differentiated into local reaction patterns and general conditions or associations, as described below.

Local Reaction Patterns

Papulo-Nodular Pattern (fig. 1)

Tattoos may show papular or nodular thickening and elevation in certain areas, in contrast to other similarly coloured areas of the tattoo that have a normal appearance. Elevations may be round and elongated and may appear confluent, and often appear where the density of pigment is high as a result of 'pigment overload' with injection of too much ink. Elevations are often chronic but may resolve over several months. Papules, which are eroded by scratching, may release their excess pigment and heal, leaving a guttate white spot. The background appears to be an agglomeration of black pigment nanoparticles, i.e. carbon black, forming large bodies in the dermis. The bodies are visible in raw biopsy samples seen by the naked eye. The skin may recognise the bodies as foreign and attempt to expel them via the transepidermal route. However, most material is held back in the dermis by the basement membrane, situated immediately under the epidermis. Papulo-nodular reactions may have other causes, such as needle trauma or instillation of too much ink in the dermis, or more than the skin is able to hold without inflammation. The papulo-nodular pattern is very common and especially noted in black tattoos and black linings. It is not an allergic reaction.

Plaque-Like Pattern (fig. 2)

These reactions show flat thickening and elevation of the entire tattoo at any site in the tattoo where the problem colour was inserted. Large adherent scales may or may not be present. Inflammation, with lymphocytes, is often major and may extend into the surrounding non-tat-

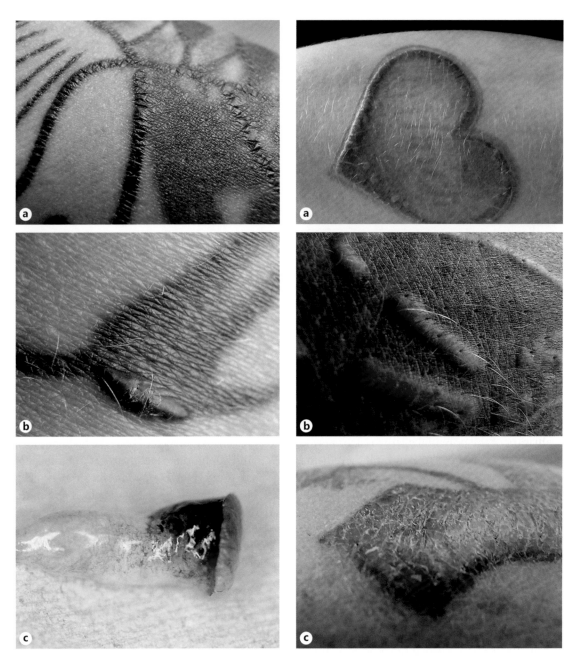

Fig. 1. Papulo-nodular pattern. **a** Elevated black lines with irregular and confluent thickening, in contrast to a normal black tattoo without any change. **b** Nodular elevation spontaneously ready to release excess pigment. **c** Raw punch biopsy of a nodule with visible agglomeration of black pigment particles, which originally were nano-sized.

Fig. 2. Plaque-like pattern. **a** Flat elevation of the entire tattoo where lilac ink was instilled. **b** Flat elevation of a red tattoo. **c** Flat elevation and major thickening limited to a red tattoo and sharply demarcated towards normal skin. **a–c** All have some adherent scaling and minor hyperkeratosis, which traditionally might be labelled 'lichenoid'.

tooed skin, and is concentrated in the outer dermis. Histology may show interface dermatitis or any of the traditional histologic patterns, which may overlap in the same biopsy. Epidermal changes with some degree of hyperkeratosis are typical. If the tattoo is a line, such as in tattooed texts, the entire line will be affected. Plaque-like reactions are primarily seen in red tattoos or in nuances of red and are a manifestation of allergy. Green and blue tattoos may also show this pattern as a result of allergy. There may be a visible colour shift from blue to green or from green to blue as the allergic reaction appears.

Excessive Hyperkeratotic Pattern (fig. 3)

These reactions exhibit inflammation, thickening, and elevation that is major and dominated by massive hyperkeratosis and cornification of the surface, which acquires a structure resembling sandpaper. The entire area dyed with the particular problem colour exhibits the same abnormality. The elevated surface is rather flat, and the pattern might be considered as a plaque-like reaction with an excessive epidermal response to the underlying inflammation. The thickened epidermis may become necrotic and ulcerate. Occasionally, epidermal folding and notches may appear on histology. The notches may go deep and result in epidermal inclusions and fistulas embedded deeply in the dermis. The histologic picture ultimately may be distinct, seen under the microscope as pseudoepitheliomatous hyperplasia. The excessive hyperkeratotic pattern appears in red tattoos and nuances of red. The pattern is considered to indicate allergy, complicated by significant leakage of the basement membrane, escape of the culprit pigment to the epidermis, severe inflammation, and a prominent proliferative response of the epidermis that manifests as excessive hyperkeratosis. In raw punch biopsies, the hyperkeratosis is seen as a whitish layer on top of the underlying dermis, which is colourful due to the red pigment.

Ulcero-Necrotic Pattern (fig. 4)

Aggressive inflammation is directly followed by tissue necrosis and ulceration at any site in the tattoo where the culprit colour was instilled into the skin. Ulceration may affect the full thickness of the dermis and may approach the subcutaneous fat. Necrosis may even extend further into deep tissues if the culprit pigment is disseminated down to the underlying muscle fascia, for example. Necrosis may even affect the regional lymph nodes holding the same pigment. This pattern, especially seen in red tattoos, is a manifestation of a strong allergy. The allergy and haptenisation, seemingly involving tissue components, may progress to autoimmunity, with an attack on non-tattoo sites of the skin integument, including inflammatory reactions, vasculites, bullous reactions, and generally delayed wound healing throughout the skin. The condition may be self-limiting and may heal over a period of several months. Surgical excision is risky and relatively contraindicated.

Lymphopathic Pattern

Excess pigment particles flow into the lymph and into the lymph vessels to a regional node, where the particles are maintained and may visibly stain the node. Tattoo pigment injected deep into the dermis may also flow into the surrounding skin and produce a visible stain in the direction of the lymph flow. This may result in damage and blockage of distal lymph vessels, with soft tissue swelling and clinically significant lymphoedema. The condition is permanent and shares traits with podoconiosis, a disease among Africans who, via fissures in their bare feet, have microparticles of soil rich in bentonite clay implanted into their tissues. This results in damage and blockage of the lymphatics, eventually resulting in major oedema of the legs, i.e. elephantiasis. Occasionally, weeks after tattooing, tattooed individuals may have swollen and tender regional lymph nodes, although normally without any sequelae other than pigment deposits in the lymph nodes.

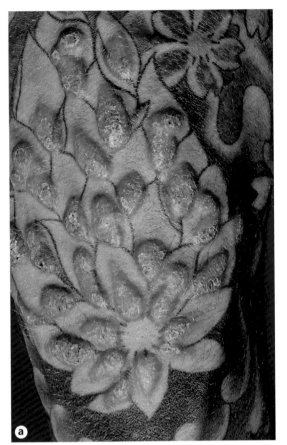

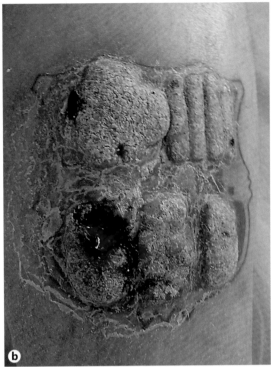

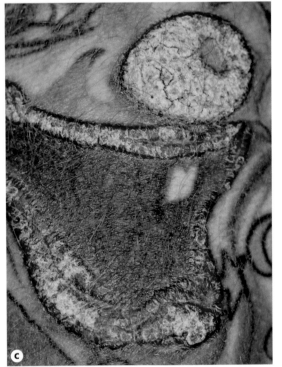

Fig. 3. Excessive hyperkeratotic pattern. **a** Distinct and prominent thickening at all sites tattooed red, with excessive hyperkeratosis. **b** Reaction entirely dominated by hyperkeratosis, with a sandpaper-like appearance of the surface, which was flat and exhibits a loss of all skin markings. At a local site, poor nutrition, and ulceration appeared after the hyperkeratosis had loosened. **c** Detail of excessive hyperkeratotic lesions.

Neuro-Sensory Pattern

Tattoo reactions and, in particular, allergic reactions often itch a lot and reduce quality of life to a degree comparable to reduction by widespread pruritic skin diseases, even though tattoo reactions typically affect only quite a small area [17]. Tattoos may induce severe and invalidating discomfort, itch and pain, without noticeable clinical changes. The histology of the skin is normal or exhibits minor lymphatic infiltration of the dermis only. It is assumed that chemical(s) in the ink, from the pigment, or released split products may stimulate the C-fibres of the sensory nerves. The sensory change may affect the dermatome or the body regions. Peripheral neuropathy, a herniated vertebral disc, and syringomyelia may be the differential diagnoses. The condition, which may be more frequent in tattoos of the forearm and wrist, has been reported as complex regional pain syndrome [18]. Surgical removal of the tattoo pigment by dermatome may produce radical relief.

Scar Pattern

Normal tattoos often exhibit mild fibrosis as a sequela of the tattoo needle trauma. Tattooing, with thousands of needle injections at the mid-dermal level, represents massive needle trauma that may result in the development of hypertrophic scars or keloids. Regions such as the chest, the shoulders, and the upper arms are predisposed to abnormal scarring. The risk increases if the needle injections reach the lower dermis and if the tattoo needle is damaged or poor in quality. Electric coil machines appear less risky than rotary machines, which may mill the skin. The risk of inducing a scar obviously depends on the experience and skill of the tattooist. Surprisingly, persons who have prominent keloids for some reason may be tattooed without any abnormal scar formation if the tattooing is performed in the very outer dermis, outside the critical anatomical sites and with care not to traumatise.

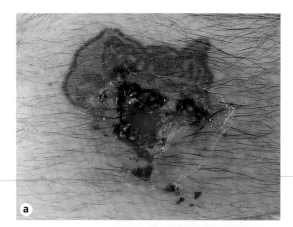

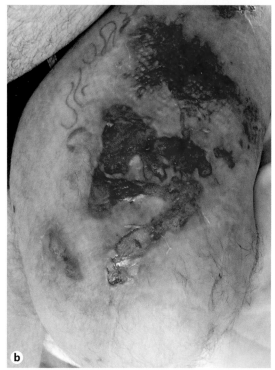

Fig. 4. Ulcero-necrotic pattern. **a** Ulceration and necrosis exclusively in the red part of a tattoo. The individual had similar necrotic elements in his normal, non-tattooed skin that started as vasculitis-like elements. Healing was spontaneous. **b** Aggressive ulceration and necrosis in a large tattoo on a leg, necessitating sequential amputations to the femur level. However, a reaction and recurrent ulceration were still present. The non-tattooed skin was also affected.

General Conditions and Associations

Tattoo-Provoked Illness
Tattooing may occasionally induce skin afflictions and provoke flares of known skin diseases. The needle trauma of tattooing, with histamine release, routinely produces an urticarial reaction that may be advanced and induce a general flush. Tattooing may be followed by long-lasting urticaria, requiring medical diagnosis and treatment. Eczema, which may be severe and due to a new allergy acquired with the tattoo, such as allergy to paraben preservatives or methylisothiazolinone. The development of allergy to latex proteins originating from the tattooist's gloves and instilled into the skin with the tattoo needle is a serious complication, with a risk of anaphylaxis upon some later exposure to latex. Tattooing is apparently not a clinically relevant inducer of allergy to nickel and chromate VI, despite trace elements of nickel being present in nearly every tattoo ink product.

It is widely unknown whether tattooing and tattoos may trigger or influence other medical diseases or be associated with general diseases specific to tattoos other than autoimmunity, as discussed above. An association with sarcoidosis or, rather, a general sarcoid reaction pattern in the body tissues is known [19].

Existing Skin Disease and Tattoo Reaction
Urticaria factitia is not congruous with tattooing and may cause major flares and flushing. Atopic skin may also be prone to tattoo-related problems and may more easily become infected since atopic skin often is colonised with staphylococci. Tattooing may also induce local chronic skin diseases such as necrobiosis lipoidica. However, the vast majority of non-infectious skin diseases are not influenced by tattooing. The well-known exception is psoriasis, which may flare up after any mechanical trauma, including a new tattoo, as described by Köbner more than a century ago, generally known as

the Köbner phenomenon [20]. Another chapter of this book reviews contraindications for tattooing.

Psycho-Social Disability
The disparity between tattoo enthusiasts, who proudly wish to display their tattoos to the world, on the one hand and all of those who silently disregard tattoos on the other hand is still very real. The clash may easily reduce job opportunities and end private and professional careers. Many tattooed individuals experience stigmatisation and barriers, especially if tattooed on the face, the neck, or the hands. Many tattoos cannot be removed, even if the best laser technology at the time is applied. Persons who have biker emblems on their skin are in a special class of physical risk. It cannot be denied that social disability can be a consequence of tattooing. The negative impact of an unwanted tattoo on psyche and quality of life is real and a significant complication.

The above shortlist of adverse reaction patterns and conditions associated with tattooing is not exhaustive, and additional manifestations of risks may occur and be depicted in the medical literature.

Infectious Complications

Tattoo needle penetration of the skin barrier may introduce a range of microorganisms into a person, particularly if the needle is not sterile or is shared among persons, resulting in a range of infections (fig. 5) [21, 22]. Microorganisms may also find their way into the body during the healing phase of a tattoo. Bacterial infections may include not only infections with Staphylococcus, Streptococcus, Pseudomonas, and Clostridium species and even tetanus but also infections with atypical bacteria, such as commensal mycobacteria; tuberculosis; and leprosy. Fungal, parasitic, and spirochaetal (namely, syphilis) in-

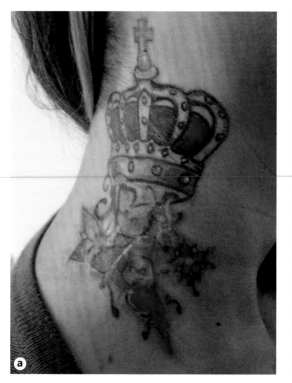

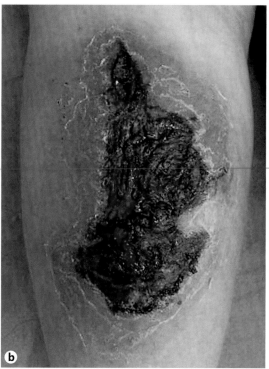

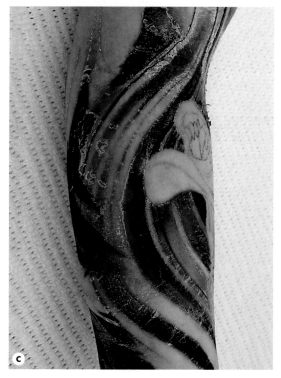

Fig. 5. Infectious complications of tattooing.
a Staphylococcal infection seemingly introduced with yellow tattoo ink. **b** Pyogenic infection in an entire tattoo, starting in the green part of the tattoo and possibly introduced with the green tattoo ink (for sequential photos, see cover of book). **c** Bacterial infection of soft tissue of the arm. Patients **a**, **b**, and **c** were treated with intravenous antibiotics and recovered without sepsis or other complications.

fections may be inoculated. Viral infections include hepatitis B and C; human immunodeficiency virus (HIV); herpes; and viruses causing local infection, such as warts, molluscum, and condylomata.

Infective microorganisms may originate from the tattooed person; the parlour; the tattooist; the needle or the instruments; or, last but not least, the tattoo ink stock product or contaminated water used by the tattooist for dilution of the ink. A recent study showed that, in accordance with other studies, as many as 10% of new inks were contaminated with bacteria that are pathogenic to humans and the label 'Sterile' on a product was not reliable [10]. The spontaneous resistance of tattooed individuals to infectants introduced by a tattoo needle must be high. Most tattooed individuals are young and in good health. Fortunately, we have not observed a very high incidence of bacterial infections following tattooing, although precise data on the incidence and prevalence of infection related to tattooing are not available. Persons having weaknesses and impaired immune systems must be especially vulnerable. Some infections are rare, endemic, or historical, albeit still being a potential treat.

Exposure of the population to pathogenic microorganisms is dynamic and may always change over time. There is presently and will continue to be a special threat from staphylococci resistant to antibiotics and bacteria, *Escherichia coli* with acquired transfer resistance carried by DNA segments, or extended-spectrum beta-lactamase resistance. There is a group of bacteria, 'flesh-eating bacteria', which cause deep wounds and necrotising fasciitis. The infection is life-threatening and may require acute surgery, with wide excision and even amputation. Aggressive strains of *E. coli* from food may cause severe casualties and death, as recently seen in Germany, and *E. coli* can be found in new tattoo inks. Bulk contaminated tattoo inks represent a hitherto and unforseen major potential risk for spread epidemic infection across national borders.

In today's clinic, pyogenic infections with staphylococci, streptococci, Pseudomonas, and *E. coli* and transfer of hepatitis B and C are the main risks associated with tattooing practices.

Infections may be superficial and may manifest as impetigo and pyogenic infection. Abscess formation may develop and require surgical incision. Profound infections may present as erysipelas or as soft-tissue infection, i.e. cellulitis, with swelling of the distal or the entire limb. Oral or intravenous antibiotic treatment is required. Bacteria may pass into the bloodstream and cause sepsis, with high fever, poor general condition, affliction and impairment of vital organs, and ultimately death, unless antibiotic treatment is given and effective in the particular case. Exceptional cases of death from tattooing occur even today. Bacteria from tattooing may also enter the blood, infect the heart valves, and result in cardiac insufficiency. There is clearly a need for early and efficient treatment of bacterial infection, if possible after isolation of the causative microorganism, which also requires culture from the culprit ink. The need for tracing the route of infection to the origin is often neglected. Proper treatment also includes prevention of new cases infected by the same source.

Mycobacterial infections develop slowly. They are often caused by contaminated tap water used for the dilution of ink. Such infections are quite rare but need special diagnostic sampling and treatment. Mycobacterial infections typically develop into local outbreaks in the neighbourhood of a parlour.

From a preventive point of view, visiting 'star' tattooists, who travel around with their tools and inks, presents a special risk of spread of infection, just as tattooing at festivals and conventions may do.

The threat of hepatitis virus B and C remains. In contrast to HIV, these viruses require only a small inoculum to infect a person. Hepatitis remains frequent among drug users. Tattooists' use of gloves and disposable needles helped to reduce this risk. Hepatitis due to tattooing is easily overlooked since this infection may develop slowly and may go unnoticed and since hepatic failure may take decennia to develop. HIV transferred by tattooing may not be noticed and linked to a tattoo since the person may have other risk exposures related to various sexual contacts.

Life-Threatening Hazards

In the past, it was recognised that infections introduced with a tattoo could kill the tattooed individual. The French marine was aware of amputations and death among the mariners and prohibited the mariners from being tattooed [23]. Today death from tattooing is exceptional albeit still a potential risk. As mentioned above the risk may vary over time and abruptly become real. Tetanus infection is today very rare, and populations normally are vaccinated.

Allergic reactions of tattoos are mostly delayed and do not threaten or shorten life unless the allergy is strong, necrotising, or associated with autoimmunity affecting normal tissues.

Syncope while being tattooed may potentially occur due to pain, epilepsy, or cardiac dysfunction or arrest, therefore, the tattooist must be aware of such risk and not tattoo predisposed persons.

There is a rare and special risk associated with allergy to latex protein. Latex particles from the tattooist's gloves can elicit anaphylactic shock in the already-sensitised consumer right as the session starts. During tattooing, tattooists can introduce multiple latex particles from the gloves into the skin and initiate allergic sensitisation of the customer, who, upon some later latex exposure, may unexpectedly and suddenly enter a state of life-threatening anaphylaxis. Some fruits can cross-react with latex and provoke anaphylaxis. Latex gloves also may provoke delayed type allergy causing hand eczema as an occupational disease affecting the tattooist.

References

1 De Cuyoer C, Perez-Cotapos M-L: Dermatologic Complications with Body Art. Tattoos, Piercings and Permanent Make-Up. Berlin-Heidelberg, Springer Verlag, 2010.

2 Goldstein N: Tattoos. J Dermatol Surg Oncol 1979;5:846–916.

3 Jacob CI: Tattoo-associated dermatoses: a case report and review of the literature. Am Soc Derm Surg 2002;28:962–965.

4 Kazandjieva J, Tsankov N: Tattoos: dermatological complications. Clin Dermatol 2007;25:375–382.

5 Kaatz M, Elsner P, Bauer A: Body-modifying concepts and dermatologic problems. Clin Dermatol 2008;26:35–44.

6 Mataix J, Silvestre JF: Cutaneous adverse reactions to tattoos and piercings. Acta Dermosifilogr 2009;100:643–656.

7 Kluger N: Cutaneous complications related to permanent decorative tattooing. Expert Rev Clin Immunol 2010;6: 363–371.

8 Desai NA, Smith ML: Body art in adolescents: paint, piercings and perils. Adolesc Med 2011;22:97–118.

9 Wenzel SM, Rittman I, Landthaler M, Bäumler W: Adverse reactions after tattooing: review of the literature and comparison to results of a survey. Dermatology 2013;226:138–147.

10 Høgsberg T, Saunte DM, Frimodt-Møller N, Serup J: Microbial status and product labelling of 58 original tattoo inks. J Eur Acad Dermatol Venereol 2013;27:73–80.

11 Baumgartner A, Gautsch S: Hygienic-microbiological quality of tattoo- and permanent make-up colours. J Verbr Lebensm 2011;6:319–325.

12 Kluger N, Koljonen V: Tattoos, inks and cancer. Lancet Oncol 2012;13:e161–e168.

13 Klügl I, Hiller K-A, Landthaler M, Bäumler W: Incidence of health problems associated with tattooed skin: a nation-wide survey in German-speaking countries. Dermatology 2010;221:43–50.

14 Høgsberg T, Carlsen KH, Serup J: High prevalence of minor symptoms in tattooos among a young population tattooed with carbon black and organic pigments. J Eur Acad Dermatol Venereol 2013;27:846–852.

15 Hutton Carlsen K, Serup J: Photosensitivity and photodynamic events in balck, red and blue tattoos are common: a 'Beach Study'. J Eur Acad Dermatol Venereol 2013, DOI: 10.1111/jdv.12093.

16 Serup J, Hutton Carlsen K: Patch test study of 90 patients with tattoo reactions: negative outcome of allergy patch to baseline batteries and culprit inks suggests allergen(s) are generated in the skin through haptinization. Contact Dermatitis 2014;71:255-263.

17 Hutton Carlsen K, Serup J: Patients with tattoo reactions have reduced quality of life and suffer from itch: Dermatology Life Quality Index and Itch Severity Score measurements. Skin Res Technol 2014, DOI: 10.1111/srt. 12164.

18 Morte PD, Mgee LM: Hyperalgesia after volar wrist tattoo: a case of complex regional pain syndrome? J Clin Neuromuscular Dis 2011;12:118–121.

19 Morales-Calaghan AM, Aguilar-Bernier M, Martinez-Garcia G, Miranda-Romero A: Sarcoid granuloma on black tattoo. J Am Acad Dermatol 2006;55:71–73.

20 Köbner H: Zur aethiologie der psoriasis. Viertel Jahresschrift für Dermatologie und Syphilis 1876;3:559–561.

21 Long GE, Rickman LS: Infectious complications of tattoos. Clin Infect Dis 1994;18:610–619.

22 Kluger N: Complications infectiouses cutanées assciées au tatouage permanent. Médicine et Maladies Infectieuses 2011;41:115–122.

23 Berchon E: Histoire Médicale du Tatouage. Paris, J-B Bailliè et Fils, 1869.

Prof. Jørgen Serup, MD, DMSc
Dermatology D41, Bispebjerg University Hospital
Bispebjerg Bakke 23
DK–2400 Copenhagen NV (Denmark)
E-Mail joergen.vedelskov.serup@regionh.dk

Serup J, Kluger N, Bäumler W (eds): Tattooed Skin and Health.
Curr Probl Dermatol. Basel, Karger, 2015, vol 48, pp 61–70 (DOI: 10.1159/000369188)

Complications of Cosmetic Tattoos

Christa De Cuyper

Department of Dermatology, AZ Sint-Jan, Brugge, Belgium

Abstract

Cosmetic tattoos, which are better known as permanent make-up, have become popular in the last decades. This same procedure can be used to camouflage pathological skin conditions, to mask scars and to complete the aesthetic results of plastic and reconstructive surgeries. The risks and complications of tattooing procedures include infections and allergic reactions. Scarring can occur. Fanning and fading of the colorants and dissatisfaction with colour and shape are not unusual. Different lasers can offer solutions for the removal of unwanted cosmetic tattoos, but complications due to the laser treatment, such as paradoxical darkening and scarring, can arise.

© 2015 S. Karger AG, Basel

Introduction

Since the 19th century, several reports have illustrated the medical applications of tattooing for aesthetic purposes [1–3]. The introduction of eyelid tattooing in 1984 represented a new start of facial cosmetic tattooing [4]. The main purpose of cosmetic tattooing is to enhance natural beauty and to increase physical appeal. The majority of subjects choose cosmetic tattooing because it offers an easy alternative to conventional make-up.

Technique and Materials

Cosmetic tattooing, which is also called micropigmentation, is usually performed with an electrical tattoo device or a tattoo pen with a rotating or oscillating disposable needle (fig. 1). Small droplets of specific permanent make-up (PMU) tattoo ink are implanted into the superficial layer of the dermis in contrast with decorative tattooing, in which the deposition of pigment occurs deeper within the dermis. Some PMU devices are programmed for specific indications. A good knowledge of anatomy is important to ensure for good results. Single-use ink caps are advised, and registration of the colours used can be helpful for later corrections. Prepared inks are available on the market, but some

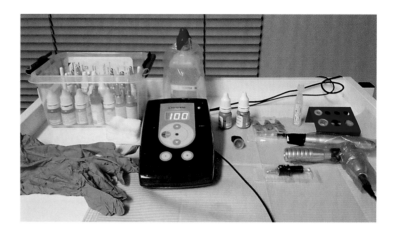

Fig. 1. Tattoo (PMU) device.

professionals make their own mixtures to obtain optimal colours to match a client's favourite make-up. The elimination of pigment can occur during the first days of healing. After healing, the remaining pigment particles are stored in dermal macrophages and fibroblasts. The nature of the material used and the level of implantation influence the quality and stability of the results. Because the level of application of PMU is more superficial than that in decorative tattooing, the spontaneous elimination of the colorant and fading may occur within years.

Indications

PMU is an excellent replacement for conventional make-up and a practical solution for people with an active lifestyle because it is time saving and always looks perfect and fresh [5] (table 1). Some choose this procedure because they have a physical impairment complicating the application of temporary make-up. Eyeliner or blepharo-pigmentation, lip liner and eyebrow colouring are very popular. When it is properly applied by an experienced technician, PMU can be more natural and realistic in appearance than conventional make-up. Medical indications include corneal reconstruction and nipple-areola complex

Table 1. Indications for cosmetic tattoos/PMU

Replacement of conventional make-up
Medical reasons:
– patients with allergies to conventional make-up
– disabled persons (arthrosis-arthritis)
– trembling hands (Parkinson disease)
– poor vision/contact lenses
– hay fever
Camouflage and correction of:
– scars (accidental and surgical)
– nipple-areola complex reconstruction
– birthmarks
– alopecia/vitiligo

reconstruction after breast reduction or breast cancer surgery [3] (fig. 2). Tattooing may help to camouflage scars, birth marks, vitiligo and alopecia and also offers a solution for patients with allergies to conventional cosmetics [6] (fig. 3).

Risks and Complications

Tattooing in general is not without risks [7] (table 2). The major risk of complications and dissatisfaction is caused by the performing of the

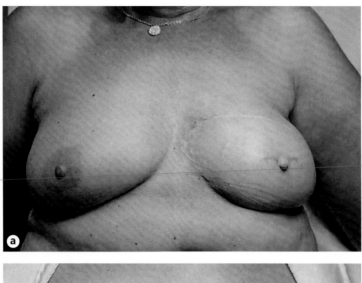

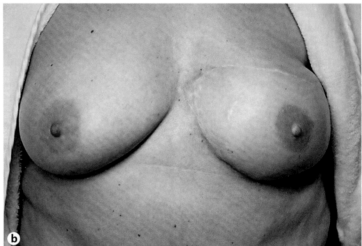

Fig. 2. Nipple-areola complex reconstruction before (**a**) and after (**b**) (courtesy of Rika Dubelloy).

procedure by an inexperienced person under poor hygienic circumstances and with materials of dubious origin. Side effects can be related to the procedure and the aftercare and also to the instruments and compositions of the inks used [8]. Short-term side effects include mild swelling and crusting, which are usually dealt with by clients and tattooists and not reported. However, when more important problems, such as infections and allergic reactions, arise, medical advice is required [9]. The US Food and Drug Administration (FDA) registered only 5 reports of adverse reactions associated with PMU from 1988 to 2003. Beginning in 2003, the FDA received more than 150 reports of adverse events occurring in persons who had undergone PMU procedures, including some severe and long-term disfiguring complications. Symptom durations have ranged from 5.5 months to more than 3 years. More adverse reactions have been linked with a specific product line, suggesting an increased risk associated with the use of these inks. This product line was recalled from the market in September 2004 [10].

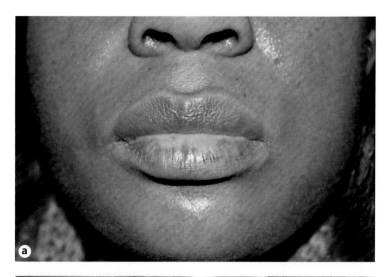

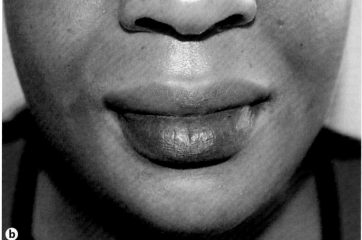

Fig. 3. Vitiligo lip correction before (**a**) and after (**b**) (courtesy of Rika Dubelloy and Finishing Touches).

Infections

When performed under correct hygienic conditions and with sterile materials, the occurrence of bacterial infection is rare. Inks can be contaminated before or after bottles are opened [11]. In recent years, several cases of atypical mycobacterial infections in decorative and cosmetic tattoos have been reported [12–14]. Histological and microbiological confirmations are helpful to exclude other granulomatous conditions, such as sarcoidosis, foreign body reactions and allergic granulomatous manifestations and to identify the responsible pathogen [15–17]. Source identification is a very important issue [12]. The registration of inks in a client's file can help to identify contaminated batches. Recently, a voluntary recall of tattoo ink, tattoo needles and tattoo kits distributed by White & Blue Lion due to pathogenic bacterial contamination was announced by the FDA [18].

Viral and mycotic infections are extremely rare. Unsterile equipment and needles can transmit all types of blood-borne infections, such as

Table 2. Complications of tattooing

Bleeding (several minutes to one hour)
Crusting (2–3 days)
Swelling (2–5 days)
Infections
    Localized
     – bacterial (emerging mycobacterial infections)
     – viral (herpes simplex)
    Systemic (blood-borne diseases)
     – hepatitis
     – human immunodeficiency virus
    Allergic reactions
     – eczematous
     – lichenoid
     – granulomatous
Hypertrophic scars/keloids
Sarcoidosis
Loss of eyelashes
Eyelid necrosis
Ectropion
MRI complications
Dissatisfaction
    Unnatural aspect
    Colour
    Shape
    Fading
    Fanning
    Distortion

hepatitis and human immunodeficiency virus. Preventive screening of body art practitioners and vaccination for hepatitis B are advised. The risk of herpes simplex reactivation on the lips induced by the procedure should be taken into account (fig. 4).

Allergy

The pigments and dyes used in tattoo and PMU inks are relatively inert and are usually well tolerated. Allergic reactions to colorants are rare, but when they occur, they may be particularly troublesome because the pigments can be difficult to remove. The majority of allergic reactions that have been reported have been related to red inks. Hypersensitivity reactions can have different clinical and histological presentations, including lichenoid, psoriasiform, eczematous, lymphomatoid and granulomatous reactions. Clinical aspects and histopathologies are often suggestive of a delayed-type allergy (fig. 5). Skin testing, however, has produced very disappointing results [19]. *In vivo* haptenisation of the colorant could be the explanation [20]. Contact dermatitis to other ingredients and additives or to the materials used during and after the procedure, such as topical antibiotics, can also occur. Photosensitivity of tattoos is probably the reason why more adverse reactions have been reported in tattoos in sun-exposed areas, such as the hands and face [7, 21].

Other Complications

In general, cosmetic tattooing causes little discomfort, and side effects are rare, although complications, such as eyelid necrosis, the loss of eyelashes, secondary cicatricial ectropion, hypertrophic scars and keloids, have been reported [1, 13]. To reduce the risk of ocular injury, protective eye shields can be used during the procedure [22]. The possibility of the Koebner effect in patients with a pre-existing skin disorder, such as psoriasis, must be considered. There have been reports of people with tattoos and permanent make-up experiencing swelling or burning in the tattooed areas when undergoing magnetic resonance imaging. This has been reported only rarely and has not been associated with any lasting effects. Pigments may also interfere with the quality of the image, particularly in the eye area [23]. The extremely rare association of skin cancer with tattoos in general and with PMU in particular seems to be a coincidence rather than a causative relation [24, 25].

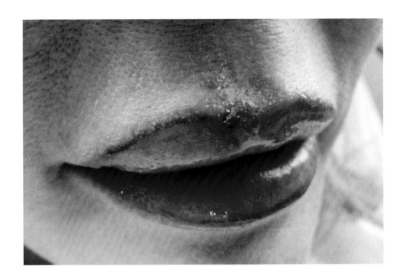

Fig. 4. Herpes simplex of the lip (courtesy of Jørgen Serup).

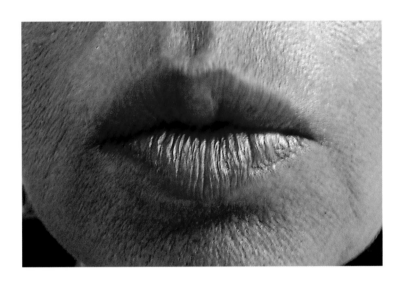

Fig. 5. Allergic reaction of PMU lip liner (courtesy of Jørgen Serup).

Dissatisfaction

Some people have unrealistic expectations and are unhappy with their cosmetic results. Customers should be informed that tissue augmentation, botulin toxin injection and plastic surgery of the face can change the appearance and lead to the distortion of PMU.

The most common complications and patient dissatisfaction, however, result from the misap-plication of colorants, pigment migration and pigment fanning [5, 26]. In these situations, the advantage of being permanent becomes the greatest disadvantage (fig. 6).

Treatment of Complications

Medical complications should be treated with specific case-related measures. Localised bacterial in-

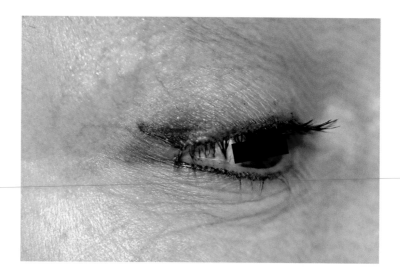

Fig. 6. Dissatisfaction. Unnatural aspect of eyeliner and fanning of the pigment.

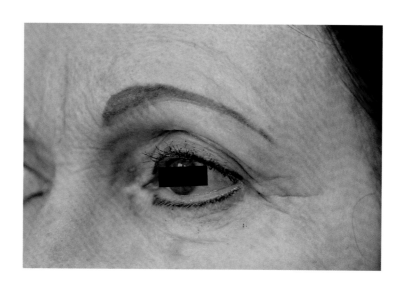

Fig. 7. Dissatisfaction with the colour and shape of eyebrow PMU.

fections require antiseptic or antibiotic treatment to minimise the risk of scarring. For severe infections, systemic antibiotics are needed. Allergic manifestations can be treated with topical applications or infiltration with corticosteroids [19]. The combination of intralesional injections of steroids and 5-fluorouracil has been used to treat foreign body reactions and may be considered. The resolution of a lip-enhancing tattoo reaction by topical tacrolimus treatment has been documented by Wylie [27]. Granulomatous reactions are often problematic because the causative material is difficult to remove. Systemic therapy with corticosteroids and cyclosporine can be used but rarely provides satisfactory results. Chronic reactions sometimes require more invasive techniques, including surgical dermabrasion or pigment removal with ablative lasers [28–30]. Objectionable tattoos can be camouflaged with conventional make-up. Over time, most cosmetic tattoos fade spontaneously.

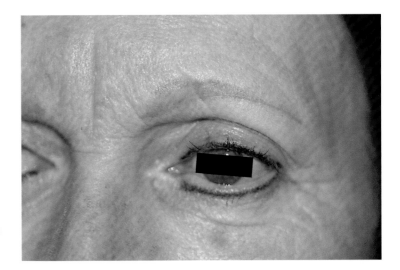

Fig. 8. Results of partial clearing after treatment with a combination of a QS Nd-Yag 532 and QS Nd-Yag 1064 laser.

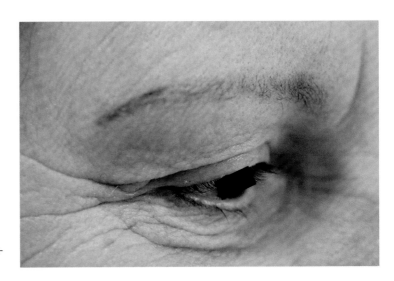

Fig. 9. Darkening of PMU after treatment with a QS Nd-Yag 532 laser.

Some people attempt to cover an unwanted tattoo with a new one with flesh tones, which seldom gives satisfactory cosmetic results because skin-toned pigments tend to look unnatural due to the fact that they lack the skin's natural translucence. Moreover, the dark underlying colours are difficult to hide. Medical advice is sought by people who want their tattoos removed. Successful treatments with tretinoin and with penta-monogalloylglucose have been reported but have not been confirmed by large studies [31, 32]. Non-specific removal

techniques, such as surgery and dermabrasion, are available but have risks of scarring and residual textural and pigmentary changes. The best cosmetic results can be obtained using pigment lasers, but even this technique has its risks, and the complete clearing of the tattoo cannot be guaranteed [33] (fig. 7, 8). Flesh tones and red tattoos containing ferric oxide may show immediate darkening when treated with short pulse lasers [33–36]. This is probably caused by the reduction of red-brown-coloured ferric oxide to black-coloured

De Cuyper

ferrous oxide (fig. 9). In our experience, the dark colour can often be subsequently removed using another appropriate wavelength [5]. Paradoxical darkening can also occur in tattoos containing titanium dioxide. The topical application of perfluorodecalin may be helpful for the reduction of laser-induced whitening, allowing for more laser passes per treatment session and improving the outcome [37]. In some recalcitrant cases, dermabrasion techniques with a carbon dioxide laser can offer a solution [28]. Pico-second lasers could be more effective but are still under investigation.

Conclusion

Although cosmetic tattooing is a common and popular procedure and is usually well tolerated, complications can occur. One problem associated with this procedure lies in the lack of uniform legislation worldwide and the lack of control of the production of the substances used. The availability of correct information about the associated risks as well as the performance of the procedure by a well-trained professional can minimise complications and dissatisfaction.

References

1 Vassileva S, Hristakieva E: Medical applications of tattooing. Clinics Dermatol 2007;25:367–374.
2 Van der Velden EM, Defrancq J, Ijselmuiden OE: Review: dermatography: a review of 15 years of clinical applications in surgery. Int J Cosm Surgery Aest Dermatol 2001;3:151–159.
3 Fahradi J, Maksvytyte GK, Schaefer DJ, et al: Reconstruction of the nipple-areola complex: an update. J Plast Reconstr Aesthet Surg 2006;59:40–53.
4 Angres G: Eyeliner implants: a new cosmetic procedure. Plast Reconstr Surg 1984;73:833–836.
5 De Cuyper C: Permanent makeup: indications and complications. Clin Dermatol 2008;26:30–34.
6 Seité S, Deshayes P, Dréno B, et al: Interest of corrective makeup in the management of patients in dermatology. Clin Cosm Invest Dermatol 2012;5:123–128.
7 Wenzel SM, Rittmann I, Landthaler M, et al: Adverse reactions after tattooing: review of the literature and comparison to results of a survey. Dermatology 2013;226:138–147.
8 Pérez-Cotapos ML, De Cuyper C, Cossio L: Tattooing and scarring: technique and complications; in De Cuyper C, Pérez-Cotapos ML (eds): Dermatologic Complications with Body Art: Tattoos, Piercings and Permanent Make-Up. Berlin, Springer Heidelberg, 2010, pp 29–41.
9 Ortiz AE, Alster TS: Rising concern over cosmetic tattoos. Dermatol Surg 2012; 38:424–429.

10 Straetemans M, Katz LM, Belson M: Adverse reactions after permanent-makeup procedures. N Engl J Med 2007; 356:26.
11 Hoegsberg T, Saunte DM, Frimodt-Møller N, et al: Microbial status and product labelling of 58 original tattoo inks. J Eur Acad Dermatol Venereol 2013;27:73–80.
12 Kennedy BS, Bedard B, Younge M, et al: Outbreak of Mycobacterium chelonae infection associated with tattoo ink. N Engl J Med 2012;367:1020–1024.
13 Wollina U: Nodular skin reactions in eyebrow permanent makeup: two case reports and an infection with Mycobacterium haemophilum. J Cosmet Dermatol 2011;10:235–239.
14 Guilieri S, Morisod B, Edney T, et al: Outbreak of Mycobacterium haemophilum infections after permanent makeup of the eyebrows. Clin Infect Dis 2011;52: 488–491.
15 Antonovich DD, Callen JP: Development of sarcoidosis in cosmetic tattoos. Arch Dermatol 2005;141:869–872.
16 Yesudian PD, Azurdia RM: Scar sarcoidosis following tattooing of the lips treated with mepacrine. Clin Exp Dermatol 2004;29:552–554.
17 Baumgarter M, Feldmann R, Steiner A: Sarcoidal granulomas in a cosmetic tattoo in association with pulmonary sarcoidosis. J Dtsch Dermatol Ges 2010;9: 900–902.
18 Specialty Pharma Association. Industry News. http://www.specialtypharma.org/news.asp?id=356157.

19 Wenzel SM, Welzel J, Hafner C, et al: Permanent make-up colorants may cause severe skin reactions. Contact Dermatitis 2010;63:223–227.
20 Serup J, Hutton Carlsen K: Patch test study of 90 patients with tattoo reactions: negative outcome of allergy patch tests to baseline batteries and culprit inks suggest allergen(s) are generated in the skin through haptenization. Contact Dermatitis 2014;71:255–263.
21 Jaeger C, Hartschuh W, Jappe U: Sunlight-induced granulomatous reaction to permanent lip liner. Hautarzt 2005;56:63–65.
22 Konuk O, Evereklioglu C, Handur A, et al: Protective eyeshield can prevent corneal trauma during micropigmentation for permanent eyeliner. J Eur Acad Dermatol 2004;18:642–643.
23 Tope WD, Shellock FG: Magnetic resonance imaging and permanent cosmetics (tattoos): survey of complications and adverse events. J Magn Reson Imaging 2002;15:180–184.
24 Kluger N, Koljonen V: Tattoos, inks, and cancer. Lancet Oncol 2012;13:e161–e168.
25 Ortiz A, Yamauchi PS: Rapidly growing squamous cell carcinoma from permanent makeup tattoo. J Am Acad Dermatol 2009;60:1073–1074.
26 Lee IW, Ahn SK, Choi EH, et al: Complications of eyelash and eyebrow tattooing: reports of 2 cases of pigment fanning. Cutis 2001;68:53–55.
27 Wylie G, Gupta G: Lip-enhancing tattoo reaction resolving with topical tacrolimus. Clin Exp Dermatol 2008;33:505–506.

28 Fitzpatrick RE, Lupton JR: Successful treatment of treatment resistant laser-induced pigment darkening of a cosmetic tattoo. Lasers Surg Med 2000;27:358–361.

29 Mafong EA, Kauvar AN, Geronimus RG: Surgical pearl: removal of cosmetic lip-liner tattoo with pulsed carbon dioxide laser. J Am Acad Dermatol 2003;48:271–272.

30 Ibrahimi OA, Syed Z, Sakomoto FH, et al: Treatment of tattoo allergy with ablative fractional resurfacing: a novel paradigm for tattoo removal. J Am Acad Dermatol 2011;66:111–114.

31 Van der Velden EM, Oostrom CAM, Roddi R, et al: Dermatography with penta-monogalloylglucose as a new treatment for removal of color pigments in the eyebrows. Am J Cosm Surg 1995;12:3–9.

32 Chiang JK, Barsky S, Bronson DM: Tretinoin in the removal of eyeliner tattoo. J Am Acad Dermatol 1999;40:999–1001.

33 Verhaeghe E: Techniques and devices used for tattoo removal; in De Cuyper C, Pérez-Cotapos ML (eds): Dermatologic Complications with Body Art: Tattoos, Piercings and Permanent Make-Up. Berlin, Springer Heidelberg, 2010, pp 91–105.

34 Anderson RR, Geronimus R, Kilmer SL: Cosmetic tattoo ink darkening. A complication of Q-Switched and pulsed-laser treatment. Arch Dermatol 1993;129:1010–1014.

35 Chang SE, Kim KJ, Choi JH: Areolar cosmetic tattoo ink darkening: a complication of alexandrite laser. Dermatol Surg 2002;28:95–96.

36 Jimenez G, Weiss E, Spencer JM: Multiple color changes following laser therapy of cosmetic tattoos. J Dermatol Surg 2002;28:177–179.

37 Reddy KK, Brauer JA, Bernstein L, et al: Topical perfluorodecalin resolves immediate whitening reactions and allows rapid effective multiple pass treatment of tattoos. Lasers Surg Med 2013;45:76–80.

Christa De Cuyper, MD
Meiboomstraat 15
BE–8370 Blankenberge (Belgium)
E-Mail christa.decuyper@telenet.be

De Cuyper

Serup J, Kluger N, Bäumler W (eds): Tattooed Skin and Health.
Curr Probl Dermatol. Basel, Karger, 2015, vol 48, pp 71–75 (DOI: 10.1159/000369644)

Chronic Tattoo Reactions Cause Reduced Quality of Life Equaling Cumbersome Skin Diseases

Katrina Hutton Carlsen · Jørgen Serup

Department of Dermatology, 'Tattoo Clinic', Bispebjerg University Hospital, Copenhagen, Denmark

Abstract

Tattoos are often associated with mild complaints, but some people develop complications that may require medical treatment, and the burden of these events has hitherto been neglected. To understand the dimensions and the psychological symptomatology of adverse events both the sensory and affective impacts, including the effect on quality of life, should be studied. Itch severity and influence on quality of life can be measured objectively. The Itch Severity Scale and Dermatology Life Quality Index scoring systems have been applied to different dermatological diseases. When ISS and DLQI scores were applied to patients with chronic tattoo reactions, tattoo complaints and impact on quality of life that were comparable to patients presenting cumbersome dermatological disease such as psoriasis, eczema and pruritus, which often show widespread effects to the skin, were uncovered. In conclusion, chronic tattoo reactions should be ranked as a cumbersome dermatological disease and, accordingly, given priority attention and qualified treatment by the public health care system.

© 2015 S. Karger AG, Basel

Introduction

Signs and symptoms of tattooed skin deviating from normal skin may be mild and acceptable, i.e. at the level of complaint or, when more severe and cumbersome, considered a complication, both of which may require medical treatment. The concept of disease goes beyond the objective signs and findings; it also includes the subjective experience and its influence on patients' lives.

Itch, stinging and pain are the most frequent reported tattoo complaints [1, 2]. Sun-induced reactions, especially in dark colours, are reported in one of five tattooed individuals, with swelling and itching being the most frequent complaints.

The chronic complications are dominated by allergic reactions, which may develop within weeks, months or years. Allergic reactions especially occur in red tattoos. Patients presenting clinically with allergic reactions are patch tested with common allergens, textile dyes, a battery of suspect tattoo ink stock products and their individual suspect inks, all of which result in an overall negative outcome [3]. The putative allergens are not directly present in the ink stock products but are formed inside the dermis over a longer period.

In this chapter, we will review the subjective symptoms associated with chronic tattoo complaints, i.e. reactions when the tattooed person may seek help from a medical professional. How do these symptoms intrude on patients' lives? What effects do they play on quality of life?

Measurements of Itch and Quality of Life

Different methods are employed to measure the burden of disease and the impact on quality of life. In the field of dermatology, the Itch Severity Scale (ISS) and the Dermatology Life Quality Index (DLQI) are mainly used.

The ISS is a questionnaire designed for the patient [4]. It was devised by Majeski et al. [5] to measure both the sensory and the affective dimensions of itch and is composed of the following 7 topics:

(1) description; (2a) sensory; (2b) affective; (3) body area; (4) intensity; (5) effect on mood; (6) effect on sexual desire/function, and (7) effect on sleep.

DLQI, which was introduced by Finlay and Khan, is a questionnaire including the following topics and elements. (1) and (2): Symptoms and feelings; (3) and (4): daily activities; (5) and (6): leisure; (7): work and school; (8) and (9): personal relationships, and (10): treatment [6, 7].

Both scoring systems are self-explanatory and can easily be completed by an adult patient. They have also both been evaluated on dermatological patients and concluded to be valid [8, 9]. Higher scores in the ISS and DLQI systems indicate a greater impact on the patients' lives. By utilizing the same methods for interpreting patients' experiences with disease, a comparison of different disease populations can be performed and the best therapy can be implemented.

Skin Disease and Quality of Life

Itch is a great burden for many dermatological patients influencing their psyche and, thereby, their ability to cope with disease. The ISS has been used to evaluate patients with pruritus, genital pruritus and nephrogenic pruritus as well as atopic dermatitis, psoriasis and urticaria [5, 8], which revealed ISS scores from 7.4 to 13.4 (table 1). Besides intensive itching, the patients also experienced depressive symptoms, anxiety and sleep impairments, which in some cases had a substantial effect on their daily life.

The DLQI has also been utilized on patients with hand eczema, pruritus and neurodermatitis and has demonstrated a moderate effect on patients' lives [4, 10, 12]. Psoriasis and atopic dermatitis have a big effect on patients' lives (table 1) [11–14].

Tattoo Complications and Quality of Life

Patients with tattoo reactions were often reported to experience itch/stinging at an extreme level when at its worst that commences all hours of the day (morning/afternoon/evening/night) [15].

Patients with tattoo reactions revealed an average ISS score of 7.2, with a range from 0 to 21 [15]. The influence of itch is presented in figure 1.

Itch was associated with concern in 48% of cases, irritation in 18% of cases, depression in 20% of cases, anxiety in 43% of cases, and concentration problems in 48% of cases. Itch also affected patients' sleep, ranging from problems falling asleep to sleep disturbance.

Interestingly, the grade of the symptom was independent of the size of the afflicted area.

The average DLQI score was 7.4 [15]. Tattoo problems had a moderate effect on patient's quality of life, and the results of the influence of tattoos on daily living are presented in figure 2. Symptoms and feelings had the greatest impact

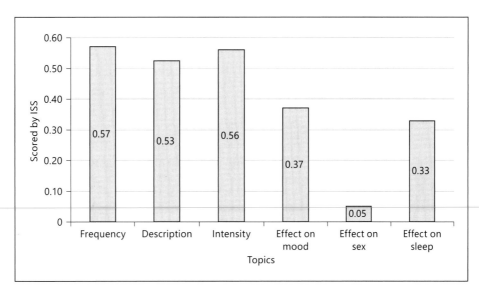

Fig. 1. The extent of tattoos causing itch, measured by the Itch Severity Scale (ISS).

Table 1. Dermatological diagnoses scored by the Itch Severity Scale (ISS) and the Dermatology Life Quality Index (DLQI)

Diagnoses	DLQI score, in total	ISS, in total	Number of participants (n)	Reference
Hand eczema	8.0	–	416	Agner et al. [10]
Pruritus	8.8	–	40	Zachariae et al. [4]
	–	9.7	83	Zachariae et al. [8]
		7.4	93	Majeski et al. [5]
Genital pruritus	–	8.6	12	Zachariae et al. [8]
Nephrogenic pruritus	–	8.5	11	Zachariae et al. [8]
Atopic dermatitis	–	9.5	20	Zachariae et al. [8]
	10.7		415	Kim et al. [11]
Neurodermatitis	9.34	–	150	An et al. [12]
Psoriasis	13.32	–	250	An et al. [12]
	–	7.5	20	Zachariae et al. [8]
	13.1	–	57	Karelson et al. [13]
	10.0		250	Tang et al. [14]
Urticaria	–	13.4	20	Zachariae et al. [8]

on patients' lives, including itching, soreness, pain and/or stinging symptoms. More than half of the patients experienced varying degrees of embarrassment/self-consciousness due to their tattoo reactions. Tattoo reactions also influenced daily activities, e.g. housekeeping in 38% of cases, choice of clothing in 53% of cases and leisure, e.g. sport activities, in 40% of cases. Personal relationships, including sex, were only mildly influenced (13%).

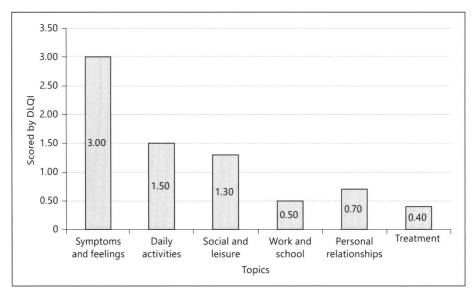

Fig. 2. Tattoos' influence on daily living, measured by the Dermatology Life Quality Index (DLQI).

Conclusion

Patients with chronic tattoo reactions are heavily burdened by itch, while stinging and pain have a moderate impact on their daily lives. The ISS and DLQI scores are comparable to those of cumbersome and widespread dermatological diseases, e.g. psoriasis, eczema and chronic pruritus. Chronic tattoo reactions should be ranked as a cumbersome dermatological disease and given priority attention and qualified treatment by the public health care system.

References

1 Hutton Carlsen K, Serup J: Photosensitivity and photodynamic events in black, red and blue tattoos are common: a 'Beach Study'. J Eur Acad Dermatol Venereol 2013, DOI: 10.1111/jdv.12093.
2 Høgsberg T, Hutton Carlsen K, Serup J: High prevalence of minor symptoms in tattoos among a young population tattooed with carbon black and organic pigments. J Eur Acad Dermatol Venereol 2012;27:846–852.
3 Serup J, Hutton Carlsen K: Patch test study of 90 patients with tattoo reactions: negative outcome of allergy patch test to baseline batteries and culprit inks suggests allergen(s) are generated in the skin through haptenization. Contact Dermatitis 2014;71:255–263.

4 Zachariae R, Claus O, Zachariae C, Lei U, Pedersen AF: Affective and sensory dimensions of pruritus severity: associations with psychological symptoms and quality of life in psoriasis patients. Acta Derm Venereol 2008;88:121–127.
5 Majeski CJ, Johnson JA, Davidson SN, Lauzon CJ: Itch Severity Scale: a self-report instrument for the measurement of pruritus severity. Br J Dermatol 2007; 156:667–673.
6 Finlay AY, Khan GK: Dermatology Life Quality Index (DLQI): a simple practical measure for routine clinical use. Clin Exp Dermatol 1994;19:210–216.

7 Finlay AY, Khan GK: Dermatology Life Quality Index: information & conditions concerning use. 1992. http://www.dermatology.org.uk/quality/dlqi/quality-dlqi-info.html (accessed November 8, 2014).
8 Zachariae R, Lei U, Haedersdal M, Zachariae C: Itch severity and quality of life in patients with pruritus: preliminary validity of a Danish adaptation of the Itch Severity Scale. Acta Derm Venereol 2012;92:508–514.
9 Zachariae R, Zachariae C, Ibsen H, Mortensen JT, Wulf HC: Dermatology life quality index: data from Danish inpatients and outpatients. Acta Derm Venereol 2000;80:272–276.

10 Agner T, Andersen KE, Brandao FM, Bruynzeel DP, Bruze M, Frosch P, Goncalo M, Goossens A, Le Coz CJ, Rustemeyer T, White IR, Diepgen T; EECDRG: Hand eczema severity and quality of life: a cross-sectional, multicentre study of hand eczema patients. Contact Dermatitis 2008;59:43–47.

11 Kim DH, Li K, Seo SJ, Jo SJ, Yim HW, Kim CM, Kim KH, Kim do W, Kim MB, Kim JW, Ro YS, Park YL, Park CW, Lee SC, Cho SH: Quality of life and disease severity are correlated in patients with atopic dermatitis. J Korean Med Sci 2012;27:1327–1332.

12 An JG, Liu YT, Xiao SX, Wang JM, Geng SM, Dong YY: Quality of life of patients with neurodermatitis. Int J Med Sci 2013;10:593–598.

13 Karelson M, Silm H, Kingo K: Quality of life and emotional state in vitiligo in an Estonian sample: comparison with psoriasis and healthy controls. Acta Derm Venereol 2013;93:446–450.

14 Tang MM, Chang CC, Chan LC, Heng A: Quality of life and cost of illness in patients with psoriasis in Malaysia: a multicenter study. Int J Dermatol 2013;52: 314–322.

15 Hutton Carlsen K, Serup J: Patients with tattoo reactions have reduced quality of life and suffer from itch. Dermatology Life Quality Index (DLQI) and Itch Severity Score (ISS) measurements. Skin Res Technol 2015;21:101–107.

Katrina Hutton Carlsen
Department of Dermatology D, Bispebjerg University Hospital
Bispebjerg Bakke 23
DK–2400 Copenhagen NV (Denmark)
E-Mail katrinahuttoncarlsen@hotmail.com

Serup J, Kluger N, Bäumler W (eds): Tattooed Skin and Health.
Curr Probl Dermatol. Basel, Karger, 2015, vol 48, pp 76–87 (DOI: 10.1159/000369189)

Contraindications for Tattooing

Nicolas Kluger

University of Helsinki and Helsinki University Central Hospital, Dermatology, Helsinki, Finland

Abstract

Tattooing is getting increasingly popular among the young. However, not everyone is suited to getting tattooed. Indeed, it is not rare for patients with a chronic skin disease or another systemic condition to be eager to get a tattoo. They perceive tattooing as a harmless, risk-free procedure. Therefore, some patients may not seek medical advice before the procedure. Some also fear a judgmental approach by their physician, who may try to discourage them. Lastly, the tattooist does not have either the training or the education to properly advise a customer about his/her condition. Therefore, it is important that any physician be able to provide adequate counselling regarding the possibility of getting tattooed and under which conditions. Even though an exhaustive list is impossible to address, the main issues include chronic skin disorders, pigmented lesions of the skin, (congenital) heart disease, immunosuppressive diseases and treatments, blood clotting disorders, and pregnancy/breastfeeding. © 2015 S. Karger AG, Basel

The contraindications for tattooing are by far one of the most important questions regarding customers' safety. This question is also paradoxically the most underrepresented in terms of medical publications. In our experience, too many physicians tend to quickly judge and contraindicate tattooing for patients, without any real data to support such a position. From our point of view, there is no strict contraindication to getting a tattoo done; however, there is definitely a certain number of situations in which individuals who want to get a tattoo should first seek medical advice to determine whether or not they can get one and, if so, under which conditions they can get it. In our daily experience, we are often contacted by professional tattooists or patients, usually with common skin conditions such as psoriasis, atopic dermatitis, or eczema, to find out whether the patients' skin is suited to being tattooed. However, we have also had to answer questions about more uncommon situations and patients with rarer conditions, such as cirrhosis, renal graft, angiomas, the Sutton phenomenon, von Willebrand disease, or even pseudoxanthoma elasticum or xeroderma pigmentosum!

Therefore, it is impossible to be fully exhaustive regarding all skin and systemic conditions to consider when deciding whether or not someone can get a tattoo. This chapter intends to summarize the most frequent situations and questions that a physician may have to deal with. From our perspective, every physician should know about these situations and be able to deliver correct and honest information to a patient who wants to get a tattoo.

Skin Diseases

Chronic Skin Disorders

The main risk for patients with chronic skin disorders when getting tattooed, which is often a matter of concern for them, is the development of the very same lesion at the site of the tattoo, e.g. the Köbner phenomenon [1]. Advising our patients with chronic skin disorders who want to get a tattoo is challenging. With the multitude of possible skin disorders, no one can predict whether a specific condition may lead to Köbnerization. The risk of Köbnerization for one disease varies from one patient to another. Meanwhile, some patients use tattooing as a way to camouflage skin lesions (scars, extended vitiligo, etc.) and/or to regain control of their body and cope with their (disfiguring) disease (fig. 1, 2). The potential beneficial effects of tattooing should not be neglected. Therefore, advice about disease should be given on a case-by-case basis, especially if the 'well-being' benefits are underlined.

According to the Boyd-Nelder classification, only three diseases do Köbnerize (psoriasis, lichen planus, and vitiligo) [2, 3] (fig. 3, 4). However, by experience, the Köbner phenomenon may complicate any dermatological disease, which may be localized to a site of previous trau-

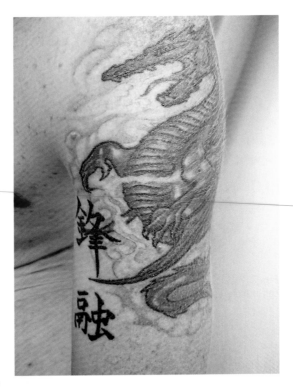

Fig. 1. Tattoo on a young patient with neurofibromatosis type 1.

ma. It is therefore not surprising that a wide number of dermatologic conditions have been described as arising on tattoos, even though such cases are usually anecdotal (table 1) [1].

It is not uncommon for us to be contacted by customers, patients, or tattooists about a condition and questioned about the 'risk' of developing a reaction to a tattoo. Overall, from our point of view, chronic skin disorders per se are not strict contraindications for tattooing. However, honest information should be given to the customer about his/her risk so that he/she can decide freely to get a tattoo or not. First, the risk of the Köbner phenomenon is rather unpredictable in terms of to whom it will occur and at which point. The Köbner phenomenon may occur between days and years afterward. Moreover, during the whole life of the bearer, there is a risk that someday, during a flare of the skin disease, a rash may occur on the

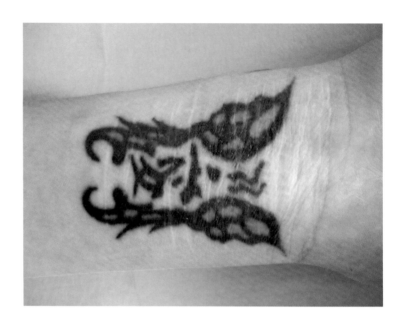

Fig. 2. Tattoo on the wrist to hide self-inflicted scarifications.

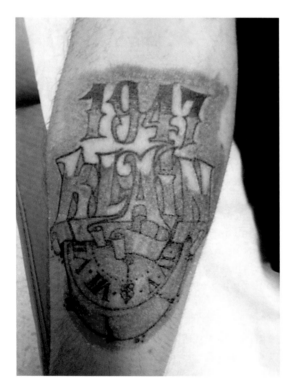

Fig. 3. Psoriasis patch on a recent tattoo in a patient with psoriasis guttata (courtesy of Dr. Levy-Rameau, Montpellier, France).

tattoo. The Köbner phenomenon is rarely 'complete', involving the whole tattoo; it may occur only on a part of the tattoo. Patients with a past history of the Köbner phenomenon on trauma sites, scars, or tattoos are more at risk. For instance, it is known that the Köbner phenomenon is an 'all-or-none' phenomenon in psoriatic patients (patients have it or do not). The risk of Köbnerization is higher if the disease is currently active. Therefore, tattooing should be delayed until the skin is clear of any (or any new) lesions and is quiescent. Based on the previous reasons, we simply discourage the so-called 'tattoo test spot on a hidden skin area' of a patient to test whether or not a patient is prone to Köbnerization. There is absolute uncertainty about the criteria for positivity or negativity (the tattoo ink quantity used in the test, the tattoo color, the delay of positivity, etc.). Not only would negative results be falsely reassuring but there is also a risk of sensitizing the customer to a tattoo ingredient. Even though tattoos have been used to cover mucosal vitiligo, tattooing on the edge of a vitiligo patch may trigger extension of the vitiligo. Moreover, the final visible result of a colored tattoo is not the same on

Kluger

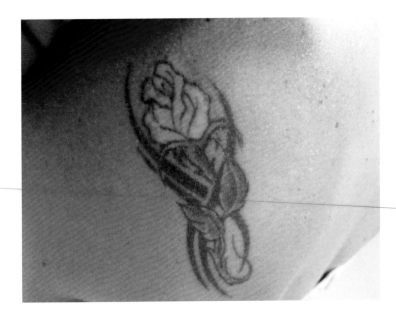

Fig. 4. Vitiligo patch restricted to a part of a tattoo (courtesy of Dr. Giacchero, Nice, France).

Table 1. Nonexhaustive list of skin disorders that have been reported on tattoos [1]

Sarcoidosis
Psoriasis
Discoid and subacute lupus
Cutaneous vasculitis
Darier's disease
Lichen planus
Lichen sclerosus and atrophicus
Granuloma annulare
Necrobiosis lipoidica
Perforating collagenosis
Morphea
Pyoderma gangrenosum

---

vitiliginous skin as on normal skin due to the lack of melanin. The physician should take into account that the treatment may include immunosuppressive therapy, such as for instance tumor necrosis factor (TNF)-alpha blockers for psoriasis, which leads to other potential issues (cf. below). In the case of skin lesions occurring on a tattoo, the treatments are exactly the same as if the disorder occurred on plain skin.

However, not every skin condition requires caution. For instance, whereas keloids are a strict contraindication for body piercings, they are not a contraindication for professional tattooing. Indeed, keloids on tattoos have been reported in specific situations: (i) tattoo burns after improper use of a laser for hair removal (on a tattooed area) [4] and (ii) ethnic tattoo scarifications in Africa. Similarly, one may think intuitively that tattooing a patient with epidermolysis bullosa may lead to blisters. This is not the case in our experience, with a few patients having undergone tattooing with no blisters. Cutaneous sarcoidosis can manifest with sarcoid papules and nodules on a tattoo [5]. However, rather than a complication, the tattoo acts as an indicator of the disease rather than a trigger. Patients with a past history of sarcoidosis are not contraindicated for tattooing, taking into account possible systemic immunosuppressive treatments (cf. below). Systematic screening for sarcoidosis before tattooing in customers with a family history of sarcoidosis is overexaggerated and has no relevance.

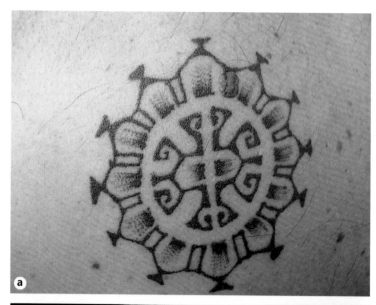

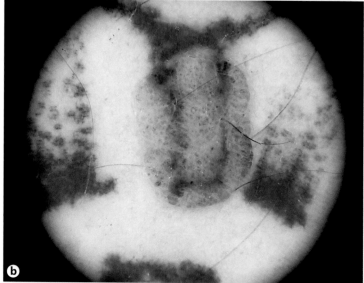

Fig. 5. Tattoo on the back with drawings performed on a naevus (**a**) and its aspects on dermatoscopy (**b**) (courtesy of Dr. Comte, Paris, France).

Naevus and Other Pigmented Lesions

Professional tattooists are generally aware that they should not tattoo on any pigmented lesion. However, experience shows that this is not always the case, even nowadays (fig. 5).

After tattooing, a traumatized tattooed naevus may be altered and display clinical changes and atypical histological features that can raise con-

cern about malignancy, such as pagetoid spread, cytologic atypia, and dermal mitosis [6]. Changes may even be delayed for years afterward due to a possible autograft phenomenon [7]. Even though a whether a single or persistent traumatic event can be a causative factor for melanoma remains debated, a clinical change in a naevus on a tattoo should prompt its immediate and complete

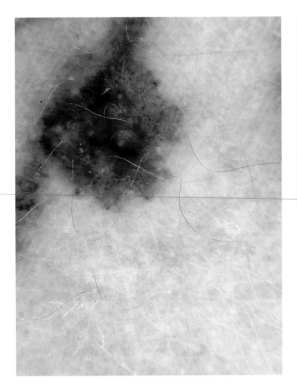

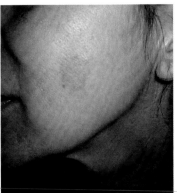

Fig. 7. Facial lentigo that was tattooed to camouflage it (courtesy of Dr. Colonna, Porto-Vecchio, France).

Fig. 6. Dermoscopic aspect of a naevus on a tattoo. Notice the excess pigmentation on the upper part due to the dermal pigments.

excision, along with a microscopic analysis [6]. The correct assessment of the patterns of a pigmented lesion by dermatoscopy is hindered by the presence of exogenous colored particles [8–10] (fig. 6).

As a general rule, no naevus or any pigmented lesion should be tattooed (fig. 7). A sufficient amount of space should be left if a naevus finds itself in the way of the tattoo. There is no rule for how much space should be given, but a minimum of 0.5–1 cm (no less) is necessary, as a nevus can still extend with time. The tattooist should avoid tattooing 'just on the edge' (fig. 8). We recommend that patients with a personal history of melanoma avoid tattoos because of the theoretical risk of a second melanoma arising on a tattoo, whose diagnosis would be delayed [8]. However, a 'small' and 'light' tattoo with bright colors on a

carefully selected area could be allowed. Young patients with a familial history of melanoma, numerous naevi, or atypical mole syndrome who are considering getting a tattoo should have a specialized consultation with a dermatologist, with a full check-up, before getting tattooed. The best location for a tattoo could be discussed, and atypical lesions could be removed before tattooing. A patient should avoid getting a tattoo in an area with lots of naevi. Customers and tattooists must know that covering a naevus with tattoos will, on the one hand, disturb its clinical surveillance and, on the other hand, possibly trigger clinical changes that will necessitate surgical excision and useless alteration of the tattoo. These customers should either avoid being tattooed on a location with a naevus and/or insist on having a tattoo whose drawings will spare the pigmented lesions.

Systemic Diseases

Heart Conditions

Infective endocarditis (IE) after tattooing is rather uncommon, especially when compared with piercing [11]. The prevalence of congenital heart disease is estimated to be 1% overall in the general population. It is likely that a similar

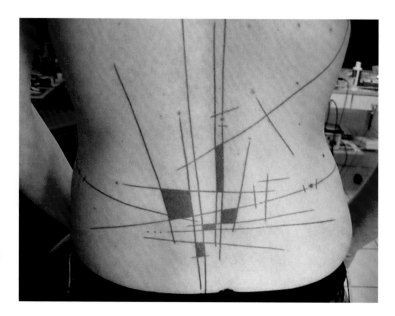

Fig. 8. Example of a tattoo sparing naevi, with sufficient space, but also artistically incorporating the naevi into the tattoo (courtesy of Dr. Werber, Toulouse, France).

percentage of customers presenting to a body-art professional would have a (diagnosed or undiagnosed) congenital heart disease [12, 13]. In 1999, Cetta et al. reported that a minority of patients with congenital heart disease (5%, 8/152) had received a tattoo without antibiotic use and had no infectious adverse events [14]. However, a few cases of IE after tattooing have been reported among patients with congenital heart disease during the past few years [15–19]. In three of those cases, the patients did not seek advice before tattooing [15, 17, 19], while in one, the patient was unaware of his condition [18].

IE is associated with bacteremia, potential dissemination, and multiple septic emboli [18]. In the context of tattooing, IE is associated with *Staphylococcus* species inoculation [15, 17, 19], which occurs either during the tattooing procedure because of a lack of hygiene, a mistake during the disinfection procedures, or the use of contaminated material, or possibly during the healing phase because of a lack of hygiene/proper after-care [12]. It is important, though, to rule out any other possible cause of IE before considering the tattoo as the culprit (dental procedure, intra-

venous drug intake, etc.). In the absence of another identified cause, a recent tattoo can be considered as the cause [19]. IE leads to a need for intravenous antibiotics and valvular replacement [17, 18]. To our knowledge, heart transplantation has not been reported thus far after tattoo-related IE.

Patients with congenital heart diseases may not perceive the risk of IE during tattooing [15]. They may be reluctant to share their wish of getting a tattoo with their physician, as the physician may not approve based on experience [14].

As a congenital heart disease may go unnoticed [12, 18], any unusual symptom occurring within weeks after tattooing (fever, chills, malaise, night sweats, or dyspnea) should prompt examination for a heart murmur and possible IE. An asymptomatic tattoo, devoid of any local sign of infection, should not rule out the diagnosis of IE [18, 19].

We recommend the following to prevent IE after tattooing [12, 13]:

(i) Patients with congenital heart diseases should be educated about the risk of IE during tattooing and body piercing procedures.

(ii) Any (future) customer with a known history of a cardiac murmur, even if only mentioned in childhood or some distant past history, should delay the procedure and seek for medical advice, followed, if necessary, by further specialized explorations.

(iii) Any patient with a known congenital heart disease should warn the general practitioner/cardiologist about the procedure, ask for updated data, and discuss possible prophylactic antibiotics.

(iv) The tattooist should be warned of the heart condition by the customer, and the procedure should be performed with the maximum asepsis (for instance, using fresh, new bottles of ink for tattooing).

The role of antibiotic prophylaxis in such invasive nonmedical procedures remains debated [13, 14]. Therefore, prophylaxis needs to be discussed on a case-by-case basis with the physician in charge. Lastly, the intake of antithrombotic treatment for a heart condition and the risk of bleeding during tattooing are other issues that should be addressed (cf. below).

Diabetes

Diabetes is one of the most common diseases worldwide. Type 1 diabetes is the most common type of diabetes in children and adolescents, but type 2 diabetes is increasing among the young [20]. It is therefore not uncommon that a diabetic patient may be interested in getting a tattoo. As a matter of fact, medical alert tattooing, e.g. a medical tattoo identification, is getting popular, at least among some patients with diabetes, in order to alert others about their condition in case of emergency [21]. There are no specific guidelines regarding the tattooing procedure in diabetic customers. According to the stage of evolution of the diabetes, the patients may be exposed to an increased risk of infection and delay of healing. To date, reports of tattoo-related complications in diabetic patients are quite rare. To the best of our knowledge, only a case of erysipelas of the lower limb was reported in a patient with type 2 diabetes [22]. It is not clear to what extent diabetes was directly involved in this complication.

Naturally, out of caution, we suggest that any diabetic patient should warn his/her physician about his/her wish for a tattoo. The tattooist should also be aware of such a condition. Diabetes should be controlled by the time of the tattooing procedure, as assessed by hemoglobin A1c, and the skin area where the tattoo will be applied should be devoid of any skin lesion. Some authors suggest avoiding tattooing the feet or the lower limbs because of the risk of diabetes-induced neurovascular disease [23]. We think that this contraindication seems rather excessive and should be discussed on a case-by-case basis, according to the presence or absence of micro- or macroangiopathy. Moreover, as the tattoo session may last several hours, the customer should take measures to prevent possible hypoglycemia.

Lastly, *granuloma annulare* and *necrobiosis lipoidica* are rare dermatologic conditions that have been sometimes associated with diabetes. As a matter of fact, several cases of granuloma annulare and necrobiosis lipoidica on tattoos have been reported in nondiabetic patients [24–26]. Diabetes could be an additional risk factor for such local complications on tattoos.

Inherited and Acquired Blood Disorders

Transient bleeding during tattooing inevitably occurs as the needles puncture the papillary dermis. During the procedure, the tattooist wipes out the suffusion of blood, and the bleeding usually stops rapidly. As the tattoo is wrapped with a plastic film for a few hours up to overnight, it is not unusual to find secretions and drops of bloods when removing the film. A discrete purpura may sometimes be seen under the tattooed area as red cells deposit in the dermis. Extensive ecchymosis under the tattoo is rare but possible and can raise concern for the customer if he/she has not been warned [27]. The evolution is spontaneously favorable, with resorption of the ecchymosis, and the skin color will follow the local bilirubin production. No cataclysmic or life-threatening bleeding or compressive hematoma has been reported after 'professional' tattooing to date.

However, young patients with inherited blood disorders (IBDs, such as hemophilia or von Willebrand disease) and also older patients with acquired blood disorders (such as thrombopenia) or receiving an anticoagulation or an antithrombotic treatment (heparin, anti-vitamin K, or simply aspirin) may want to get a tattoo. As for congenital heart diseases, these patients do not always correctly perceive the potential risk of bleeding. They may neglect, either unconsciously or on purpose, to mention their condition to the tattooist. Moreover, the tattooist may not ask about or consider such a risk. Khair et al. recently showed that having an IBD did not prevent half of the respondents in their study from getting tattooed or pierced [28]. It is clear that there are some patients with an IBD or an acquired blood disorder who undergo tattooing. We have the experience of a young patient with von Willebrand disease who underwent two tattoos, with no complication.

On the Internet, it is widely known and accepted that tattoos are contraindicated for patients with blood disorders. Thus, some patients are being refused tattoos 'systematically' because of an IBD. From our point of view, such a strict position should be moderated, and systematically refusing tattooing to such patients remains debatable. The patients may feel 'different' because they (think that they) cannot get tattooed. We know by experience that, at least for some individuals, tattooing has a positive effect in terms of ego bolstering and is part of a coping strategy as a way to regain control of their own body, as for diabetes, as stressed above [21].

Nowadays, the following is therefore important: (i) health care providers (nurses and physicians) should understand the medical issues associated with tattooing, have a nonjudgmental approach, and be able to correctly inform patients about the risks; (ii) patients should discuss their wish to get tattooed with their physician; (iii) tattoo artists should systematically delay the procedure and refer such patients to their physicians, and (iv) these patients must be considered for prophylactic treatment before such a procedure [29].

For patients presenting with antithrombotic coagulation, the reason why they are receiving such treatment, with a mechanical valve and cardiopathies among the indications, should be investigated, and then, the risk of endocarditis should be discussed. Temporary withdrawal of the treatment for the tattoo session should be discussed with the physician in charge [29].

Immunosuppressive Conditions and Therapies
Nowadays, the risk of infections after tattooing has greatly improved, thanks to the education of tattooists and their conformity to standard procedures of hygiene and asepsis. Infections mainly occur due to a lack of such procedures, especially in cases of amateur, home-made tattoos or if performed by unlicensed tattooist [30]. Infection may also occur in cases of severe immunodeficiency. Several years ago, Tendas et al. reported the case of a young, 24-year-old Italian who developed an *ecthyma gangrenosum* on a recent tattoo during an acute myeloid leukemia relapse [31]. We did not find any case of severe infection after tattooing in patients under immunosuppressive therapies [32]. We have the personal experience of young patients who were tattooed while under immunosuppressive therapies (oral corticosteroids, methotrexate, TNF-alpha blockers). According to the patients, the anti-TNF-alpha drugs were responsible for increased fatigue, diminished stamina after the session, a delay in tattoo healing, and secondary cutaneous infection after a session due to an after-care error. Moreover, one of our patient developed psoriasis on her tattoo, as a TNF-alpha blocker was given for this indication [32].

Patients with human immunodeficiency virus are exposed to the same complications as any other individuals whose immunity is at acceptable levels. A tattoo reaction has been reported during immune restoration in a single case [33]. Moreover, patients with human immunodeficiency virus specifically develop leishmaniasis on tattoos due to the tropism of this parasite for macrophages [34, 35].

When an immunosuppressive treatment is initiated in a young patient, the physician should inquire about the patient's potential wish for a tattoo. Increased awareness should be encouraged among those who already have tattoos, as they may be more likely to get a new one and may not perceive the risk. The level of immunosuppression related to the therapies, the disease itself, and the potential comorbidities (such as diabetes) have to be taken into account. A nonjudgmental approach is mandatory to allow a better understanding of the situation by the patients and better adherence to potential contraindications. The reasons for contraindications should be explained to the patient, stressing that they are temporary and related to the risk of severe infections. A tattoo can always be reconsidered when the treatment is withdrawn or at a maintenance level. In contrast, it remains reasonable to delay/avoid any tattoo when the disease is active and the treatments are currently at high dosages [32]. Systematically advising patients against a tattoo under mild immunosuppressive treatment is not supported by experience or data in the literature [36]. Lastly, patients may develop other complications on tattoos, such as the Köbner phenomenon on a tattooed area, if the immunosuppressive treatment is given again for a skin condition (psoriasis, sarcoidosis, chronic cutaneous lupus, etc.). The role of etanercept in an anecdotal case of a granulomatous tattoo reaction has been speculated [37].

If permission for a tattoo is granted, the patient should choose a tattooist who respects the rules of asepsis and hygiene in his/her parlor. The tattooist should know about the condition of the patient so that he/she can take the maximum precautions to avoid potential inoculation, such as using new tattoo bottles for the patient, performing a shorter session, paying attention to any unusual local symptoms before a new session, and consulting the patient immediately in the case of such symptoms [32].

Pregnancy and Breastfeeding
To date, no complication regarding the infant has been reported after a mother has undergone tattoo session(s) *during* pregnancy or breastfeeding [38]. Tattooists, parturient patients, and breastfeeding mothers are unlikely to perform/get tattoos during that specific period. However, some of us have experience with a pregnant woman or a breastfeeding mother insisting on getting tattoos [39]. Moreover, parturient women may undergo sessions at the very beginning of their pregnancy, while still unaware of it. Others may omit mentioning that they are breastfeeding when presenting to the tattooist. Overall, the prevalence of such situations is totally unknown. For the mother, the complications are the same as for any other individuals getting a tattoo. For the fetus, the risks of transmission of infection and toxic chemicals through the placenta and the milk have never been evaluated. Inoculation of microorganisms and local infection after tattooing and inoculation of blood-transmitted diseases remains low in parlors respecting strict hygiene procedures. Potential bacterial dissemination, although always possible, is exceptional. Moreover, maternal bacterial infections are rarely transmitted to their infants through breast milk. Temporary cessation of breastfeeding may be proposed for a limited time. Antibiotics are usually not a contraindication for breastfeeding but have to be chosen carefully during pregnancy. Some of the chemicals found in tattoo inks (heavy metals, amines, etc.) can be transferred through the human placenta [39]. There are few data regarding breast milk, and the potential systemic distribution of tattoo ingredi-

ents or by-products in the circulation and therefore possibly through the placenta during pregnancy or in the milk is not known. However, the existence of nanoparticles (<100 nm) in tattoo inks reopens this question. The risks of undergoing tattooing *during* pregnancy or breastfeeding are unclear and rather theoretical. However, because a tattoo can always be performed afterward, we suggest delaying any tattooing procedure until the end of pregnancy/breastfeeding. Additionally, the risk to fetal development in heavily tattooed mothers is not known either. The risk related to tattooing as a potential environmental occult source of toxic chemicals for the fetus should be thoroughly investigated. Of note, we have the experience of 25 tattooed women in France who are also professional tattooists who had 36 pregnancies within the context of their professional activities. The favorable outcomes of the pregnancies in our series are rather reassuring in terms of the possible diffusion of tattoo ink particles through the placenta (data unpublished, under submission).

References

1 Kluger N: Cutaneous complications related to permanent decorative tattooing. Expert Rev Clin Immunol 2010;6:363–371.

2 Weiss G, Shemer A, Trau H: The Koebner phenomenon: review of the literature. J Eur Acad Dermatol Venereol 2002;16:241–248.

3 Rubin AI, Stiller MJ: A listing of skin conditions exhibiting the koebner and pseudo-koebner phenomena with eliciting stimuli. J Cutan Med Surg 2002;6:29–34.

4 Kluger N: Sarcoidosis on tattoos: a review of the literature from 1939 to 2011. Sarcoidosis Vasc Diffuse Lung Dis 2013;30:86–102.

5 Kluger N, Hakimi S, Del Giudice P: Keloid occurring in a tattoo after laser hair removal. Acta Derm Venereol 2009;89:334–335.

6 Kluger N, Catala D, Thibaut I: Naevus and tattooing: a matter of concern. J Eur Acad Dermatol Venereol 2008;22:767–768.

7 Persechino S, Caperchi C, Bartolazzi A: Melanoma mimicry on a tattoo: an autograft hypothesis. J Am Acad Dermatol 2007;57:S122–S123.

8 Kluger N, Thomas L: The dragon with atypical mole syndrome. Arch Dermatol 2008;144:948–949.

9 Gall N, Bröcker EB, Becker JC: Particularities in managing melanoma patients with tattoos: case report and review of the literature. J Dtsch Dermatol Ges 2007;5:1120–1121.

10 Pohl L, Kaiser K, Raulin C: Pitfalls and recommendations in cases of laser removal of decorative tattoos with pigmented lesions: case report and review of the literature. JAMA Dermatol 2013;149:1087–1089.

11 Armstrong ML, DeBoer S, Cetta F: Infective endocarditis after body art: a review of the literature and concerns. J Adolesc Health 2008;43:217–225.

12 Kluger N: Bacterial endocarditis and body art: suggestions for an active prevention. Int J Cardiol 2009;136:112–113.

13 Tse DM, Khan S, Clarke S: Bacterial endocarditis and body art: active prevention or antibiotic prophylaxis. Int J Cardiol 2010;139:297–298.

14 Cetta F, Graham LC, Lichtenberg RC, Warnes CA: Piercing and tattooing in patients with congenital heart disease: patient and physician perspectives. J Adolesc Health 1999;24:160–162.

15 Satchithananda DK, Walsh J, Schofield PM: Bacterial endocarditis following repeated tattooing. Heart 2001;85:11–12.

16 Shebani SO, Miles HF, Simmons P, Stickley J, De Giovanni JV: Awareness of the risk of endocarditis associated with tattooing and body piercing among patients with congenital heart disease and paediatric cardiologists in the United Kingdom. Arch Dis Child 2007;92:1013–1014.

17 Tse D, Khan S, Clarke S: Bacterial endocarditis complicating body art. Int J Cardiol 2009;133:e28–e29.

18 Akkus NI, Mina GS, Fereidoon S, Rajpal S: Tattooing complicated by multivalvular bacterial endocarditis. Herz 2014;39:349–351.

19 Orton CM, Norrington K, Alam H, Alonso-Gonzalez R, Gatzoulis M: The danger of wearing your heart on your sleeve. Int J Cardiol 2014;175:e6–e7.

20 Canivell S, Gomis R: Diagnosis and classification of autoimmune diabetes mellitus. Autoimmun Rev 2014;13:403–407.

21 Kluger N, Aldasouqi S: The motivations and benefits of medical alert tattoos in patients with diabetes. Endocr Pract 2013;19:373–376.

22 Ahluwalia R, Mills A, Cuthbertson D: An 'Avatar' infection: associated cellulitis in a type 2 diabetes patient following decorative tattooing. Practical Diabetes 2011;28:292.

23 Glassy CM, Glassy MS, Aldasouqi S: Tattooing: medical uses and problems. Cleve Clin J Med 2012;79:761–770.

24 Bethune GC, Miller RA, Murray SJ, Walsh NM: A novel inflammatory reaction in a tattoo: challenge. Am J Dermatopathol 2011;33:740–741, 749.

25 Kluger N, Godenèche J, Vermeulen C: Granuloma annulare within the red dye of a tattoo. J Dermatol 2012;39:191–193.

26 Wood A, Hamilton SA, Wallace WA, Biswas A: Necrobiotic granulomatous tattooreaction: report of an unusual case showing features of both necrobiosis lipoidica and granuloma annulare patterns. Am J Dermatopathol 2014;36:e152–e155.

27 Kluger N: Acute complications of tattooing presenting in the ED. Am J Emerg Med 2012;30:2055–2063.

28 Khair K, Holland M, Pollard D: The experience of girls and young women with inherited bleeding disorders. Haemophilia 2013;19:e276–e281.

29 Kluger N: Tattooing, piercing and inherited coagulation disorders. Haemophilia 2013;19:e358–e359.

30 Kluger N, Saarinen K: *Aspergillus fumigatus* infection on a home-made tattoo. Br J Dermatol 2014;170:1373–1375.

31 Tendas A, Niscola P, Barbati R, Abruzzese E, Cuppelli L, Giovannini M, Scaramucci L, Fratoni S, Ales M, Neri B, Morino L, Dentamaro T, De Fabritiis P: Tattoo related pyoderma/ectyma gangrenous as presenting feature of relapsed acute myeloid leukaemia: an exceptionally rare observation. Injury 2011;42:546–547.

32 Kluger N: Tattooing and piercing: an underestimated issue for immunocompromised patients? Presse Med 2013.

33 Silvestre JF, Albares MP, Ramón R, Botella R: Cutaneous intolerance to tattoos in a patient with human immunodeficiency virus: a manifestation of the immune restoration syndrome. Arch Dermatol 2001;137:669–670.

34 Colebunders R, Depraetere K, Verstraeten T, Lambert J, Hauben E, Van Marck E, Maurer T, Bañuls AL, Dujardin JC: Unusual cutaneous lesions in two patients with visceral leishmaniasis and HIV infection. J Am Acad Dermatol 1999;41:847–850.

35 Kluger N: Leishmaniasis in Spanish tattoos. Enferm Infecc Microbiol Clin 2010; 28:667.

36 O'Connor MB, Phelan MJ: Should rheumatology patients on immunosuppressive medications be advised against getting tattoos? Ir Med J 2012;105:124.

37 Bachmeyer C, Blum L, Petitjean B, Kemiche F, Pertuiset E: Granulomatous tattoo reaction in a patient treated with etanercept. J Eur Acad Dermatol Venereol 2007;21:550–552.

38 Kluger N: Body art and pregnancy. Eur J Obstet Gynecol Reprod Biol 2010;153: 3–7.

39 Kluger N: Can a mother get a tattoo during pregnancy or while breastfeeding? Eur J Obstet Gynecol Reprod Biol 2012; 161:234–235.

Nicolas Kluger
Departments of Dermatology, Allergology and Venereology, Institute of Clinical Medicine
University of Helsinki, Skin and Allergies Hospital, Helsinki University Central Hospital
Meilahdentie 2, PO Box 160
FIN–00029 HUS, Helsinki (Finland)
E-Mail nicolaskluger@yahoo.fr

Serup J, Kluger N, Bäumler W (eds): Tattooed Skin and Health.
Curr Probl Dermatol. Basel, Karger, 2015, vol 48, pp 88–96 (DOI: 10.1159/000369191)

Laser Tattoo Removal, Precautions, and Unwanted Effects

Yvonne Eklund · Agneta Troilius Rubin

Centre for Laser and Vascular Anomalies, Department of Dermatology, Skane University Hospital, Malmö, Sweden

Abstract

Laser tattoo removal uses the physical properties of photoselective thermolysis in order to remove tattoo pigment. The technique has gradually improved over the years with the development of Q-switched lasers, with overall good results and a relatively low degree of adverse effects. However, lasers cannot always erase the unwanted tattoo completely, and there are still risks of unwanted effects such as scarring, pigment changes, ink darkening, and potential aggravation of latent skin conditions. This chapter will discuss the precautions that have to be taken and what pitfalls to avoid before starting the procedure of laser tattoo removal.

© 2015 S. Karger AG, Basel

Introduction

Tattoos have been part of human culture for thousands of years, with a wide range of patterns and symbolic values. Earlier in the history of mankind, tattooing was not as mainstream a feature as it has become today, with millions of people having tattoos or planning on getting one. The quest for expressing your individual identity seems to be central. However, many tattoo customers have regrets about their tattoo sooner or later in life, and this leads to an increasing worldwide demand for effective and safe ways of tattoo removal [1].

Since 1993, at our hospital department, we have removed different kinds of tattoos, mainly with a quality-switched, or Q-switched (QS), pulsed laser. In order to qualify for our laser treatment regime, patients have to fulfil certain criteria since financing of the sessions is subsidised with public means. The tattoos removed have varied, including stigmatising symbols and patterns (fig. 1), tattoos associated with an earlier criminal life, and medical tattoos. Additionally, some patients, and especially women, have had tattoos forced upon them by a dominant partner. Cosmetic tattoos with extreme disfiguration have also been accepted for treatment. Furthermore, all patients with traumatic tattoos have been offered laser treatment, as well as those who have developed different allergic reactions to the tattoo ink.

Early Tattoo Removal and Non-Specific Wavelength Lasers

Over the years, different chemical abrasions and surgical techniques have been used for tattoo removal, but with many side effects, and especially scarring and pigment retention. Heating and

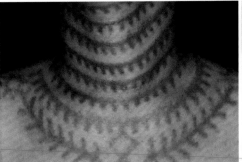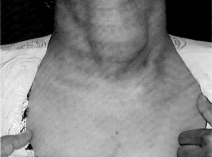

Fig. 1. Shamanistic tattoo for medical effect of goitre. Skin type V. Before and after several QS Nd:YAG laser 1,064 nm treatments. Postinflammatory hyperpigmentation to a certain degree on the neck where it was treated only 3 times. Photos: Dr A Troilius Rubin.

burning the skin in order to get rid of tattoo pigment have been used for centuries, including using fire, charcoal, and cigarettes. In the 1980s, removing tattoos in a more controlled manner, with heat, was tried with an infrared coagulator. Still, scarring was common due to the non-specific heat damage of dermal tissue [2]. Try-outs with lasers started, such as with argon lasers, but since the wavelengths were non-specific for the tattoo ink and instead largely absorbed by melanin and haemoglobin, the procedure often ended up with the same problem as earlier, causing scarring. Another alternative at this time was the carbon-dioxide laser (CO_2 laser), with vaporisation of the upper skin layers as its major mechanism in order to clear away the tattoo ink by transepidermal migration. However, there were great differences in depth during one and the same session, which often resulted in thick scarring and residual pigment [3].

Principles of Q-Switched Laser in Tattoo Removal

Anderson and Parrish's principle of selective photothermolysis in 1983 revolutionised the treatment of tattoos. They proposed that if a wavelength was well absorbed by the target and the pulse width was equal to or shorter than the tar-

get's thermal relaxation time, the heat generated from the laser would be confined to the target [4]. Considering that ink particles are very small and will hold heat in just a fraction of a second, one must use extremely short pulses. With the introduction of so-called QS lasers in the 1990s, with specific wavelengths that were well absorbed by ink particles and with a pulse duration of only nanoseconds, there was a golden standard for laser tattoo removal. Increasing evidence has also shown that there seems to be an important mechanism of photo-acoustic waves created by heat differences in the skin, contributing to the effect [5].

The most common colour of a tattoo is black, and following that are blue, green, red, yellow, and orange. All of these colours have different wavelength absorption, ranging from about 420 to 800 nm (table 1). A suitable laser with a specific wavelength is chosen according to this principle (table 2). However, nowadays, especially in professional tattoos, there is a wide range of colour mixes, making it sometimes a challenge to foresee the pigment reaction to a chosen laser wavelength. This problem is particularly seen in so-called cover-up tattoos placed on an earlier tattoo.

If the right wavelength and adjustable parameters such as spot size and fluence are chosen, the heat accumulation in the target colour will result in fragmentation of the ink, with the surrounding

Table 1. Absorption spectrum of the different tattoo pigment colours, measured in nanometres

Colour	Maximum absorption, nm
Black	600–800*
Blue-green	656–808
Permanent green	570–800
Red-violet	500–570
Orange	420–540
Yellow	470–485

* Black absorbs over the entire spectrum, with no specific peak (adapted from Verhaeghe 2010 [6]).

Table 2. QS lasers with their specific wavelengths and colour targets

Wavelength, nm	Laser	Colours
532	Nd:YAG laser	Red, orange, (brown, yellow)
694	Ruby laser	Black, blue, green, (purple, brown)
755	Alexandrite laser	Black, blue, green, (brown)
1,064	Nd:YAG laser	Black, blue, (brown)

The colours in brackets indicate some but less satisfactory absorption than for the other chromophores (adapted from Verhaeghe 2010 [6] and Karsai and Raulin 2011 [21]).

tissue spared [6]. Immediately after the laser treatment, an expected whitening of the skin will be seen, and this is usually a sign of good light absorption by the ink. The reaction represents dermal and epidermal vacuolisation due to localised steam formation and is often accompanied by normal pinpoint bleeding to a moderate degree, as a sign of slight epidermal disruption. The skin will heal within the next 2–7 days. In order to avoid bacterial infection, we recommend application of antiseptic ointment or dressing during this period. In the weeks following the laser procedure, there will be a gradual clearing of the tattoo

pigment by immune cells, such as macrophages and lymphocytes, via the lymph nodes. However, where the ink goes after the lymph nodes is not yet established, which means that a full comprehension of all immunological pathways involved is still lacking. Therefore, there have been questions about the safety of the ink particles regarding their potential toxicity, both before and after laser treatment, and their allergenic and carcinogenic properties [7, 8]. These fears have made a few physicians quit removing tattoos with lasers.

Initial Consultation

The patient should be thoroughly informed about what laser treatment of a tattoo actually comprises. There is a common misconception among the public that it is easy to remove a tattoo. Multiple laser treatments are always required, and many times, it is not possible to remove the tattoo completely, especially for multilayered, re-tattooed ones. It is important that the patient receives information on this concept and that an estimation of the number of laser sessions needed is made at the initial consultation. Otherwise, there will be a risk of poor treatment adherence, with the patient underestimating the effort and time required to clear a tattoo. In 2009, the Kirby-Desai scale was presented as a practical tool for assessing the number of laser sessions needed. In short, a darker skin type; dense tattoo ink; professional, complex tattoos with many colours; and distal tattoos on the extremities will require many laser treatments [9]. In some cases, up to 20 sessions or more are needed. Amateur tattoos are usually easier to remove, with fewer numbers of treatments, because of the irregularity of the depths of the pigment and the lower amount of pigment used.

In a substantial percentage of patients, there will be some residual pigment resisting further laser removal, depending on the factors mentioned above. It might be tempting to be more aggressive in treatment parameters or to use shorter treatment intervals, but since tattoo ink is cleared by dermal macrophage cells several weeks after each laser procedure, it is of utmost importance that there is a treatment interval of at least 6–8 weeks. Shorter treatment intervals have been reported to interfere with immune cell activity and may even increase the risk of scarring and ink retention [10]. If the tattoo has many features that will make full clearance impossible, it may be wiser to discourage the patient from any laser treatment at all. In order to avoid disagreement over the result or other issues, photos should be taken before starting the laser sessions and also during the treatment period.

Medical Evaluation

Because of the theoretical systemic spread of fragmented ink particles after laser treatment, we never treat pregnant or lactating women. Additionally, patients with severe diabetes are discouraged from QS laser treatment due to their diminished wound healing and higher risk of complicated infections. With regard to the safety of personnel, human immunodeficiency virus or hepatitis could be a risk factor. However, to our knowledge, no cases of patient-laser surgeon transmission have yet been reported. Furthermore, some medications might interfere with a successful result, such as retinoids, which are reported to increase the potential for scarring in some cases, although other reports do not fully support this [11]. Earlier gold injections against arthritis can result in hyperpigmentation (chrysiasis), even if the gold was given years ago [12]. It is also of value to know if the patient has any allergies, considering that it sometimes will be necessary to orally or topically treat the patient with medication. Questioning about earlier scarring is important since this can reveal whether the patient has a tendency to form hypertrophic scars or keloids. If an increased risk of scarring is suspected, information should be given, and as a precaution, a corticosteroid ointment and silicon dressing could be applied after each laser procedure.

General Precautions

Even though the rates of adverse effects are low with QS lasers, there are still some general risks that have to be considered before starting laser treatment. For example, a laser machine is not safe to use if the treating personnel does not have the proper education and experience. Even if photoselective thermolysis is the goal of tattoo removal, the wrong choice of wavelength, fluence, or pulse width will not reach this goal and will instead cause dermal damage and long-term side effects. Parameter settings that work well and safely in one patient might be wrong in another due to differences in skin texture and pigmentation. There are also risks of treating a tattoo with too many pulses on a single occasion since it can lead to a too-intense tissue reaction. In one rare case, this reaction led to a compartment syndrome of the forearm. For this reason, newer methods (such as the R20 method) that comprise multiple passes on the same occasion for better tattoo clearing should, according to our opinion, perhaps not be performed at distal parts of extremities [13, 14]. Even in the hands of an experienced laser surgeon, it is sometimes best to perform treatment first on a small test surface, especially if there are uncertainties about the right choice of wavelength and the response of the ink particles.

Dermatological Assessment

There is a necessity of having professional skills in the medical field since there are dermatological reactions, nevi, and tumours found within a tattoo in some cases. This needs to be evaluated before treatment. For example, psoriasis, lichen, and vitiligo can be exacerbated by tattooing (Koebner phenomenon) and potentially also by the procedure of lasing. Other histological reactions in tattoos might be reactions to the pigment itself, and these can be granulomatous or lichenoid, and sometimes even pseudolymphomas might develop [15]. All of this can be a diagnostic challenge. Additionally, different tumours can occur within a tattoo, such as basalioma, squamous cell carcinoma, and malignant melanoma. Whether this is a coincidence or actually caused by the tattoo is not established. A general rule is to never put a tattoo over a pigmented lesion and, before tattoo removal, to always excise a nevus or tumour in order to acquire a histopathological diagnosis [16, 17]. Finally, infectious complications should be avoided, and if there are signs of an active skin infection, whether bacterial or viral, laser treatment should be postponed and the infection treated. Additionally, if the tattoo is near an area with inactive intermittent herpes infection, e.g. the mouth, one should consider herpes prophylaxis in order to avoid reactivation.

Scarring

The risk of developing scars from laser tattoo removal is generally reported to be low, or just a few percent [18]. However, using too-high energy fluence and a too-large spot size increases the risk of deeper thermal injury, with potential scarring as a consequence. If exaggerated inflammation post-laser is noticed, a cooling device can be used, together with the application of a potent corticosteroid ointment. In a reported series of treatment-resistant tattoos, as many as 18.8–25% developed scarring, probably due to more intense treatment [16]. If there is a need to penetrate deeper, a larger spot size should be tried first, instead of increasing the fluence, in order to get less light scattering in the skin and hence less damage [19]. However, there are risks even with this strategy. Although the right parameters might be used, with an adequate tissue reaction, it is well established that with multiple laser sessions, the risk of fibrosis as well as hypopigmentation or postinflammatory hyperpigmentation will gradually increase [10].

Dyspigmentation

Hyper- and hypopigmentation as adverse effects of laser tattoo removal are more common than scarring [20]. Hyperpigmentation might follow inflammation or numerous laser treatments. It is more common in darker skin with more melanin and can often develop even after an adequate laser reaction. Hyperpigmentation can often be managed with longer intervals, letting the pigment gradually fade. It can often be a benefit to prescribe a bleaching agent, such as hydroquinone 2–4%. In all cases, ultra-violet exposure should be avoided. The risk of hypopigmentation will increase not only with too-high fluences and subsequent inflammation but also if shorter wavelengths are used since this means potential competing absorption by the melanosomes in the basal layer of the epidermis. Consequently, in order to avoid hypopigmentation in dark-skinned patients, longer wavelengths and lower fluences are preferable. If hypopigmentation is seen, longer treatment intervals would be of value so that the skin and its melanosomes have time to recover. Most of the time, loss of pigment is transient, but it may persist for several months or years. However, some authors report permanent loss of melanin pigment in up to 10% of all cases [21].

Ink Retention and Paradoxical Ink Darkening

Black and blue pigments are often the easiest tattoo pigments to remove, while moderate success is seen with green. A poorer outcome is specifically seen with white, purple, turquoise, yellow, orange, and flesh-toned colours. Sometimes, instead of a QS laser, a pulsed dye laser (510 nm) can be used to treat pigment on the red-yellow spectrum, with good results described; however, it is not the first-line choice since its pulse duration is considerably longer [21, 22].

Paradoxical ink darkening might occur after QS laser treatment, especially in tattoos containing

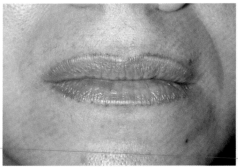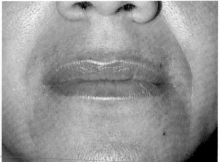

Fig. 2. Paradoxical ink darkening to the left. Treated successfully with QS Nd:YAG laser 1,064 nm to the right. Photos: Dr A Troilius Rubin.

titanium dioxide, such as white ink, which is often used to add brilliance to other tattoo inks. Ink darkening might also develop due to the ferric oxide in flesh-toned cosmetic tattoos, often used as permanent make-up. The mechanism is probably due to a chemical reduction of the pigment with the laser light [23]. A trial session would be valuable in such cases since this ink darkening may be irreversible. After the immediate whitening is gone, about 10–20 min post-treatment, an evaluation of a possible colour change can be made. Even if a chemical reduction does occur, according to our experience and other reports, switching to a QS laser with an appropriate wavelength will often remove the darkened pigment (fig. 2) [24, 25]. Some authors suggest using a CO_2 laser in treating flesh-toned cosmetic tattoos or altered ink as a good alternative, taking advantage of the mechanism of transepidermal pigment migration [26]. In some cosmetic tattoos, such as permanent eyeliner, it is quite common to see fanning of the ink downwards, into the lower eyelid. This is usually easy to remove with a QS laser and does not need more than 1–2 treatments.

Traumatic Tattoos

Traumatic tattoos are the result of accidents in which pigmented particles get embedded in the skin. These can arise from abrasive damage, e.g.

asphalt from a bicycle accident, or a penetrating force, such as a graphite pencil. Unfortunately, a quite common cause of traumatic tattoos is explosions from fireworks and gun powder (fig. 3). This situation constitutes a specific risk since the material can explode during laser treatment and create pitted scars in the skin of the patient [27]. Therefore, these cases should always be treated with caution. Success in clearing the traumatic tattoo will depend on the depth and on the particle size. Deeply embedded material may not be erased completely, and the patient should be informed of this. Harder materials, e.g. asphalt and car paint, will need more treatments, while softer materials, e.g. dirt and mascara, need less [28]. If the particles are too large, the laser will not be sufficient to target them with its short pulses. In such situations, an ablative laser, such as an Erbium:YAG or CO_2 laser, could be beneficial [29].

Allergic Reactions

If the patient has an allergy to the tattoo, this will appear as a typical allergic dermatitis or as either a granulomatous or a lichenoid reaction within specific colour areas [15]. In our experience, most common is an allergic reaction to red pigment, but an allergy to all sorts of colours can develop,

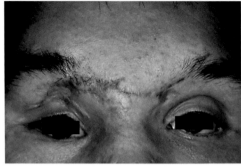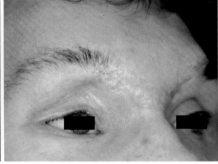

Fig. 3. Traumatic tattoo due to gun powder. Six sessions of QS Nd:YAG laser 1,064 nm. Photos: Dr A Troilius Rubin.

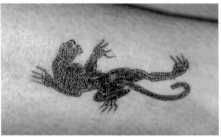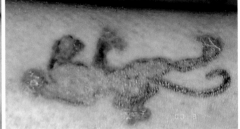

Fig. 4. Allergic reaction to red tattoo ink probably induced by the laser after two sessions of QS Nd:YAG laser 532 nm. Photos: Dr A Troilius Rubin.

with the least common being to black. Sometimes, it takes a long time, up to a year or so, to develop an allergy. This is due to chemical changes in the ink over time, with sunlight being an important factor. Laser treatment itself can also, in rare cases, induce allergy to the fragmented ink (fig. 4) [30, 31]. As mentioned earlier, after QS laser treatment, tattoo ink is cleared by cells that transport the ink fragments via the lymphatic system. Consequently, there is a potential risk of a systemic reaction to the ink particles after laser treatment, especially if there has been a local allergic reaction. Being prepared for such a reaction is therefore essential. The reports on clinical reactions following laser treatment have so far been mainly composed of mild or moderate allergic dermatitis, although generalised reactions have

also been described in some published cases [32]. To avoid a systemic reaction, some laser surgeons recommend a CO_2 or Erbium:YAG laser instead of, or before, QS laser treatment [33]. However, in our department, we have successfully treated at least ten patients with a localised allergic reaction to tattoo ink with a QS Nd:YAG laser. Several patients received intralesional corticosteroids or were prescribed daily application of a potent corticosteroid ointment in order to suppress most of the localised allergic reaction 1–2 months before laser treatment. At the time of treatment, all patients received an oral antihistamine one hour before laser treatment and were also kept under close surveillance during and 4 hours after the session. So far, there have not been any systemic allergic reactions during or after the procedure.

Newer Treatments and Future

Today, there are already promising studies and ongoing usage of the next generation of QS lasers, using pulses in the range of picoseconds, which are reported to create even better results in clearing a tattoo. This is attributed to the shortening of the pulse, matching the thermal relaxation time of the tattoo ink better and generating more effective photo-acoustic waves [5, 34]. However, these new machines are currently very costly, and it is too early to tell if they are worthwhile for their improved capacity for clearing tattoo ink. Hence, more studies are needed.

Newer techniques are combinations of already-known modalities, such as pretreating the skin with a fractional CO_2 laser or an Erbium:YAG laser and then directly treating the tattoo with a QS laser [35]. Another combination is the fractional QS laser (which is also new) with a QS laser with a full beam [5, 36]. Furthermore, in order to lessen the degree of scattering and to increase the penetration of light, it is possible to use diascopy (compression of the skin with a glass plate) during the QS laser session. In our experience, this seems to lead to a better effect of clearing deeper pigment. There are also reports on transdermal application of glycerol for the same effect [37].

For the future, one of the most important things is the development of safer tattoo pigment. Considering the large number of tattooed people who want to remove a tattoo, it would be so much easier if the pigment were made of nontoxic, biodegradable particles. However, this means that a tattoo will not 'be for life' and will therefore lose its symbolic value for many tattoo admirers. Should permanent ink be the overall choice of the tattoo community, it would be of great advantage if this ink had well-known absorption wavelengths, thereby making it easier to remove with a QS laser. Five years ago, a new tattoo ink was marketed in the United States, designed as microbeads of polymethylmethacrylate containing bioresorbable ink with specific laser wavelengths (InfinitInk; Freedom, Inc., N.J., USA). We will hopefully see more of this and of such initiatives in the future. In the meantime, the next important step is the development of lasers. For example, it would be of help to have lasers that can emit a large variety of wavelengths for treating all of the different ink colours that exist today while, at the same time, being able to penetrate deeper. Even if we do achieve all of the above improvements that are wished for, it would be very favourable if the public were given better information on the limitations of laser tattoo removal before getting a tattoo.

References

1 Laumann AE, Derick AJ: Tattoos and body piercings in the United States: a national data set. J Am Acad Dermatol 2006;55:413–421.

2 Colver GB: The infrared coagulator in dermatology. Dermatol Clin 1989;7:155–167.

3 Kent KM, Graber EM: Laser tattoo removal: a review. Dermatol Surg 2012;38:1–13.

4 Anderson RR, Parrish JA: Selective photothermolysis: precise microsurgery by selective absorption of pulsed radiation. Science 1983;220:524–527.

5 Luebberding S, Alexiades-Armenakas M: New tattoo approaches in dermatology. Dermatol Clin 2014;32:91–96.

6 Verhaeghe E: Chapter 7: Techniques and Devices Used for Tattoo Removal; in De Cuyper C, Pérez-Cotapos ML (eds): Dermatologic Complications with Body Art: Tattoos, Piercings and Permanent Make-Up. Heidelberg, Springer-Verlag, 2010, pp 91–105.

7 Ferguson JE, Andrew SM, Jones CJ, August PJ: The Q-switched neodymium: YAG laser and tattoos: a microscopic analysis of laser-tattoo interactions. Br J Dermatol 1997;137:405–410.

8 Bäumler W, Eibler ET, Hohenleutner U, Sens B, Sauer J, Landthaler M: Q-switch laser and tattoo pigments: first results of the chemical and photophysical analysis of 41 compounds. Lasers Surg Med 2000;26:13–21.

9 Kirby W, Desai A, Desai T, Kartono F, Geeta P: The Kirby-Desai Scale: a proposed scale to assess tattoo-removal treatments. J Clin Aesthet Dermatol 2009;2:32–37.

10 Kirby W, Chen CL, Desai A, Desai T: Causes and recommendations for unanticipated ink retention following tattoo removal treatment. J Clin Aesthet Dermatol 2013;6:27–31.

11 Alissa A: Concomitant use of laser and isotretinoin, how safe. Grapevine, American Society for Laser Medicine and Surgery, 2011.

12 Almoallim H, Klinkhoff AV, Arthur AB, Rivers JK, Chalmers A: Laser induced chrysiasis: disfiguring hyperpigmentation following Q-switched laser therapy in a woman previously treated with gold. J Rheumatol 2006;33:620–621.

13 Rheingold LM, Fater MC, Courtiss EH: Compartment syndrome of the upper extremity following cutaneous laser surgery. Plast Reconstr Surg 1997;99:1418–1420.

14 Kossida T, Rigopoulos D, Katsambas A, Anderson RR: Optimal tattoo removal in a single laser session based on the method of repeated exposures. J Am Acad Dermatol 2012;66:271–277.

15 Bassi A, Campolmi P, Cannarozzo G, Conti R, Bruscino N, Gola M, Ermini S, Massi D, Moretti S: Tattoo-associated skin reaction: the importance of an early diagnosis and proper treatment. Biomed Res Int 2014;2014:354608.

16 Karsai S, Krieger G, Raulin C: Tattoo removal by non-professionals – medical and forensic considerations. J Eur Acad Dermatol Venereol 2010;24:756–762.

17 Pohl L, Kaiser K, Raulin C: Pitfalls and recommendations in cases of laser removal of decorative tattoos with pigmented lesions: case report and review of the literature. JAMA Dermatol 2013; 149:1087–1089.

18 Bernstein EF: Laser treatment of tattoos. Clin Dermatol 2006;24:43–55.

19 Choudhary S, Elsaie ML, Leiva A, Nouri K: Lasers for tattoo removal: a review. Lasers Med Sci 2010;25:619–627.

20 Klein A, Rittmann I, Hiller KA, Landthaler M, Bäumler W: An Internet-based survey on characteristics of laser tattoo removal and associated side effects. Lasers Med Sci 2014;29:729–738.

21 Karsai S, Raulin C: Laser treatment of tattoos and other dyschromia; in Raulin C, Karsai S (eds): Laser and IPL Technology in Dermatology and Aesthetic Medicine. Berlin/Heidelberg, Springer Verlag, 2011, pp 189–210.

22 Stafford TJ, Tan OT: 510-nm pulsed dye laser and alexandrite crystal laser for the treatment of pigmented lesions and tattoos. Clin Dermatol 1995;13:69–73.

23 Kirby W, Kaur RR, Desai A: Paradoxical darkening and removal of pink tattoo ink. J Cosmet Dermatol 2010;9:149–151.

24 De Cuyper C: Permanent makeup: indications and complications. Clin Dermatol 2008;26:30–34.

25 Fitzpatrick RE, Lupton JR: Successful treatment of treatment-resistant laser-induced pigment darkening of a cosmetic tattoo. Lasers Surg Med 2000;27:358–361.

26 Mafong EA, Kauvar AN, Geronemus RG: Surgical pearl: removal of cosmetic lip-liner tattoo with the pulsed carbon dioxide laser. J Am Acad Dermatol 2003; 48:271–272.

27 Taylor CR: Laser ignition of traumatically embedded firework debris. Lasers Surg Med 1998;22:157–158.

28 Troilius A: Effective treatment of traumatic tattoos with a Q-switched Nd:YAG laser. Lasers Surg Med 1998;22: 103–108.

29 Kunzi-Rapp K, Krähn GM, Wortmann S, Peter RU: Early treatment of traumatic tattoo by erbium-YAG laser. Br J Dermatol 2001;144:219–221.

30 Serup J, Hutton Carlsen K: Patch test study of 90 patients with tattoo reactions: Negative outcome of allergy patch test to baseline batteries and culprit inks suggests allergen(s) are generated in the skin through haptenization. Contact Dermatitis 2014;71:255–263.

31 Vasold R, Naarmann N, Ulrich H, Fischer D, König B, Landthaler M, Bäumler W: Tattoo pigments are cleaved by laser light-the chemical analysis in vitro provide evidence for hazardous compounds. Photochem Photobiol 2004;80: 185–190.

32 Yorulmaz A, Onan DT, Artuz F, Gunes R: A case of generalized allergic contact dermatitis after laser tattoo removal. Cutan Ocul Toxicol, DOI: 10.3109/ 15569527.2014.933972.

33 Ibrahimi OA, Syed Z, Sakamoto FH, Avram MM, Anderson RR: Treatment of tattoo allergy with ablative fractional resurfacing: a novel paradigm for tattoo removal. J Am Acad Dermatol 2011;64: 1111–1114.

34 Brauer JA, Reddy KK, Anolik R, Weiss ET, Karen JK, Hale EK, Brightman LA, Bernstein L, Geronemus RG: Successful and rapid treatment of blue and green tattoo pigment with a novel picosecond laser. Arch Dermatol 2012;148:820–823.

35 Weiss ET, Geronemus RG: Combining fractional resurfacing and Q-switched ruby laser for tattoo removal. Dermatol Surg 2011;37:97–99.

36 Luebberding S, Alexiades-Armenakas MR: Fractional, nonablative Q-switched 1,064-nm neodymium YAG laser to rejuvenate photoaged skin: a pilot case series. J Drugs Dermatol 2012;11:1300–1304.

37 McNichols RJ, Fox MA, Gowda A, Tuya S, Bell B, Motamedi M: Temporary dermal scatter reduction: quantitative assessment and implications for improved laser tattoo removal. Lasers Surg Med 2005;36:289–296.

Yvonne Eklund, MD
Department of Dermatology, Skane University Hospital
SE–205 01 Malmö (Sweden)
E-Mail Yvonne.Eklund@skane.se

Serup J, Kluger N, Bäumler W (eds): Tattooed Skin and Health.
Curr Probl Dermatol. Basel, Karger, 2015, vol 48, pp 97–102 (DOI: 10.1159/000369187)

Nano-Scale Observations of Tattoo Pigments in Skin by Atomic Force Microscopy

Colin A. Grant[a] · Peter C. Twigg[a] · Desmond J. Tobin[b]

[a]Department of Medical Engineering, Faculty of Engineering and Informatics, [b]Centre for Skin Sciences,
Faculty of Life Sciences, University of Bradford, Bradford, UK

Abstract

In this study, we have shown how particles in carbon black tattoo ink accumulate in the human skin dermis using fine-resolution atomic force microscopy, with which a single ink particle in the collagenous network can be imaged. This information further demonstrates that tattoo inks are nano-particles. Further, we have deposited a commercially available tattoo ink on a glass slide and calculated a range of volumes for single ink particles.

© 2015 S. Karger AG, Basel

Introduction

The skin, which is the body's largest organ, is positioned at the interface between the external environment and internal anatomical structures, and as such, it provides a barrier against a range of environmental hazards [1]. Recent trends in the 21st century have shown an increase in the number of people with one or more tattoos or body art, some covering large regions of the skin's surface. Tattoo inks consist of a solid pigment dispersed in an aqueous medium that acts as a carrier and is usually a combination of an alcohol and water. Neither tattoo ink manufacturers nor tattoo artists who concoct their own ink have revealed the components or their precise proportions in their inks. Solid pigments for black ink are usually made from carbon black; however, a study of 58 inks of 6 different colours has shown that these pigments are predominantly less than 100 nm in diameter [2]. Nano-particles (defined as particles under 100 nm in size) are generally found to be more chemically reactive due to their high surface-to-volume ratios and are potentially cytotoxic because they may be able to pass through cell membranes.

For many centuries, microscopes have been invaluable instruments used by scientists, especially in the biological sciences. However, the resolution of light microscopes is limited due to diffraction, and electron microscopes require vacuum conditions. The atomic force microscope (AFM) was first created in the 1980s, invigorating the microscopy field [3]. The AFM possesses a long silicon (or silicon nitride) cantilever/probe assembly (fig. 1a) with a sharp probe on the underside of the cantilever with a half-cone angle of approximately 36°, and it

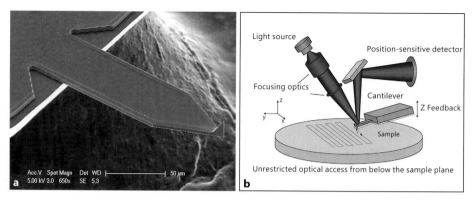

Fig. 1. a Scanning electron microscopy image of AFM silicon cantilever OMCL-AC160TS-R3 (diagram courtesy of Olympus Corporation, Japan). **b** Schematic of mechanism of surface scanning with an AFM (diagram courtesy of Oxford Instruments Asylum Research, USA).

typically has a spherical radius of approximately 10–20 nm.

Intricate details of how an AFM works can be found elsewhere [4]. In brief, a laser is aligned to the back of the cantilever/probe assembly, which itself is angled downward at approximately 12° (fig. 1b). Then, the cantilever/probe assembly is oscillated at its resonant frequency by a piezoelectric motor. The oscillating probe is brought into intermittent contact with a sample surface and is scanned over an area of interest, from a few nanometres up to a maximum of 100 μm. Changes in oscillation amplitude due to surface topography deflect the laser beam and bring about a change in signal at the photo-detector. This is a feedback channel that ultimately changes the vertical (Z) distance between the tip and sample, resulting in a surface image with contrast based on height, amplitude (error) or phase lag, which can reveal structures not present in the height image.

Advanced AFM instruments using low temperatures and high vacuum conditions have been used to image atoms [5] and even molecular bonds [6, 7]. However, an AFM can work under both air and aqueous conditions, and with the appropriate equipment, it can run at a wide range of temperatures of up to ~300°C. This makes it ide-

al for investigations of biological or anatomical samples under representative physiological conditions. Further, the cantilever/probe assembly can be used both as a tool for surface visualisation and as an indentation device to extract material properties from a surface of interest. For example, it has been recently demonstrated that the elasticity of a single collagen fibril is reduced by 3 orders of magnitude simply by hydrating a sample [8] and that collagen properties can be tuned by varying the aqueous media [9]. The discrete, periodic banding patterns of collagen fibrils have different static and dynamic mechanical properties [10]. Finally, surface images of skin scar tissue have shown a high degree of orientation of collagen fibrils as a result of wound healing with variations in the mechanical properties of the tissue in comparison with healthy skin [11]. In this study, for the first time, we utilise this microscopy technique to evaluate tattooed skin samples.

Methods

Cryo-Sectioning Tissue
A sample of tattooed skin was obtained from the forearm of a 62-year-old male. Full consent was obtained from the ethics committee of the clinic and the

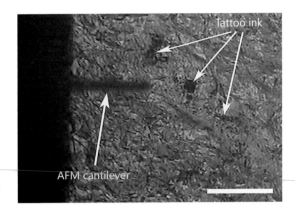

Fig. 2. Top-down optical microscope image of an AFM cantilever in the proximity of tattoo ink agglomerates in a dermis skin section. Scale bar, 200 μm.

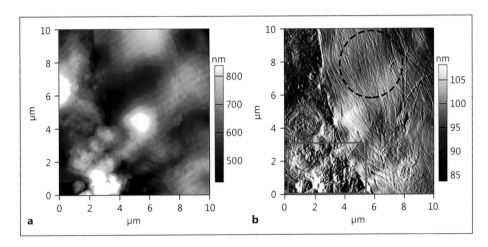

Fig. 3. A 10-μm AFM image of a (**a**) height image and a corresponding (**b**) amplitude image.

university for the use of this tissue. The tattooed skin sample was collected in buffered saline and stored upon arrival at the laboratory in a –80°C freezer. The skin sample was placed in a cryostat (Leica CM1860) and adhered to a metal chuck using an optimum cutting temperature embedding compound (Agar Scientific, Essex, England). Thin sections of dermal skin (5 μm) were collected onto poly-lysine-coated microscope slides and stored at –80°C until analysis.

Atomic Force Microscopy
The microscope slides containing the cryo-sectioned tissue sample were placed on the sample stage of an MFP-3D AFM (Asylum Research, Santa Barbara, Calif., USA) and imaged in air in intermittent contact

mode using Olympus AC160 silicon probes (k ~40 N/m, tip radius ~10 nm). A suitable area of interest at the periphery of the tattoo ink aggregates was located using an AFM optical camera (10×) before engaging on the surface and imaging (fig. 2). All images were processed using AFM software based on IGOR Pro platform (Wavemetrics, USA).

A 10-μm AFM scan image is shown in figure 3, in which (a) is the height image, and (b) is the amplitude or error image. The skin in this region of interest is clearly undulating with a large vertical data scale, which causes the nano-particles to be very difficult to discern.

However, from the amplitude image, a number of observations can be made. The right-hand side of the

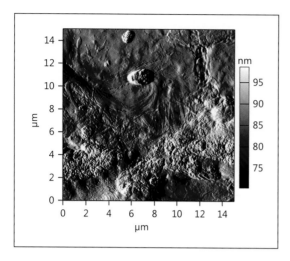

Fig. 4. A 15-μm amplitude image showing the greater density of ink pigment aggregates within the collagenous network.

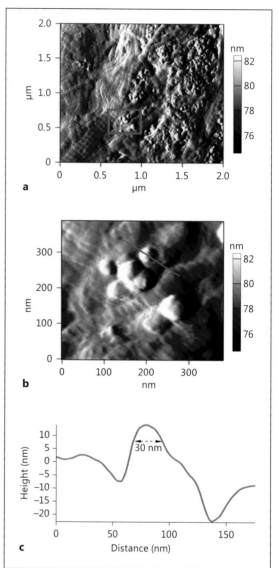

Fig. 5. a A 2-μm amplitude image showing thinly dispersed ink pigments. **b** A 400-nm scan region from the red square, resolving a primary particle. **c** A line section over a primary pigment particle, showing the profile of the surface.

amplitude image shows the strong orientation of the collagen fibrils, which is known to occur following wound healing or trauma [11] (in this case, receiving a tattoo). There are a number of small individual ink particles in the region of the highly oriented collagen fibrils, which are shown within the dashed circle in the amplitude image (fig. 3b) and are not visible in the corresponding height image (fig. 3a). Further, at the bottom left of figure 3b in the red rectangle, there are 'clumps' of aggregated ink particles that can be seen better in the amplitude image compared with the height image.

With a larger field of view, as shown in figure 4, clumps of tattoo pigment aggregates can be seen together with a large accumulation of pigment that dominates the lower half of the 15-μm image. It should be noted that because the tattooed dermis was cryo-sectioned at 5 μm, the tattoo pigment clusters are located at the sectioned tissue surface as well as sub-surface. The skin surface appears unscathed by the cryo-sectioning; otherwise, there would be shear-induced damage to the tissue.

The AFM has an impressive resolution capability in the z (vertical) direction down to the Angstrom level. Figure 5a shows a 2-μm AFM amplitude image of clusters of tattoo ink pigment particles dispersed within the collagen network. Figure 5b reveals a single ink particle with a diameter of 30 nm, as measured

from a line profile (fig. 5c) within a cluster of ink particles. Because the use of an AFM involves surface metrology, the particle shown is likely to be embedded in the collagen network and may be larger than calculated. Unfortunately, the age/duration of the

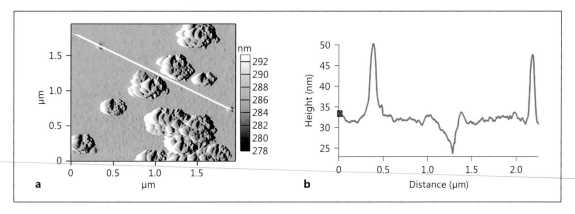

Fig. 6. a A 2-µm amplitude scan of tattoo ink on a glass slide. **b** A line section along the black, dashed line linking particle 1 and particle 2.

tattoo and the identity of the ink(s) used on the arm of the 62-year-old subject are not known, although the surface colour was monochrome (blue/black). The ink pigments in the skin are likely to have diffused/repositioned over time since the original tattoo event because it is known that deposited ink pigments are typically not stationary and are subjected to the cell-mediated non-self immune response of the body.

To demonstrate the validity of the AFM images of the ink pigments deposited in the dermal collagenous networks, we imaged a commercially available tattoo ink (Scream Black, Tattoo World UK) at the primary particle level as a control. The tattoo ink was diluted (1:1,000), and a 100-µl droplet was placed on a poly-lysine-coated glass slide. Following 10 minutes of deposition time, the ink was washed off of the surface and gently dried with a stream of nitrogen and then placed under an AFM. The resulting AFM scan of the dispersed ink particles is shown in figure 6a. Despite being a different black tattoo ink source, there was a striking similarity in the accumulation of the pigments on the skin and the glass substrate (c.f. fig. 3b, 4, 5a, b with fig. 6).

A line section over two individual particles on the glass surface is shown in figure 6b, in which the heights of the particles are 17 and 16 nm, respectively, and the widths are 68 and 42 nm, respectively. Assuming that these two single pigments are representative and have near-circular geometries, these dimensions indicate a volume of ink pigment particles of between 1,385 and 3,631 nm^3. Putting these values into context, a spherical nano-particle of 100 nm in diameter would have a volume of 523,599 nm^3. We hypothesise that single, isolated, primary nano-particles in the dermis could well be the origin of allergic responses due to the higher reactivity of smaller-sized nano-particles compared with the agglomerated particles found in tattoo skin. Nanomaterials are known to exhibit different properties from their bulk counterparts; the smaller the particle, the larger the fraction of atoms at the surface and the larger the binding energy per atom, resulting in surface atoms that are less stable (i.e. more reactive) than bulk atoms [12].

Conclusion

This preliminary study has shown that the AFM can resolve ink nano-particles from sections of tattooed human skin. The size of the individual tattoo ink particle in the dermal network, as resolved by an AFM, was approximately 30 nm. The clusters of ink attached to the glass substrate in the control experiment showed a striking similarity to the agglomerated ink pigments found in tattooed skin. With ink pigments on glass, line profiles can be used to measure surface area and height, revealing the volume of a single ink pigment.

References

1 Tobin DJ: Biochemistry of human skin-our brain on the outside. Chem Soc Rev 2006;35:52–67.

2 Høgsberg T, Loeschner K, Löf D, Serup J: Tattoo inks in general usage contain nanoparticles. Br J Dermatol 2011;165: 1210–1218.

3 Binnig G, Quate CF, Gerber C: Atomic force microscope. Phys Rev Lett 1986; 56:930–933.

4 Santos NC, Castanho MARB: An overview of the biophysical applications of atomic force microscopy. Biophys Chem 2004;107:133–149.

5 Giessibl FJ: AFM's path to atomic resolution. Materials Today 2005;8:32–41.

6 Gross L, Mohn F, Moll N, Liljeroth P, Meyer G: The chemical structure of a molecule resolved by atomic force microscopy. Science 2009;325:1110–1114.

7 Gross L, Mohn F, Moll N, Schuler B, Criado A, Guitián E, Peña D, Gourdon A, Meyer G: Bond-order discrimination by atomic force microscopy. Science 2012;337:1326–1329.

8 Grant CA, Brockwell DJ, Radford SE, Thomson NH: Effects of hydration on the mechanical response of individual collagen fibrils. Appl Phys Lett 2008;92: 3902–3904.

9 Grant CA, Brockwell DJ, Radford SE, Thomson NH: Tuning the elastic modulus of hydrated collagen fibrils. Biophys J 2009;97:2985–2992.

10 Grant CA, Phillips MA, Thomson NH: Dynamic mechanical analysis of collagen fibrils at the nanoscale. J Mech Behav Biomed Mater 2012;5:165–170.

11 Grant CA, Twigg PC, Tobin DJ: Static and dynamic nanomechanical properties of human skin tissue using atomic force microscopy: effect of scarring in the upper dermis. Acta Biomater 2012;8: 4123–4129.

12 Roduner E: Size matters: why nanomaterials are different. Chem Soc Rev 2006; 35:583–592.

Dr. Colin A. Grant
Polymer IRC Labs, Faculty of Engineering & Informatics, University of Bradford
Bradford BD7 1DP (UK)
E-Mail c.grant@bradford.ac.uk

Serup J, Kluger N, Bäumler W (eds): Tattooed Skin and Health.
Curr Probl Dermatol. Basel, Karger, 2015, vol 48, pp 103–111 (DOI: 10.1159/000370012)

Manufacturing of Tattoo Ink Products Today and in Future: Europe

Ralf Michel

TIME – Tattoo Ink Manufacturer Europe, Neuburg am Rhein, Germany

Abstract

The article describes the European market situation and the legal framework in Europe. It shows the state-of-the-art production under ISO 9001:2008 quality management and describes the future of tattoo ink production based on good manufacturing practice guidelines for tattoo inks. © 2015 S. Karger AG, Basel

Definition of Tattooing and Permanent Make-Up

'Tattooing is a practice whereby a permanent skin marking or design (a 'tattoo') is administered by intradermal injection of products consisting of colorants and auxiliary ingredients' [1].

'A permanent make-up (PMU) consists of colorants and auxiliary ingredients which are injected intradermally for the purposes of enhancing the contours of the face' [1].

The following text addresses the use of tattoo ink for both purposes because both products are regulated in the same way.

European Market Situation

Most inks being used for tattoos are manufactured outside of Europe (estimated at 70–80%). American products used by professional artists are dominating the market, and inks from Asia are mainly distributed to non-professionals.

Permanent make-up inks are mainly manufactured in Europe (estimated at 70–80%), and only a few products are imported from America and Asia [2].

European manufacturers of inks are mainly located in England, Germany, France, Italy and Spain. There are approximately 30 companies that produce tattoo inks in Europe. Many permanent make-up inks are private-label products manufactured in Germany or Italy.

Legal Situation and Market Control

The resolution ResAP(2008)1 on the requirements and criteria for the safety of tattoos and permanent make-up (superseding resolution ResAP(2003)2 on tattoos and permanent make-up) can be considered as state-of-the-art for the manufacturing of tattoo inks.

Only a few European countries have adopted national regulations on tattoo inks (Netherlands, Germany, France, Spain, Sweden, Switzerland, and Norway), and some are using the resolution to control tattoo inks (Italy, Slovenia, Denmark and Austria). Denmark and Austria have well-prepared national regulations based on ResAP(2008)1 but are awaiting further steps of the European Commission.

Currently, manufacturers of tattoo inks have to follow many national regulations. In countries with national regulations, ink manufacturers are controlled by the authorities, and in other countries, such as the United Kingdom, there is no control at all.

In Spain, the agency controlling medical products (Agencia Española de Medicamentos y Productos Sanitarios) is responsible for tattoo inks, and these products need to be homologated. The rules of this homologation are not clear, and there are only a few homologated products. Most artists in the tattoo industry use non-homologated products. This information shows that over-regulation cannot create a safer market for consumers.

ResAP(2008)1 could only be a first step towards the regulation of tattoo inks. There is a scientific knowledge gap with regard to the process of tattooing and what happens when inks enter the body. For this reason, cosmetic regulations are used to create prohibited ingredient lists. In general, no ingredients that are forbidden for use in cosmetic products can be used in tattoo inks. All other ingredients that are not regulated in cosmetics can be used. Some colourants that are allowed in cosmetics but have been identified as dangerous for tattoos have been added to the prohibited list.

Current Situation in Europe

Manufacturers in continental Europe have reformulated their inks and avoid ingredients that are banned for use in tattooing according to ResAP(2008)1. Some companies have established a system of raw material management, defining and controlling the quality of raw materials used in their products.

A risk assessment should be performed according to ResAP(2008)1, but in fact, there is currently no guideline for the risk assessment of tattoo inks, and there is still a scientific gap.

An ad hoc group on the safety of tattoos and permanent make-up of P-SC-COS of the Council of Europe presented a draft version, entitled 'Towards a Toxicological Risk Assessment of Tattoo Chemicals and Inks' [3], which can be used as a guideline for the risk assessment of tattoo inks in the near future and also describes the existing scientific gap.

The biggest problems in the past were the microbiological contamination of inks and the presence of carcinogenic aromatic amines and carcinogenic polycyclic aromatic hydrocarbons (PAHs).

Inks manufactured today in countries with national regulations are much safer than they were 10 years ago. The microbiological quality of today's products is good, and the contamination of inks is a minor problem now compared with the beginning of this century. Inks are delivered sterile and are formulated to remain in microbiologically stable conditions after opening.

Pigment Yellow 74 has been associated with many reports of o-anisidine, which is a carcinogenic aromatic amine in tattoo inks. Most

European manufacturers have now replaced this pigment. Both resolutions, ResAP(2003)2 and ResAP(2008)1, have significantly improved ink quality with regard to carcinogenic aromatic amines, and they are currently found in very few inks manufactured in Europe.

PAHs are present in most carbon black pigments on the market. There are very few pigments available that fulfil the requirements for tattoo inks, and it is difficult for manufacturers to find them and choose the best one for their inks. Many European producers of tattoo inks have solved this problem within the last years, but there are still products on the market that do not comply with the recommendations of ResAP(2008)1.

Problems for Ink Manufacturers Today

Trying to follow the resolutions and national regulations in Europe is associated with the following problems for manufacturers:

Lack of Harmonised Analytical Methods
National laboratories and most ink manufacturers use a microwave digestion method, and most manufacturers of permanent make-up inks use a cosmetic method for analysing nickel in aqueous solutions. The results obtained with these two methods have been surprisingly different. Using the cosmetic method, ink has been found to be 'nickel free', but with the microwave digestion method, 60 ppm or more of nickel have been detected. There is an easy explanation for this discrepancy, which is that the 'products containing nickel around 60 mg/kg are based on iron oxides' [4].

The same problem occurs with PAH analyses, which depend on the solvent, temperature and time. Using the method of the US Food and Drug Administration according to requirement 21 CFR Section 178.3297, it is possible to manufacture black carbon-based inks (which comprise more than 98% of all black inks on the market) according to the demands of the resolution. Using another method might result in the detection of higher pigment levels.

The same problems occur with analyses of carcinogenic aromatic amines. Using the wrong method will result in negative findings when in fact pigments are able to separate into forbidden compounds.

Lack of Guidelines for Risk Assessment
There is currently no clear way to make a risk assessment, and manufacturers only collect available data for raw materials.

Lack of Guidelines for Good Manufacturing Practice (GMP)
Is the cosmetic GMP the correct guideline, or should the GMP for the manufacturing of sterile pharmaceuticals be followed? In 2005, TIME published a draft GMP guideline stating that tattoo inks should be treated comparable to class 2b medical device products (implantable devices and long-term surgically invasive devices) [5].

Finally, the market situation itself makes it difficult to apply changes to manufacturing processes. Without common regulations throughout Europe and for imported products, competitors have very low costs compared to European manufacturers in regulated countries. The pigments that are currently used to create inks are much more expensive, and the quality management system required to manufacture a safe product is costly and includes the management of raw materials and additional analyses. The current market prices of tattoo inks do not allow for full compliance with GMP production guidelines.

Ink Production Today and Quality Management

Figure 1 shows a simplified flow chart depicting how to manage ink production under ISO 9001: 2008, starting with the delivery of raw materials. Not shown in the figure is the purchasing process,

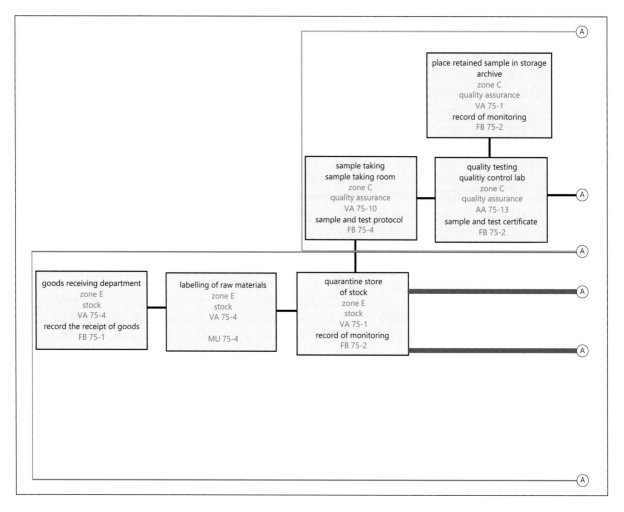

Fig. 1. Flow process chart – good manufacturing practice of tattoo inks.

including the definition of quality parameters for the raw materials.

The process must be described in process instructions (marked VA) and work instructions (marked AA). Forms are defined (marked FB) and used for documentation.

It is necessary to designate one person to be responsible for each step, and the same person must not carry out production and quality management.

For production in a cleanroom, a zone is used to indicate the conditions. This manner of pro-duction is for non-sterile inks. The sterilisation of inks occurs after the filling and sealing of the final container. The zones are defined according to the GMP of sterile medicinal products. Zone E is lo-cated outside of the cleanroom.

The first step is the receipt and labelling of the raw material and the first check of documents. The material is stocked in a quarantine store. From the quarantine store, it is transferred to a sampling room, where samples are taken for analysis and testing and retained for documen-tation.

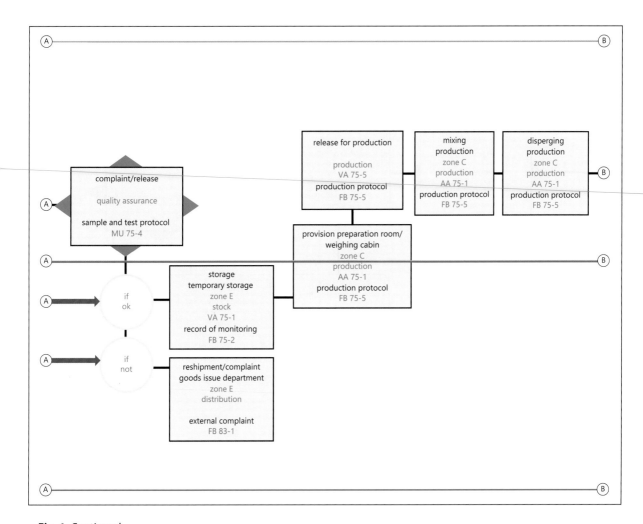

Fig. 1. Continued.

After quality control, the raw material is stocked in a raw material store if all tests have been passed. If the raw material does not pass the tests, it is returned to the supplier or discarded.

In the preparation room (weight cabin), all ingredients are checked again and weighed according to the manufacturing protocol. Then, the ink is mixed and dispersed, following the work instructions. In-process controls guarantee a constant quality of the manufactured product. The ink is than checked again, and if it complies with the standards and reference samples, it is sent to the filling department. If the ink does not comply with the internal standard, it is quarantined.

The next step is the filling and sealing of the product. Sterilisation is carried out during this step, after which the product is again quarantined unless it is released by the quality safety department with proof of sterility.

The inks are than labelled and packaged with all necessary information, including sterilisation batch data. After a final inspection of quality, including packaging and labelling, the inks are released for sale.

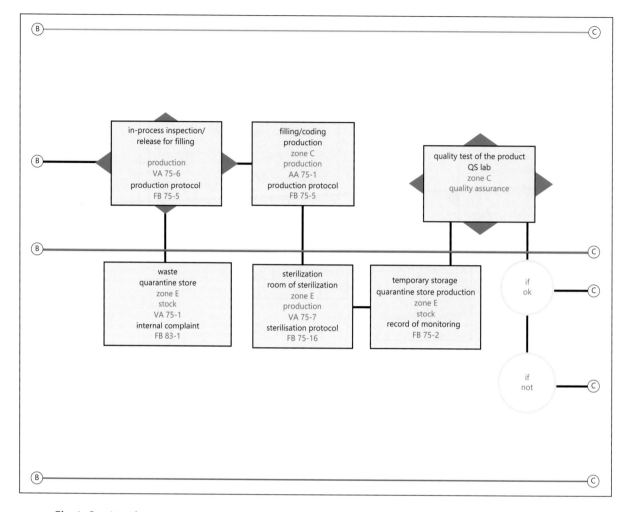

Fig. 1. Continued.

Guidelines for the GMP of tattoo inks are shown in figure 2, which depicts aspects of GMP production.

An effective quality assurance (QA) system involving management and personnel of various departments needs to be established. It is necessary to have personnel with the skills necessary to achieve QA objectives, and these individuals need regular training in the theory and application of QA and GMP.

For the personnel and premises, hygiene programmes are obligatory. Premises and manufacturing equipment need strict hygiene standards to avoid contamination and any adverse effects. Premises and equipment critical for maintaining the quality of products need appropriate validation.

Production must be organised according to GMP with pre-established instructions and procedures. Documentation and the investigation of process deviations and product defects are necessary. It is also important to have technical and/or organisational measures in place to avoid cross-contamination. The validation of new manufacturing processes and those that have

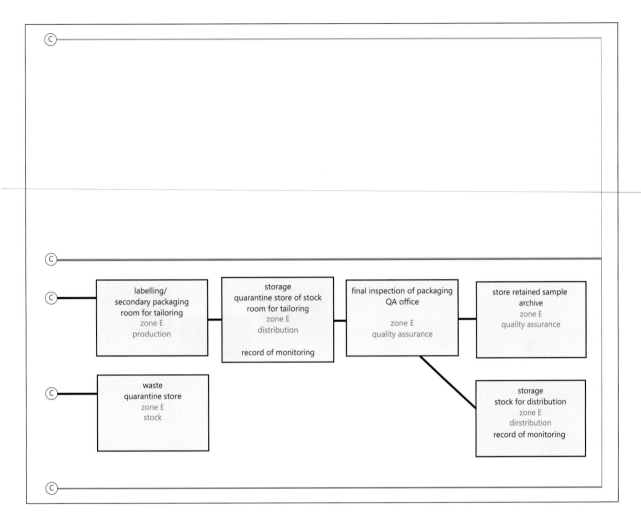

Fig. 1. Continued.

substantially changed is essential for production. Critical phases of the manufacturing process need revalidation.

The company should establish a system of documentation covering manufacturing operations and the trace history of the manufacture of each batch. For electronic or other data processing systems, it is necessary to prove that data are appropriately stored during the period of question.

For quality control and labelling, it is necessary to have a person who is qualified and independent of production. The quality control laboratory is responsible for the starting materials, packaging materials, and intermediate and finished products. Contract laboratories may be used.

The final control of the finished product before its release on the market includes the assessment of production conditions, in-process controls, manufacturing documents and conformity of specifications. Samples of the finished product for each batch retained must be stored for a minimum of 1 year after the expiration date, and samples of certain raw materials must be stored for 2 years after the release of the product.

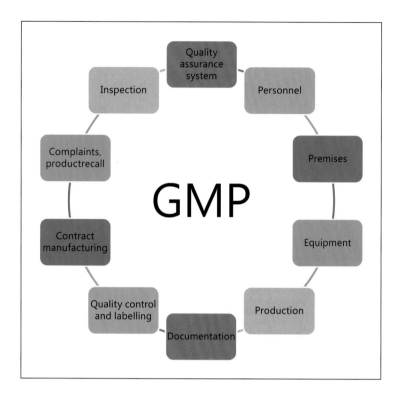

Fig. 2. Aspects of GMP production.

It is possible to use a contract manufacturer. A written contract documents the responsibility of each party, and the contract acceptor has to respect the principles and guidelines of GMP and to submit to inspections carried out by competent authorities.

After the release of the product on the market, it is necessary to examine and record complaints regarding defects in the product and to inform the competent authorities of any defect that could result in a recall or restriction on supply. A recall must be prepared for urgent actions.

Finally, states have to inspect production to ensure adherence to the principles and guidelines of GMP and to exchange information with other competent authorities. The manufacturer has to ensure that manufacturing operations are being carried out according to GMP and provide authorisation. The manufacturer also must perform regular self-inspections.

Summary

There are still many steps necessary to achieve the common regulation of tattoo inks in Europe and many questions to be answered. It must be accepted that there are still scientific gaps with regard to tattooing that need to be researched in the future. There is a lack of sufficient testing methods to get all data for a full risk assessment.

Despite these problems, it is still possible to start regulating tattoo inks. As a first step, it will be necessary to set up harmonised analytical methods. Based on these methods, the limits set in ResAP(2008)1 have to be reviewed.

With guidelines available for the safety assessment of tattoo inks by the Council of Europe, it is possible to create a first common regulation based on the Council of Europe resolution ResAP(2008)1 for all European countries and for importers.

References

1 Council of Europe: 2. Definitions; in: Resolution ResAP(2008)1 on requirements and criteria for the safety of tattoos and permanent make-up (superseding Resolution ResAP(2003)2 on tattoos and permanent make-up). Council of Europe, 2008.

2 Internal marked review by TIME – Tattoo Ink Manufacturers of Europe.

3 Council of Europe, Final draft 18–09–2014 PA/PH/COS (10) 27 2R.

4 Prior G: Tattoo Inks: Analysis, Pigments, Legislation: An Introduction to Tattoo Inks, Their Analysis, Pigments in Use, Their Chemical Classes, Present Legislation in Europe, Problems Arising from Incomplete Laws, Quantification of Pigments and Metals in the Skin. epubli GmbH, 2014, p 62.

5 TIME – Tattoo Ink Manufacturer of Europe: Good Manufacturing Practice of Tattoo Inks, 2005.

Ralf Michel
DC-TP Europe GmbH
Lotsenstrasse 10
DE–76776 Neuburg am Rhein (Germany)
E-Mail contact@time-online.eu

Serup J, Kluger N, Bäumler W (eds): Tattooed Skin and Health.
Curr Probl Dermatol. Basel, Karger, 2015, vol 48, pp 112–117 (DOI: 10.1159/000370014)

The Realistic Variables Underlying True Safety in Tattoo Pigment Manufacturing

Mario Barth

INTENZE Products, Hackensack, N.J., USA

Abstract

The regulation of the manufacture of tattoo ink products in the USA and the rest of the world is the focus of this article, which outlines the historical relationships between official and unofficial manufacturing and associated regulations, self-regulating movements within the industry and the impacts of over-regulation on the economics of ink manufacturing markets. The author, Mario Barth, highlights that changes in industry standards of production that are too rapid can cause the system to deteriorate, leading to an essentially negative shift to the underground markets. In addition, these regulations would not lead to a healthier end product because the currently considered health problems associated with tattoos (affecting 6% of tattoos performed in Germany) could be caused by multiple additional factors, such as the tattooing technique and aftercare. The pigment itself (which causes health issues in only 0.6% of tattoos) could in this equation not be optimized within an overregulated market. Further, aspects of price and revenue are analyzed in detail, showing that high quality suppliers are spending most of their efforts on passing regulations and that these regulations are not decreasing the amount of low-quality products in the general market. Finally, the notion of tattooing as 'an adult decision' is explained as another variable that has to be considered in creating regulations because the decision-making process for a tattoo (considering the price, quality and definitely the permanency) has and will have a self-regulating impact driven by the clients.

To be perfectly clear before I start, I just want to say that I am not at all opposed to the regulation of tattoo pigments. However, I do believe that there are many variables to the equation and that over-regulating pigment manufacturing is just as dangerous as having no regulations or guidelines at all. The ResAP/2008, in its original form, led to massive changes in tattoo pigment manufacturing. Tattoo pigment manufacturers are still trying to comply with these regulations as new restrictions are put in place overnight. For an inside view from the perspective of a tattoo pigment manufacturer, please continue reading.

To properly understand why the tattoo pigment manufacturing industry is welcoming proper regulation and recognizes its importance, we need to look at tattoo pigment manufacturing historically. Pigment manufacturing is as old as tattooing itself. In the beginning, pigments were merely produced by the performing artist, and they have been prepared in this way until recently.

The following quote is from a 1925 Percy Waters catalog, in which he talks about his pigment [1]:

'Use only the best colors purchased from reliable dealers. They are chemically pure and harmless to the skin, while imitation colors sold by so-called importers, are nothing more than common house paint, and likely poison. Genuine colors are seldom found among the beginners, as they, not knowing the difference, use what they are told, or perhaps buy them at a far higher price. The best colors are used by the OLD TIME TATTOOERS, who know the kind to buy as well as they know a bright colored tattoo will bring them business.'

Although it can be strongly argued that the colors used during this time period were safe and harmless and that only old-timers had knowledge of the best colors to use, this quote shows, in documented form, that the industry began to self regulate and consider product safety almost 100 years ago. It also raises a more interesting point, which can be recognized by sitting back and reading more closely between the lines, about the real issue related to the connections between artists' qualifications, supplies, knowledge and proper tattoo pigments. It is very clear that even during this early time of professional tattooing and pigment manufacturing, the educational level of the performing artist played a significant role in the behavior of the pigments. To date, not much has changed with the use of imitation colors, which are mostly produced by 'underground' tattoo pigment manufacturers. These imitation colors are used primarily but not exclusively by 'underground' or beginner tattoo artists, who out-number the professionals.

Some can argue that this is one more reason for the upcoming regulations, which aim to promote the safety of the end consumer, and they may be correct; however, the sole challenge remains in regulation which is a combination of product, education, proper use of material and the vital aftercare by the client of the tattoo, this is not considered or even remotely addressed. To state this issue as an example, a car is built with no tires, and it is placed on wooden blocks. It does not matter how great the interior and engine are, the vehicle will remain motionless, and people will walk rather than use it for its intended purpose of transportation.

It is a commonly known fact in the tattoo industry that tattoo artists, pigment manufacturers, and tool manufacturers and suppliers will and do self-regulate, and they have done an exceptional job at it over the past hundred or so years with no help from the regulating agencies. However, this does not mean that there should be no regulations; in fact, it suggests the complete opposite. It merely shows that arguably, it will be necessary to work closely together and to understand that a craft that is a thousand years old cannot be changed in a couple of years, especially by regulating pigments without truly understanding the global impact, training needed for the industry, economic feasibility, qualified control, targeted and proper enforceability and more importantly, sustainability. It does not help to regulate one part of the equation and not consider the equally important counterpart and then expect a sustainable outcome. To clarify this in more detail, consider whether it is possible to lose 40 kilos or pounds in 1 day. Although it seems impossible, it is achievable by severing all of the limbs and the head. Although it is very clear that the weight loss was accomplished, life will no longer be sustained. Thus, it is of the upmost importance to consider all variables before making a decision based solely on a theoretical thought process. Considering the example above, one outcome would ultimately result in the loss of life. It would be an easier and ultimately better choice to lose this weight over an extended period of time, which represents a healthier alternative associated with a lifestyle change. Similarly, the regulation of tattoo pigment manufacturers needs to be implemented over a significant period of time to ensure sustainability, achievable measures and the ability for all manufacturers to comply without jeopardizing the health and safety of the end consumer while still keeping a sufficient number of licensed and qualified artists. The enforcement of these regulations in an extreme fashion does not provide quality pigment manufacturers with enough time to make proper changes, giving underground artists, who lack regulations and are thus more likely to cause health concerns that are not traceable and are more difficult to treat, a chance to take over the industry. Although it seems logical to enforce stringent regulations on pigments for tattooing, without the training of artists and the education of the end consumer on the importance of aftercare, these regulations will actually achieve the opposite of their desired effects. One must understand that every human being who receives and applies these pigments and the clients taking care of the finished tattoo have many very different ways of doing so, creating countless combinations of variables. This issue also becomes very clear when a person experiences a possible reaction to a pigment.

It may be very interesting to analyze this issue. Key indicators must be examined, including how many reactions can be traced back to improper supplies, application and aftercare, and it is always easiest find fault with the pigment. Human nature makes it easy to place the blame on a product instead of considering that proper pigment use and care is equally important.

A study performed at the University of Regensburg on health problems associated with tattooed skin indicated that 6% of tattooed persons reported persistent health problems after receiving their first tattoo. On average, these persons had two to three tattoos [2], which reduces this figure [3] to 2.6% reactions per tattoo received.

In a follow-up report, Professor Richard White from the University of Worcester [4] suggested that there are four causes of adverse dermatological effects besides allergic reactions – the techniques, the instruments (needles and machines), the aftercare and the ink products.

This means that if weighted with the same importance, only 0.65% of reactions related to the 1,000,000+ tattoos done yearly in Germany have direct correlations with the ink product used.

Allergic and intolerance reactions are not separately considered within that 0.65% because they have been recently identified as the biggest contributors to personal hygienic product reactions by the German 'Industrie-Verband für Körperpflege.' This could be considered to be an additional factor disputing the 'authentic' health problems caused by tattooing pigments.

This research has provided further clarification that the over-regulation of tattoo pigments is questionable. Especially considering how time and cost intensive these changes are for manufacturers and government regulatory agencies, even more concerns are raised by analyzing the possible peak point at which a qualitative regulation becomes such an overburden that it triggers a decline in manufacturing, and it becomes easier to create uncontrolled underground pigments.

Let's take a look at another factor, the pricing structure of the industry itself. The current professional pigments per 30 ml are priced in the range of EUR 9.00–14.00. Research in the industry has shown that the most common bottle size in use is 30 ml. Quality pigment manufacturers are working very hard to deliver a product that is high quality with health and safety in mind, whereas others are more concerned with reaching the masses with a product that is lower in quality but has a higher profit margin. The retail cost of the same 30-ml bottle is the same in the 'underground' market; however, the profit margin is significantly higher, and manufacturers choose not to follow regulations, even going so far as to not label or to continuously rename a product. Current raw pigment prices have risen, and some have even increased from USD 5.00–75.00 per pound. The biggest variable, however, is the retail price, which has not changed in 25 years, leaving quality manufacturers battling with very tight margins.

Disturbingly, the legislative system focuses more on over-regulating already quality-driven companies with new, unexplained pigment prohibitions instead of creating a unified, controlled enforcing and testing system in Europe.

This situation is akin to illegal immigration. Making it harder to immigrate legally does not make illegal immigrants stop because they have no intention of being legal anyway. It just causes them to find different ways to enter into foreign countries without detection.

A very unique challenge arises in changing these prohibited pigment lists. First, without the proper documentation of several years' worth of research on the dangers of tattooing by regulating agencies, there is no clear guideline to follow. Second, there is no list of permitted pigments, which forces manufacturers to guess what they can use next. To understand the complexity of this issue in terms of production and mixing, it is necessary to consider the limited number of base pigments, which are worked into more than 200 different shades of color.

Every time there is a change in a pigment requirement for a single color, it takes approximately 6–12 months until tattoo pigment manufacturers can truly comply.

Consider the following example:

Step 1: The tattoo pigment manufacturer is informed of a new item on the prohibited list (which has received prior approval and now has been changed). It has to be understood that this information is not currently communicated proactively; instead, the manufacturer has to comply reactively because there is no proper pre-informative channel between legislative agencies and manufacturers. At this moment, it is a code-red situation, and the manufacturer has to decide which of the items in research and development could be used as a replacement. Most well-established manufacturers do preliminary testing on skin with different available pigments that are not on the prohibited list.

Step 2: The owners themselves typically act as test subjects in these cases to avoid conflicts. Let's assume that one pigment is available that is ready to be used and is not on the ban list. It will have to be sent to a third party laboratory to pass all of the regulations, which will have a turnaround of 4–6 weeks. If the sample passes, it will be ready to be intermixed with all possible shades.

Step 3: At this time, it will take at least 6 weeks to recreate shades of colors that have been previously used. It is of the upmost importance that colors are matched properly because the end consumer will be unable to make changes to the final product after it is tattooed into the skin. Never-ending variables and possibilities start to arise again. Different countries have different inhabitants with a variety of skin conditions depending on the environment (e.g. the temperature or level of sun exposure) and a wide range of skin tones, and variations in healing conditions and artist education may also be present. The manufacturer has to perform tests on several subjects, who are in most cases the owner and/or very close relatives of the company. Who else would run the risk of the permanent color changing after healing to something less desirable than expected?

Step 4: This process alone (from receiving the tattoo to its complete healing) takes a minimum of 12 weeks!

Step 5: If the pigment is now ready to be part of the full production schedule, companies must create many different shades. Let's assume that a yellow pigment is changed. There will be between 40 and 80 color tones that must be re-formulated, and the desired inventory must be created. In the real world of manufacturing, only 30% of companies worldwide can create more than 10 shades of colors per day effectively, and even more importantly, in sufficient volumes, after which they have to be labeled and packaged in many different languages, according to the requirements of the laws of each individual country. Thus, even in the best case in which everything works well, it will take a minimum of 24 weeks (yes, almost 5–6 months) to make the proper changes.

There is another factor to be considered, which is the permanency of the pigments. It should never be forgotten that a tattoo is meant to be permanent and not temporary. People with no tattoos always seem to have concerns about what happens when a tattooed person ages and whether he or she will regret the decision to become tattooed. It is of the utmost importance to realize that it is very well known in the industry that when a person decides to receive his or her first tattoo, he or she has thought about it and researched it before deciding to fully commit to permanently changing his or her body. In today's age, the myth of the drunken sailor stumbling into a dark back corner and getting tattooed from some stranger, waking up the next morning with a tattoo on his arm that he did not want is outdated. In the same way, people no longer have to ride a horse to get from New York to California. Times have changed and people have evolved. Most people who receive a tattoo in 2014 will choose a design, agree to its placement on their body, and then get through the somewhat painful and timely process of tattooing in addition to the lengthy healing process afterwards. To assume that a person receiving this mark out of his or her own free will and decision made a mistake is of great ignorance to the fact that people differ and make their own choices.

Now, why is it so important to understand the challenges for regulating the tattoo pigment industry? Why should it be of concern? Well, some could argue that it is not important, but it is extremely critical to understand the economics of tattooing at the professional versus underground level. A statistical verification by the Pew Research Center dated 12.11.2013 mentions that the average cost of a professional tattoo is USD 45.00 (EUR 35.00) [5]. The same tattoo performed underground would cost USD 25.00 (EUR 19.00). This is where the trouble starts, considering the other factors in the calculation. Let's assume that both of the artists have to pay for their supplies and rent a place of business; however, one will be controlled and one will not, one will be trained and one will not, and one will use higher quality supplies, and the other will not.

The consumer decides who will do his or her tattoo. Yes, it is still an adult decision. It is no less of an adult activity than drinking a beer or having a cigarette and most likely, there is less of a chance

of injury or even death. Both beer and cigarettes are very well regulated and both have risks, as does the act of getting tattooed. The industry itself is pushing to create more awareness of choosing properly trained artists, thereby lowering the risk of complications arising after the tattoo is finished to a figure even lower than the 2.6% stated above. Not bad for a self-regulated industry that nobody cared about 5 years ago. It will be of great necessity to include proper training, supplies and aftercare for effective regulation.

The financial impact of the past 10 years on pigment manufacturing has been dramatic if not already close to devastating. Five years ago, most pigments were created in basements, kitchens and garages, and 60% still are (remember the immigration example?). Today, leading companies have facilities with internal laboratories and cleanrooms. They follow the label requirements of the US Food and Drug Administration and make daily changes to better their products. Good manufacturing practice is standard, as is the traceability of products. The main manufacturers are proactively trying to get updated information from regulating authorities so that they can provide the necessary quality products and abide by new laws. This may not sound like a regulatory problem, but it will be when this industry deteriorates and loses another quality manufacturer to draconian regulations, which currently may be responsible for the pigment reactions of less than 1 PERCENT of persons getting tattooed this year. We all would love to have 0% risk. Unfortunately, it is not possible. Considering that most manufacturers are willing and happy to conform with upcoming regulations and that they all agree on the concerns and dangers, their rates of implementation cannot be determined without the discussion of all quality pigment manufacturers as well as regulatory agencies. Going further, it must be considered that most regulations will not be economically technically achievable outside of theory in a laboratory. In real production scenarios, industry could be forced right back to where it feels comfortable and where it will remain for another 1,000 years. These events will occur for the following reasons: some of the new proposed raw pigments are way too high in price, the color shades are completely prohibited, they are not readily available in the amounts needed, and they may not conform with the tattoo industry standard of permanency (that the color will stay the same shade under the skin after healing). Another factor to consider is that the price of a 30-ml bottle would need to increase significantly, forcing artists to find an alternative and cheaper source. At this point, there is no proposal explaining how the government will supplement the research and development to make an improved product for the better health and safety of the end consumer. A grant or some kind of assistance would possibly make this transition feasible. In addition, how will the government enforce the purchasing of tattoo pigments through licensed and regulated tattoo pigment manufacturers (including purchases made by unlicensed tattoo artists and shops)?

In conclusion, there are many factors and variables that need to be taken into consideration before such stringent laws and regulations are enforced and must be followed by quality manufacturers. Changes to regulations and laws are creating a safer environment every day for the manufacturer and end consumer, they just need to be carried out with sufficient time to make them reasonable to achieve and more importantly, to sustain on a continuous basis. Ultimately, ResAP/2008 was a great regulation in its original form. Many color companies are still working today to create an environment in which this regulation can be achieved. Many newly proposed updated and implemented additions to the original regulation have only led to ongoing chaotic changes, and they have also had dramatic negative effects on sustainability. Many companies that are willing to make changes to improve the tattoo pigment industry have taken on great financial strain to provide better conditions for the end consumer and an improved product according to ResAP/2008. With the ongoing inconsistency of unified testing methods, which is still the GIANT ELEPHANT in the room throughout Europe, in addition to the other variables mentioned, there is still a lot to be done before this is to be advocated and drastic changes are made. Currently, the odds are not in favor of the willing players in this highly important undertaking, which aims to improve the health and safety of the general public at large. One thing that we can all agree upon is that the health and safety of the person(s) getting tattooed as well as the survival of professional tattoo artists and pigment manufacturers are the most important factors.

References

1 McKay EC: Pigment. 2011. http://www.tattooarchive.com/tattoo_history/pigment.html.
2 Klügl I, Hiller KA, Landthaler M, Bäumler W: Incidence of health problems associated with tattooed skin: a nationwide survey in German-speaking countries. Dermatology 2010;221:43–50.
3 Market Research Interpretation/Intenzive Marketing International/2014. 'N=3000 –> 6%=180 indicating tattoos I N=3000 * 2,3=6900 Tattoos done on the requested persons – 180 tattoos of 6900=2,6%'.
4 Wright R: Tattoos as wounds: a clinical efficacy study of two aftercare preparations. Wounds UK 2012;8:32–40.
5 Statistic Brain: Tattoo statistics. 2013. http://www.statisticbrain.com/tattoo-statistics/.

Mario Barth
Intenze Products
15 Van Orden Place
Hackensack, NJ 07601 (USA)
E-Mail mb@starlighttattoo.com

Serup J, Kluger N, Bäumler W (eds): Tattooed Skin and Health.
Curr Probl Dermatol. Basel, Karger, 2015, vol 48, pp 118–127 (DOI: 10.1159/000369236)

Making Innovative Tattoo Ink Products with Improved Safety: Possible and Impossible Ingredients in Practical Usage

Michael Dirks

H-A-N GmbH, Esslingen, Germany

Abstract

Today's tattoo inks are no longer just simple solids in liquid suspension. Nowadays, these inks are high-tech dispersions made from finely spread pigments in a binder-solvent mixture. These so-called colour dispersions must follow the modern standards of tattooing, which are increasing every year. They must be rich in chromophoric pigments and yet fluid, they must not dry rapidly, and there should be no occurrence of any sedimentation, even during longer tattoo seasons. An innovative tattoo ink should enable long-lasting, brilliant tattoos without a negative impact on the artist's workflow and of course without endangering the consumer. The high standard in tattoos, regarding the motives and techniques, that is witnessed today could not be achieved by the artists without quality tools and modern tattoo ink. This article will give the reader a brief overview of the different ingredients of tattoo ink and of the function of binding agents and solvents in modern tattoo ink as well as describe what additives are used to achieve the desired behaviour during application. Furthermore, the article will take a look into the pigments that are used in tattoo ink and show why certain pigments are not suited for tattoo ink. The differences, advantages and disadvantages of organic and inorganic pigments will be explained.

© 2015 S. Karger AG, Basel

Tattoo Inks

Broadly speaking, tattoo inks are a suspension of non-soluable pigments in a liquid. The liquid of tattoo ink consists of two components: a binder and a solvent. The fine-dispersed pigment mixture is stabilised by additives. Preservatives can be added to prevent microbiological spoilage. Figure 1 shows a schematic of the composition of the main ingredients of tattoo ink.

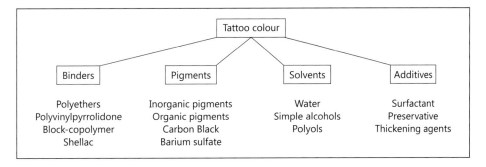

Fig. 1. Simplified representation of the composition of tattoo ink.

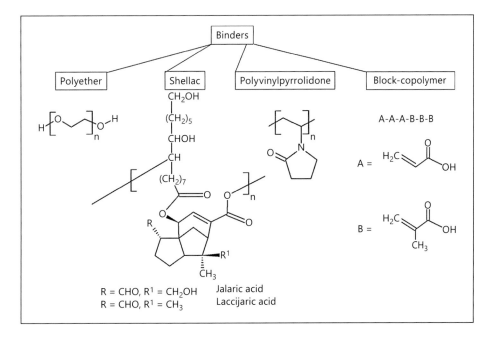

Fig. 2. Structural formulae of binding agents used in customary tattoo inks.

Binding Agents

Binding agents, or binders, are the non-volatile compounds of tattoo ink, not including pigments and filler but including additives [1]. The binder binds the pigment particles to each other and to the tattooing needle for easier injection of the ink into the skin. Figure 2 shows the most important binding agents in customary tattoo inks. Because of their high molar mass, the binding agents are limited in their bio-availability and are not seen as an acute hazard. The average molar masses can be found in table 1.

Solvents

All of the above-mentioned binders are soluble in water or are neutralised with an alkaline solution. Because of this, water is the main ingredient of

Table 1. Average molar masses of binding agents

Polymer	Molar mass
Polyethylene glycol	200–600 g·mol^{-1} (liquid); >4,000 g·mol^{-1} (solid)
Poloxamer 188	7,680–9,510 g·mol^{-1} (solid)
Polyvinylpyrrolidone	2,500–2,500,000 g·mol^{-1} (solid)
Shellac	1,500–2,500 g·mol^{-1} (solid)
Acrylate	10,000–200,000 g·mol^{-1} (solid)

Table 2. Purposes of solvents used in tattoo inks

Solvent	Purpose
Water	Solvation of binder
Ethanol	Regulates drying properties, masks smells
Isopropyl alcohol	Regulates drying properties, masks smells
Glycerin	Increasing viscosity, humectant
Propylene glycol	Humectant, increases dispersability

tattoo ink. Also, simple and polyvalent alcohols are used to define characteristics like drying properties, viscosity and dispersibility. The characteristics of solvents used in tattoo inks are shown in table 2. With the exception of water, the usage of solvents should be limited because high concentrations of alcohol can irritate the skin.

Additives

Additives are auxiliary materials that are added to exclude unwanted characteristics or to enhance wanted characteristics [2]. The concentration of additives used in tattoo inks is not higher than 5%. The used additives include the following: surfactants to adjust the surface as well as thickening and thixotroping agents and preservatives.

Surface-Active Additives (Tensides)
Tensides are used in tattoo inks to better disperse and stabilize the pigments during the production process, leading to a longer shelf life.

The power of attraction of the pigment molecules leads to cohesion, and therefore, they drive to have the smallest possible surface in a given volume. This property is known as surface tension and can lead to problems regarding interactions with other ingredients of the formulation. Fine-dispersed pigments tend to agglomerate to bigger structures and resist wetting by the binder solution if the surface tension of the substance is not adjusted with boundary layers. Compatibilisers, like tensides, are necessary for the complete removal of air from the agglomerates and complete coating of the pigment particles with the binder solution.

Thickening Agents
The only way to inhibit the reagglomeration and therefore sedimentation of inks during longer storage is to enhance its structural viscosity and thixotropy. Thixotroping agents, like silica, build up the yield point without impairing the shear conditions during processing. Figure 3 shows, in a schematic way, that the edges of silica are flat and

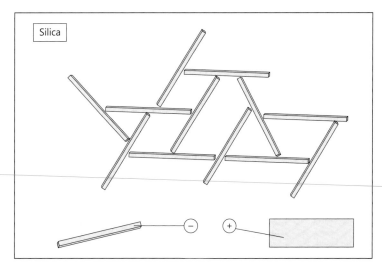

Fig. 3. Card house-like structures of silica.

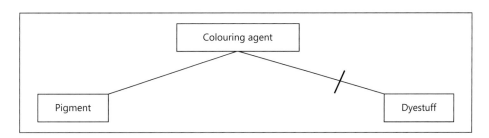

Fig. 4. Per definition, dyes and pigments are colorants.

that the molecules are arranged in a card house-like structure in idle conditions because of different surface charges.

Preservatives
As products with a high portion of water, tattoo inks must be protected against microbiological spoilage. To reduce the risk of allergic reaction, it's best practise to waive preservatives. Water-rich media provide better reproduction opportunities than water-scarce media. The water activity, as a unit for the availability of water, and not the portion of water in a medium is crucial for the reproduction of microorganisms. To deny microorganisms the opportunity to reproduce in tattoo ink, the water activity value should be <0.6 [3].

Pigments

Pigments are by definition insoluble, organic or inorganic colorants in medium, and dyes are soluble organic colorants in medium [4]. Dyes are not suitable as tattoo ink because they are soluble and will be biodegraded very fast after application. Figure 4 shows the divison of colouring agents into pigments and dyestuff. Figure 5 shows a rough division of the pigments and fillers used in tattoo inks. Every class of pigments has its advantages and disadvantages and have typical pigment impurities, i.e., inorganic impurities like heavy metals in metal oxide pigments, organic impurities like aromatic amines in organic coloured pigments, and impurities like polycyclic aromatic hydrocarbons (PAHs) in Carbon Black pigments.

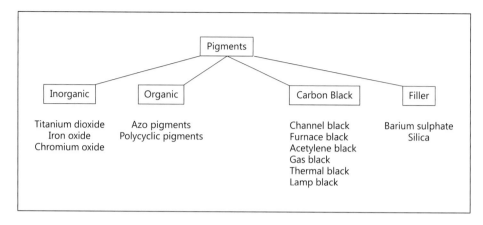

Fig. 5. Division of pigments.

Inorganic Pigments

The most-used inorganic pigments in tattoo inks are limited due to their application properties. The used pigments include iron oxide, titanium dioxide and chromium oxide green.

Titanium Dioxide Pigments
Titanium dioxide pigments show very little absorption ability and reflect almost unchanged white light because of its high scattering power. Titanium dioxide pigments have the highest refractive index of all white colorants, so they are suitable for lightening colours. Of the three known crystal modifications of titanium dioxide, Brookit has no role in the production of tattoo inks, and because of its strong photochemical activity, Anatas has only a very little role in the production of tattoo inks. As shown in figure 6, the most important crystal modification of titanium dioxide for tattoo inks is Rutil [5].

Iron Oxide Pigments
Many variants of iron oxide are used as yellow-, red- and brown-hued pigments. The characteristics of iron oxides limits their use in tattoo inks but also makes them suited for permanent make-up. Iron oxides have a dull and non-brilliant hue compared to inorganic pigments. Iron oxide pigments have a very high opacity. Figure 7 shows that, in contrast to iron oxide red, which is heat stable to temperatures up to a 1,000°C, yellow and brown iron oxides are not heat stable. In general, tattoos made of iron oxide pigments tend to change to a red hue over time. The reason for this is the tendency of iron oxide to change to the heat-stable red haematite.

Chromium Oxide Green
The chromium oxide pigments chromium oxide green (Cr_2O_3) and chromium oxide hydrate green (viridian) ($Cr_2O_3x3H_2O$) are chromatically limited to green. Their authentic characteristics and their heat stability are comparable to iron oxide pigments. During production, hexavalent chromium is reduced to trivalent chromium. Chromium oxides must be closely monitored for soluble chromium VI [5]. These pigments are only used in permanent make-up due to their dull and 'dirty' hue.

Impurities of Inorganic Pigments
As mentioned before, inorganic pigments always have unwanted and quality-diminishing impurities. Nickel, chromium, copper and cobalt are

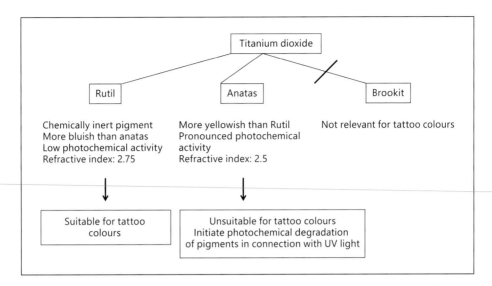

Fig. 6. The crystal modifications of titanium dioxide.

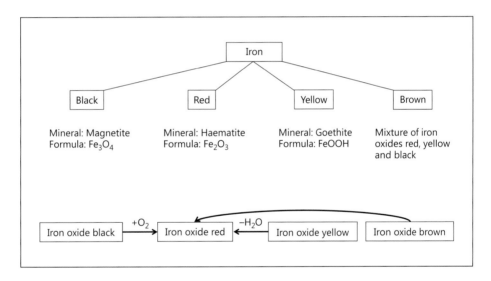

Fig. 7. Variants of iron oxide pigments.

commonly found in the analyses of iron oxide pigments, but these do not lead to allergic reactions as often as expected. Perhaps the reason is the encasing of these different metals in the spinel structure. Further research is required on this matter.

Organic Pigments

The use of organic pigments enables us to imitate almost every colour the human eye can perceive. In comparison to inorganic pigments, organic pigments are more brilliant and have high-

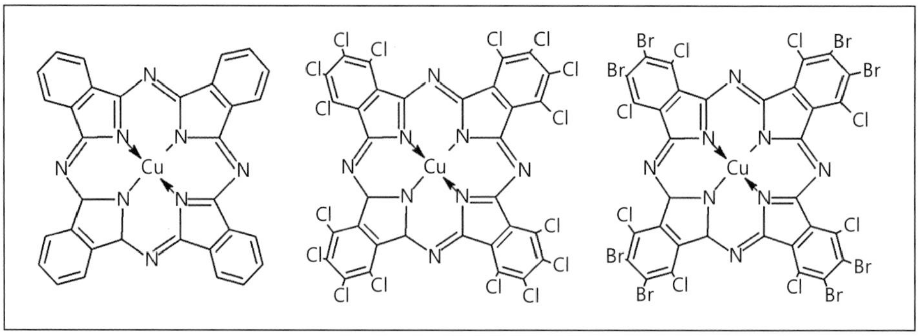

Fig. 8. The polycyclic pigments CI 74160, CI 74260 & CI 74265.

er colour strength when blended with white. The variants of these pigments cover the whole colour spectrum but have worse dispersibility than inorganic pigments. Organic pigments can be roughly divided into azo and polycyclic pigments.

Azo Pigments

Azo pigments are compounds that contain the azo group –N = N– chained to sp2-hybridised C atoms. The generic formula is

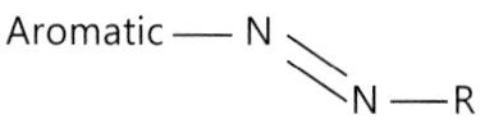

Aromatic — N
                ‖
                N — R

R = rest and Aromatic = aromatic rest.

The amount of azo groups is used to differentiate between mono and diazo compounds. Compounds with three or more azo groups are not used in any technical scenario. The most-used manufacturing process for these pigments is the azo coupling reaction [6, 7].

Polycyclic Pigments

Polycyclic pigments are not a uniform class of pigments; they are a round-up of all non-azo pigments. With the exception of triphenylmethane pigment, all polycyclic pigments have ring systems. A special case is the polycyclic metal complex of the phthalocyanine system, as shown in figure 8.

Impurities in Organic Pigments

Due to their nature, organic pigments have fewer impurities than inorganic pigments. The contamination with heavy metals is much lower compared to inorganic pigments, but due to their production process, they can contain aromatic amines as unwanted accompanying substances. Analytical findings of heavy metals like copper can be traced back to copper bound to phthalocyanine pigments.

Carbon Black

Soot, also called Carbon Black, is one of the pigments most suited for tattoo ink. Depending on the manufacturing process and curing, these pigments are very different in size and therefore are different in their dispersibilities. Often, the end prodcut is described to have an aerodynamic diameter of 0.1 micrometer. The origins for manufacturing are small spherical parts (the so-called primary particles or nodules), with a size of 15–300 nm. These particles are melted to particle aggregates with an aerodynamic diameter of 85–500 nm. As shown in figure 9, strong electric forces keep these aggregates

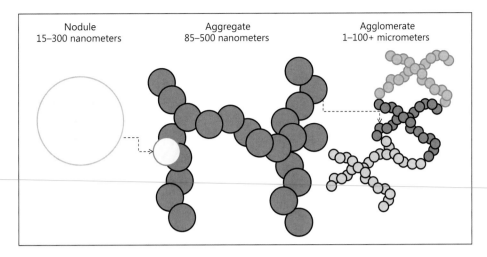

Fig. 9. Structural development of Carbon Black.

together, and when associated with other aggregates, they form agglomerates. All of this happens during the manufacturing process, and consequently, the majority of Carbon Black on the market consists of agglomerates sized 1–100 μm because these agglomerates, once formed, never break. For better handling and to minimise the occurrence of dust, Carbon Black is sold in pellets with a size of 0.1–1 mm. So, the ultrafine primary particles are only found in the production furnace [8].

Impurities of Carbon Black

Depending on the manufacturing process, Carbon Black can contain impurities in the form of PAHs.

Filler

Fillers usually consist of inorganic substances with different chemical composition and physical properties. Their main task is to fill the tattoo ink with spatial framework material to influence storage properties. The most-used fillers in tattoo inks are silica and barium sulphate.

Barium Sulphate

There are two different types of barium sulphate: the naturally occurring, so-called baryt and the synthetically manufactured blanc fixe. The latter is free of unwanted accompanying substances and matches the strict legislative regulation regarding the solubility of barium [5]. As shown in figure 10, barium sulphate is used as a flocculation partner for organic pigments. With controlled flocculation of organic pigments with barium sulphate, the properties relevant for manufacturing, for example, dispersibility, are optimised. The sediment that develops during longer storage is redispersed better, and no demixing of pigments with different densities occurs.

Measurements Taken by the Manufacturer to Ensure Consumer Safety and Satisfaction

To ensure a high standard of quality, there are two dimensions. One dimension is consistency between each batch of a certain colour, i.e., every batch of a dark green colour is the same shade of dark green. To achieve this goal, standard quality

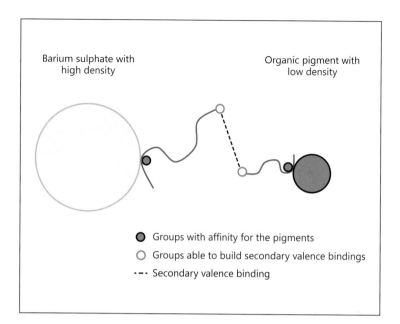

Fig. 10. Controlled flocculation (simplified, not to scale).

control processes are enforced as in every other colour-processing or colour-producing industry. The other dimension is safety. Every batch of raw materials is tested for inorganic impurities, like heavy metals, or organic impurities, like PAHs. During production, the accidental intake of nickel is prevented using only tools that have either no or very little nickel contamination. Also, all things made out of plastic that directly contact tattoo inks have to conform to the strict criteria of the numerous EU and FDA regulations. Every batch is sterilised with non-ionising gamma rays to ensure that they contain no microbiological pollution. Also, random samples are taken after sterilisation for microbiological testing to ensure that the sterilisation has worked as intended, and all pieces of the packaging are chosen with the aforementioned EU and FDA regulations in mind. Of course, all of these steps are documented to ensure traceability, which is very important, not only as a tool for guaranteeing consumer safety, but also as a tool to facilitate continuous improvement in manufacturing methods.

Conclusion and Outlook

The manufacturing of tattoo inks with better safety depends on the legislation. A general prohibition of pigments or limitation of pigments with reference to cosmetic ordinances is not suitable. As a result, pigments that have been in use for decades and are much safer than pigments that have not undergone cosmetic safety evaluations have been banned. Also, the approach for using pigments that are regulated by the ordinance for cosmetics and are allowed for use in every product is wrong because many of the allowed pigments are azo pigments and are therefore contaminated with aromatic amines. Instead of a regulation on pigments, the introduction of security dossiers for tattoo colours with no-observed-adverse-effect level and acceptable daily intake values would improve the situation. But, the scientific data needed to calculate these values is inadequate. A standardised EU legislation with validated methods of examination is desirable and would be useful.

References

1 DIN EN 971–1:1996–09, Paints and Varnishes – Terms and Definitions for Coating Materials – Part 1. Berlin, Beuth, 1996.
2 Nanetti P: Lackrohstoffkunde. Hannover, Vincentz, 1997.
3 Umbach W: Kosmetik und Hygiene. Weinheim, Wiley-VCH, 2004.
4 DIN 55943–11–1993, Colouring Materials; Terms and Definitions. Berlin, Beuth, 1993.
5 Goldschmidt A, Streitberger HJ: BASF-Handbuch Lackiertechnik. Hannover, Vincentz, 2002.
6 Zollinger H: Chemie der Azofarbstoffe. Basel, Birkhäuser, 1958.
7 Zollinger H: Diazo Chemistry. Weinheim, VCH-Verlagsgesellschaft, 1994.
8 International Carbon Black Association (ICBA): Carbon Black User's Guide – Safety, Health, & Environmental Information. ICBA, 2004.

Michael Dirks, Dipl.-Ing. (FH)
H-A-N GmbH
Eberhard Bauer Strasse 32
DE–73734 Esslingen (Germany)
E-Mail m.dirks@h-a-n.de

Serup J, Kluger N, Bäumler W (eds): Tattooed Skin and Health.
Curr Probl Dermatol. Basel, Karger, 2015, vol 48, pp 128–135 (DOI: 10.1159/000369195)

Tailored Surface Engineering of Pigments by Layer-by-Layer Coating

Lars Dähne[a] · Julia Schneider[a] · Dirk Lewe[b] · Henrik Petersen[b]

[a] Surflay Nanotec GmbH, Berlin, and [b] MT.DERM GmbH, Berlin, Germany

Abstract

We have evaluated the feasibility of layer-by-layer encapsulation technology for the improvement of dye pigments used for tattoos or permanent make-up. The formation of core-shell structures is possible by coating pigments with thin films of several different polyelectrolytes using this technology. The physicochemical surface properties, such as charge density and chemical functionality, can be reproducibly varied in a wide range. Tailoring the surface properties independently from the pigment core allows one to control the rheological behaviour of pigment suspensions, to prevent aggregation between different pigments, to reduce the cytotoxicity, and to influence the response of phagocytes in order to have similar or the same uptake and bioclearance for all pigments. These properties determine the durability and colour tone stability of tattoos and permanent make-up. © 2015 S. Karger AG, Basel

Introduction

In recent times, the desire for tattoos and permanent make-up has increased tremendously [1]. Consequently, the variety and to some degree the safety of coloured dye pigments used in tattooing have broadened remarkably. Due to the increasing importance of pigments, scientific research on pigment safety, pigment improvement, and the mechanisms of tattoo durability as well as tattoo removal has started to evolve [2]. However, due to the wide range of different pigments available and the complicated interactions between these dyes and the dermis, based on the immune response of the skin, research on these problems is still at an early stage and requires further dedicated studies.

Several health issues related to embedding different pigments into the skin are already recognised, such as toxicity, especially for heavy-metal pigments; potential cancerous risk, e.g. for the polycyclic aromatic compounds in Carbon Black [3, 4] and in azo dyes; the slow dissolution of pigments; the photoreactivity of organic dyes; and the formation of dangerous radicals by titanium dioxide (TiO_2) pigments [5]. These problems arise mainly as a result of direct contact between the dangerous compound or its surfaces with the tissue of the dermis, leading to an immune response in the body. Besides the health risks, there are also several problems in the quality of tattooing, arising mainly from insufficient long-term stability. This leads to fading and shifts of colour tones over time, which often requires a refreshment of the pigment injection. For example, as our own observations have shown, brown colour tones based on

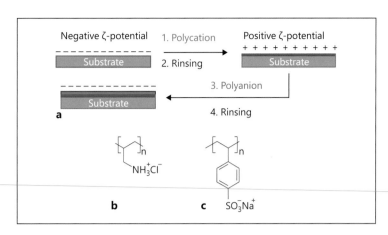

Fig. 1. a Steps 1 to 4 show the process of the layer by layer coating for planar surfaces. In steps 1 and 3 either a positively or negatively charged polyelectrolyte is adsorbed to the surface. In steps 2 and 4 the surface is washed in order to remove excess polyion. Example polycation poly(allylamine hydrochloride) (PAH, **b**) and the polyanion poly(styrenesulfonate sodium salt) (PSS, **c**).

inorganic pigments containing different iron oxides for black, red, and yellow as well as TiO_2 for white shift to a rose tone after several months due to a faster removal of yellow pigments compared with red and white ones. In contrast, for organic pigments, the colour shifts from warm brown to grey, caused by faster disappearance of red and yellow pigments. Several factors determine the instability of pigments in the skin, such as dissolution, chemical degradation, photobleaching, and enzymatic degradation or bioclearance by the phagocytes of the immune system. Phagocytes take up foreign particles according to recognition of the particles as being dangerous for the body. This recognition is based on the physicochemical surface properties and the size of the particles. After uptake of those particles, the phagocytes can leave the skin in order to remove the pigment from the organism, which leads to fading. Moreover, the cells could also encapsulate the pigments and remain in the skin, which would increase the long-term stability of the tattoos.

Some of the above-described problems can be reduced by encapsulating the pigments in polymer shells, thus preserving their size and colour but unifying and optimising their surface properties. This requires a thin, transparent, and homogeneous coating with a thickness in the nanometre range. A possible solution is encapsulation

based on layer-by-layer (LbL) technology. This self-assembly process was developed on planar surfaces approximately 20 years ago [6]. Some years later it was extended to colloidal systems [7, 8]. Nowadays, LbL technology is the subject of intensive research on many different applications, such as corrosion control, biomedical applications, and material science applications, including drug delivery, catalysis, and medicine [9].

LbL technology allows for charged surfaces to be coated with polymer films and for the thickness of these films to be controlled on the nanometre scale. This is demonstrated by coating a pigment to generate a negatively charged surface, determined by electrophoresis as the ζ-potential [10]. If an aqueous solution of a positively charged polyelectrolyte, such as poly(allylamine hydrochloride) (PAH) (fig. 1b), is applied to the pigment, the PAH will be adsorbed onto the surface due to electrostatic attraction and an increase in entropy. Not only are the negative charges on the pigment surface neutralised by the adsorption but also the ζ-potential of the pigment surface is completely reversed to a positive value. When a defined positive potential is achieved, the adsorption stops due to repulsion of further PAH molecules in the solution. After rinsing, excess PAH is removed, and the process can be repeated by assembling a polyanion, such as

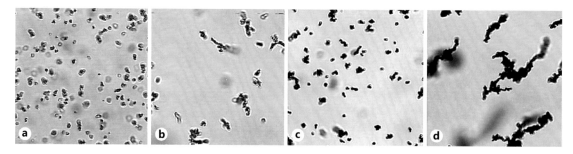

Fig. 2. Transmission microscope images of inorganic tattoo pigments (image size 40 μm × 40 μm). **a** Titanium dioxide; **b** iron oxide yellow; **c** iron oxide red; **d** aggregated iron oxide black.

poly(styrenesulfonate sodium salt) (PSS; fig. 1c), in the same manner, which changes the surface potential back to a negative value (fig. 1a). This can be repeated many times, yielding a constant increase in thickness of approximately 4 nm for each double layer of PAH/PSS. A variety of more than 50 polyanions and also polycations with quite different properties and functionalities are commercially available, giving this technology enormous potential to easily modify the surface properties of particles.

We will report pigment encapsulation in LbL films and present initial results regarding the properties of such core-shell structures and their potential for future applications in the tattoo and permanent make-up industry. Although LbL coating can be applied to all pigments, we will focus on the encapsulation of inorganic tattoo pigments, including TiO_2, iron oxide black, iron oxide yellow, and iron oxide red.

Experimental Section

Physicochemical Properties of Selected Pigments
Pigments are characterised by properties such as chemical composition, colour, size distribution, shape, porosity, surface roughness, and surface charge. The last is the determining property for pigment encapsulation. Thus, the surface charges of some tattoo pigments were determined; these

Table 1. ζ-Potentials of dye pigments used in tattoo and permanent make-up applications determined in 10 mM Tris buffer solution at pH 7 by electrophoresis using a Zetasizer from Malvern Instruments

Tattoo pigment	ζ-Potential in mV
Titanium dioxide	−45.0
Iron oxide yellow	−29.9
FD&C Yellow 6 Lake	−18.2
DSC Red 30 Lake	−30.1
Pigment Red 5	−25.1
Iron oxide red	−32.0
FD&C Red 40 Lake	+21.7
Pigment Blue 15	−30.3
Iron oxide black	−29.3
Carbon black	−24.9

are listed in table 1. Apart from the positively charged FD&C Red 40 Lake, all of them exhibit a negative surface charge. High-resolution confocal laser scanning microscopy (CLSM) has been used for analysing size distribution, porosity, and polyelectrolyte coating on the surface by means of fluorescently labelled polyelectrolytes. Transmission images of tattoo pigments (fig. 2) show that the size varies between 1 and 10 μm. There are multiple shapes, from almost spherical to needle-like. In the case of iron oxide black, the ferromagnetic properties can be detected as causing the formation of temporary aggregates between the primary pigment particles.

Dähne · Schneider · Lewe · Petersen

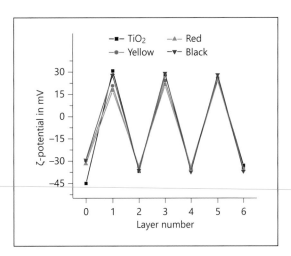

Fig. 3. Progress of surface charge of tattoo pigments with increasing number of surface layers. The ζ-potential becomes positive after adsorption of the first polycationic PAH layer. The adsorption of a second polyanionic PSS layer turns the potential back to negative, and so forth.

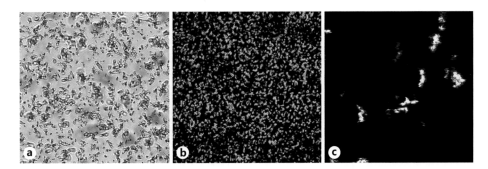

Fig. 4. Transmission and confocal laser scanning microscopy (CLSM) fluorescence images of (PAH-Rho/PSS)$_2$-coated iron oxide yellow: **a** transmission image; **b** CLSM fluorescence image (80 × 80 μm); **c** high-resolution CLSM fluorescence image (20 × 20 μm).

Physicochemical Properties of Layer-by-Layer Coatings

The four different pigments were LbL coated with 6 layers, starting with the polycation PAH and then alternating PSS and PAH. One way to control coating success is to measure the change in the ζ-potential (fig. 3). After the first layer, the charge changes to a positive value for all pigments. Following deposition of the next layer (PSS), the charge changes back to a negative value, and so on. While the surface charges of different pigments are different at the beginning, they become more equal as the layer number and film thickness increase.

The coated pigments exhibit almost no change in size compared with the uncoated ones because the layer thickness after 6 layers is around 12 nm, which is negligible in comparison to the particle diameter.

The polymer film is not visible by transmission microscopy due to the limited spatial resolution of optical microscopes. However, fluorescently labelled polyelectrolytes help to visualise the deposited polyelectrolytes in the fluorescence images of a CLSM (fig. 4). The fluorescence intensity is correlated with the adsorbed amount of polyelectrolytes. The pigments were coated with two double layers of PSS and PAH,

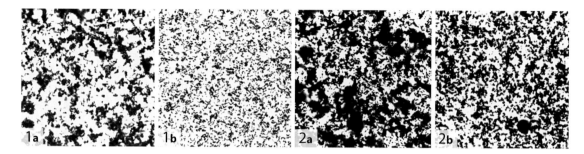

Fig. 5. Microscopy images of uncoated and coated pigments: (1) iron oxide yellow, (2) iron oxide red; **a** uncoated and **b** LbL-coated particles (PAH/PSS)$_2$; image size 80 × 80 μm.

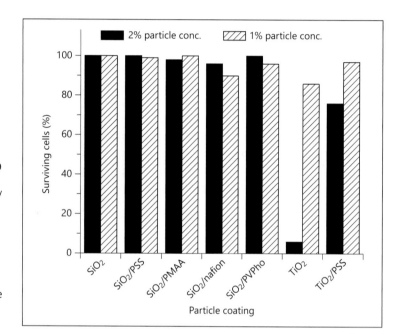

Fig. 6. Percentage of surviving RKO cancer cells after 24 h incubation with uncoated or coated (PAH/PSS/PAH/Polymer X) titanium dioxide and silicon dioxide particles whereupon the external coating was varied (X = PSS, poly(methacrylic acid sodium salt PMAA), Nafion, or poly(vinyl phosphate sodium salt)PVPho). The tests were performed at two different particle concentrations.

with PAH covalently linked to the fluorescent dye rhodamine B (PAH-Rho) at every 160th monomer position. Figure 4c shows some fluorescence in the interior of the particles, indicating the deposition of PAH-Rho inside the pores or fissures of the particles.

The deposition of LbL films on different pigment particles leads to homogeneous, chemically identical surfaces with a uniform ζ-potential, independent of the core material. Furthermore, the external surface potential can be tuned to be either negative or positive, depending on the polyelectrolyte species of the last layer.

The unification of and partial increase in the surface charge of pigments increase their repulsion and diminishes the tendency to aggregate during storage. Aqueous suspensions of uncoated and coated iron oxide yellow and red were sonicated and stored for 3 days. After shaking, CLSM images of the samples showed different size distributions for the particles (fig. 5). The uncoated particles showed a much higher degree of aggre-

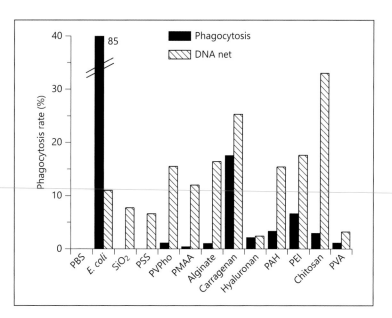

Fig. 7. Phagocytosis of LbL-coated silica particles with a 4.3 μm diameter. In addition to the percentage of ingested particles (black), the percentage of sacrificed phagocytes (patterned) forming DNA nets is shown. The x-axis indicates the external polyelectrolyte layer. Phosphate buffered saline (PBS) and *Escherichia coli* are the negative and positive control samples.

gation when compared with the coated ones. This phenomenon is even more noticeable for mixtures of different uncoated pigments, sometimes yielding strong aggregation due to large differences in their ζ-potentials. However, mixtures of coated pigments with different gravimetric densities show the undesired effect of faster phase separation. As a second consequence suspensions of coated particles can have a concentration 1.5 times higher than uncoated ones and still have the same liquid properties.

Cell Response to Layer-by-Layer Coated Particles
The equalisation of the surface properties is expected to have remarkable effects on the behaviour in the skin. Thus, initial tests have been performed in order to investigate the cytotoxicity of different LbL coatings, as well as their recognition by human phagocytes. For this purpose, different polyelectrolyte coatings have been chosen and assembled on monodisperse model particles, including silicon dioxide (SiO_2) and titanium dioxide (TiO_2). Particles of 1 μm in diameter were used for cytotoxicity tests and SiO_2 particles with 4.3 μm for phagocytosis tests. The particles were

coated with a basic layer of PAH/PSS/PAH, while the last layer was varied using different polyanions, such as poly(methacrylic acid sodium salt) (PMAA); Nafion, which is sulphonated Teflon; or poly(vinyl phosphate sodium salt) (PVPho). The cytotoxicity test was performed with RKO cancer cells that were incubated for 24 h in 1- or 2-percent-by-weight particle suspensions. The incubation was performed under very slow agitation in order to avoid particle sedimentation on the cells as well as abrasion of the cells by the moving particles. The results are shown in figures 6 and 7.

The investigations with 1 μm SiO_2 particles showed that despite the high particle concentration, the PSS- and PMAA-coated particles are well tolerated by the cells. The hydrophobic Nafion and the PVPho coatings revealed a slightly decrease of the cell tolerance (fig. 6). In contrast, uncoated TiO_2 showed a clear toxic effect that could be dramatically reduced by the encapsulation with PAH/PSS. The surprisingly high cytotoxicity of TiO_2 could have been caused by radical formation on its surface by light irradiation, which could not be fully avoided during the experiment. In addition, the high density of TiO_2, 4.3 g/cm^3, compared to 1.8 g/cm^3 for SiO_2, could have led to more sedimentation and additional mechanical stress on the cells.

The experiments with human phagocytes were performed using 4.3 μm SiO_2 particles with different LbL coatings. In the standard phagocytosis tests, the number of particles ingested by the phagocytes is correlated with their danger potential [11]. In addition to phagocytosis for some particles, we observed sacrificed phagocytes that released their DNA in order to immobilise the particles with a DNA net. The results summarised in figure 7 show both the percentage of ingested particles and the number of sacrificed phagocytes.

The results reveal that by LbL coating, the response of the immune system to particles can be strongly influenced. For instance, positively charged surfaces (PAH, polyethylenimine (PEI), and chitosan in fig. 7) showed greater phagocytosis than the negative ones (PVPho, PSS, and hyaluronan), which is in good agreement with the literature [9]. Surprisingly, the biopolymers alginate and carrageenan resulted in greater phagocytosis compared with the synthetic polymer PSS and polyvinyl alcohol (PVA).

Since the unusual DNA-net formation was assumed to be eventually caused by the large size of the particles, further investigations on smaller LbL coated particles as well as on real tattoo pigments are in progress.

Summary and Outlook

We have evaluated the feasibility of LbL encapsulation technology for the improvement of tattoo and permanent make-up pigments. It was shown that formation of core-shell structures is possible by coating pigments with thin films composed of several different polyelectrolytes. An overview of possible problems in tattooing and the possibility of addressing these problems with LbL technology is given in figure 8.

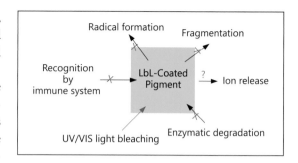

Fig. 8. Processes that are considered of importance for tattoos. The red crosses show processes that can be potentially prevented by LbL encapsulation, while photobleaching and slow dissolution probably cannot be inhibited by this method.

Physicochemical surface properties such as charge density and chemical functionality could be reproducibly varied in a wide range. The new surface properties changed the rheological behaviour of pigment suspensions remarkably, preventing aggregation between different pigments but also resulting in faster phase separation of pigment mixtures. Investigation of the response of cells and phagocytes to coated model particles showed that LbL films have the potential to reduce or even prevent the fading and shifts of colour tones of tattoos caused by phagocytosis.

Additionally, the polymer network around the pigments can prevent their fragmentation into smaller pieces. Beneficial is also the very thin and transparent polyelectrolyte shell that does not change the colour of the pigments by absorption of visible light. However, it does not efficiently absorb UV light to protect them against photobleaching. From numerous studies of the permeability behaviour of polyelectrolyte films, the following possible advantages can be derived. First, LbL polyelectrolyte films are impermeable to macromolecules such as enzymes [8], which should prevent enzymatic degradation of coated pigments. Second, the release of dissolved molecules from the pigment surface can be reduced or completely stopped if the molecules are highly charged or have a high molecular weight. Third, recent investigations on LbL membranes showed that oxygen transport is strongly hindered [12], which could also prevent chemical oxidation of pigments. Fourth, radical formation on encapsulated pigment surfaces by photochemical processes [5] will not affect human tissue cells but will instead be quenched by the polyelectrolyte shell.

Acknowledgements

We are grateful to Dr. Radostina Georgieva and Prof. Hans Bäumler (Institute of Transfusion Medicine, Charité Berlin) for the phagocytosis tests. For the cytotoxicity tests, we thank Dr. Manfred Jugold (Deutsches Krebsforschungszentrum Heidelberg). Many thanks also to Barbara Baude for the experimental work.

References

1 Bäumler W: The fate of tattoo pigments in the skin (presentation). First International Conference on Tattoo Safety, Berlin, 2013.

2 Luch A, Laux P, et al: Tattoos: is there more than 'meets-the-eye'? Tattooing from a toxicological perspective. The Lancet, submitted.

3 Sahu D, Kannan GM, Vijayaraghavan R: Carbon black particle exhibits size dependent toxicity in human monocytes. Int J Inflam 2014;2014:827019.

4 Lehner K, Santarelli F, Vasold R, König B, Landthaler M, Bäumler W: Black tattoo inks are a source of problematic substances such as dibutyl phthalate. Contact Dermatitis 2011;65:231–238.

5 Rancan F, Nazemi B, Rautenberg S, Ryll M, Hadam S, Gao Q, Hackbarth S, Haag SF, Graf C, Rühl E, Blume-Peytavi U, Lademann J, Vogt A, Meinke MC: Ultraviolet radiation and nanoparticle induced intracellular free radicals generation measured in human keratinocytes by electron paramagnetic resonance spectroscopy. Skin Res Technol 2014;20: 182–193.

6 Decher G, Hong JD, Schmitt J: Buildup of ultrathin multilayer films. Thin Solid Films 1992;210:831–835.

7 Donath E, Sukhorukov GB, Caruso F, Davis SA, Möhwald H: Novel hollow polymer shells by colloid-templated assembly of polyelectrolytes. Angew Chem Int Ed 1998;41:4019–4022.

8 Peyratout C, Dähne L: Tailor-made polyelectrolyte microcapsules: from multilayers to smart containers. Angew Chem Int Ed 2004;43:3762–3783.

9 Mercato LL, Rivera-Gil P, Abbasi AZ, Ochs M, Ganas C, Zins I, Sönnichsen C, Parak WJ: LbL multilayer capsules: recent progress and future outlook for their use in life sciences. Nanoscale 2010;2:458–467.

10 http://www.silver-colloids.com/Tutorials/Intro/pcs1.html (accessed 2001–2012).

11 Prietl B, Meindl C, Roblegg E, Pieber TR, Lanzer G, Fröhlich E: Nano-sized and micro-sized polystyrene particles affect phagocyte function. Cell Biol Toxicol 2014;30:1–16.

12 Jang WS, Rawson I, Grunlan JC: Layer-by-layer assembly of thin film oxygen barrier. Thin Solid Films 2008;516: 4819–4825.

Lars Dähne
Surflay Nanotec GmbH
Max-Planck-Strasse 3
DE–12489 Berlin (Germany)
E-Mail L.daehne@surflay.com

Serup J, Kluger N, Bäumler W (eds): Tattooed Skin and Health.
Curr Probl Dermatol. Basel, Karger, 2015, vol 48, pp 136–141 (DOI: 10.1159/000369647)

Chemical Purity and Toxicology of Pigments Used in Tattoo Inks

Henrik Petersen · Dirk Lewe

MT.DERM GmbH, Berlin, Germany

Abstract

The safety of tattoo inks has obviously increased in Europe since the existence of European Union Resolution ResAP(2008)1, which resulted in the improved quality control of pigment raw materials due to the definition of impurity limits that manufacturers can refer to. High-performance pigments are mostly used in tattoo inks, and these pigments are supposed to be chemically inert and offer high light fastness and low migration in solvents. However, these pigments were not developed or produced for applications involving long-term stay in the dermis or contact with bodily fluids. Therefore, these pigments often do not comply with the purity limits of the resolution; however, it is required that every distributed tattoo ink does not contain aromatic amines and not exceed the limits of heavy metals or polycyclic aromatic hydrocarbons. Current toxicity studies of pigments underline that no ecotoxicological threat to human health or to the environment should be expected. However, the pigment as well as its impurities and coating materials must be considered. In order to evaluate the safety of pigments according to their impurities, two different validated sample preparation methods are necessary: (1) simulation of their long-term stay in the bodily fluid of the dermis and (2) simulation of cleavage due to laser removal or ultraviolet exposure. The development of standardized, validated and well-adapted methods for this application has to be part of prospective efforts. Concerning legislation, it might be appropriate that the first regulative approaches be based on those of cosmetics.

© 2015 S. Karger AG, Basel

Introduction

Tattooing of humans has a long history and was independently developed in different areas of the world. In the early beginning, tattooing was often used for spiritual signs or for martial reasons, but currently, it is used more as body art to create individual appearance or to demonstrate the belonging to specific groups. In Germany, 10% of the population is tattooed, and because of its rising popularity, it can be expected that this number will increase within the next years. The results of surveys of a group of tattooed people pointed out that 67.5% of the people suffered skin problems like itching, burning or redness and that 6.6% reported persistent symptoms, skin papules or granuloma [1]. During studies on a red pigment, it was shown that up to 9.42 mg/cm^2 of pigment, 2.53 mg/cm^2 on average, is applied into the skin, depending on the technique and experience of the tattooist [2, 3]. In the early stages, people dispersed carbon black from campfires or pigments from other natural sources into water in order to get a pigment paste. With industrialization in the 19th century, companies started to synthesize pigments and to produce tons of raw materials to be used by the growing industries for applications like automotive coatings and interior or exterior paints. The development of new pigments for the special demands of several industrial applications is the reason for the current presence of a huge variety of different chemical structures and modifications. Therefore, pigment manufacturers sometimes offer the same pigment class for more than one application (plastics, coatings, printing, textiles). Some pigments that are in accordance with the European Union (EU) Regulation on cosmetics are also available. However because the tattoo business is small and not profitable compared to other industries, like cosmetics or industrial coatings, the pigment manufacturer doesn't make any efforts to develop and produce any specific pigments for this application. Obviously, these pigments often do not comply with the purity limits for heavy metals, harmful aromatic amines and others that are prescribed in the EU resolution ResAP(2008)1 on tattoo inks because the pigments are produced for other applications, where higher limits are tolerated. This is why tattoo ink manufacturers have to carefully choose their supplier and conduct accurate and repeating quality control on the purchased pigments. Authorities' interests in the safety of tattoo inks have increased in the past few years, and there are ongoing discussions about how the safety of pigments can be accurately evaluated. This article will give an overview about the pigments used in tattoo inks and the problems that manufacturers are facing because of the impurities and regulatory situation. This article will also give insight into quality control from the manufacturer's point of view.

Overview of Used Pigments

The selection of pigments in tattoo or permanent make-up (PMU) ink can differ because of the demand for more natural colors in PMU, but for more bright and shiny colors for tattoo inks. Generally, pigments in water-based inks have to offer high light fastness and stability against bleeding due to the permanent stay of the inks in the dermis because migration of particles in the skin or ultraviolet-induced cleavage of pigments has to be avoided. In table 1, a list of pigments that are often used in tattoo and PMU inks is shown.

Mostly, the pigments belong to the group of high performance pigments, which are supposed to be chemically inert and are distinguished with high light fastness, weather stability and low-migration properties in solvents. These properties make these pigments adequate for tattoo inks because they achieve long-lasting colors in the skin.

Current Regulatory Situation in the European Union

The first EU Resolution ResAP(2003)2 dealing with tattoo and PMU products was launched in 2003 and was replaced by the actual EU Resolution ResAP(2008)1 in 2008. Resolution ResAP(2008)1 is the most detailed regulatory document to point out requirements and criteria for the safety of tattoos and PMU. This resolution is a recommendation and has to be transferred into local law, but up to now, just a few EU countries have done so. All other countries do not entirely or adequately regulate this kind of application or the used products. Manufacturers should be encouraged to make data like the composition and the toxicological data of the substances of their product available to the competent authorities [4]. This resolution also lists the aromatic amines that should not be present in tattoos and PMU products because of their potentially harmful carcinogenic, mutagenic, reprotoxic and sensitizing properties. Some examples of

Table 1. A choice of pigments in tattoo and PMU inks [11]

Color	Name	C.I.	Chemical class	Industrial applications
	Pigment Blue 15	74160	Phthalocyanine	printing, plastics, textiles
	Pigment Green 36	74265	Phthalocyanine	automotive coatings
	Pigment Red 177	65300	Anthraquinone	plastics, automotive coatings
	Pigment Red 202	73907	Chinacridone	coatings, printing
	Pigment Red 254	56110	Diketopyrrolopyrrole	automotive coatings
	Pigment Red 22	12315	Naphthol AS	printing, textiles
	Pigment Red 210	12477	Naphthol AS	printing
	Pigment Red 101	77491	Iron oxide (Fe_2O_3)	food, cosmetics
	Pigment Orange 73	561170	Diketopyrrolopyrrole	coatings
	Pigment Orange 13	21110	Diazopyrazolone	plastics
	Pigment Yellow 138	56300	Chinophthalone	coatings, plastics
	Pigment Yellow 42	77492	Iron oxide (FeO(OH))	food, cosmetics
	Pigment Yellow 65	11740	Single Azo Yellow	coatings
	Pigment Yellow 55	21096	Double Azo Yellow	printing
	Pigment Violet 37	51345	Dioxazine	printing, coating
	Pigment Violet 12	58050	Anthraquinone	coatings
	Pigment Black 7	77266	Carbon Black	plastics, coatings, cosmetics
	Pigment Black 11	77499	Iron oxide (Fe_3O_4)	food, cosmetics
	Pigment White 6	77891	Titanium Dioxide	cosmetics, coatings

Table 2. Overview of the limits and methods for detection according to ResAP(2008)1

Element or compound	Limit, ppm	Detection method
Aromatic amines	absence	eGC-MS/LC-MS after extraction in phosphate buffer or HCl [4]
PAH	0.5	no method described
Benzene-a-pyrene	5	no method described
As, Se, Sb, Pb	2	no method described
Ba, Sn, Zn	50	no method described
Co, Cu (soluble)	25	no method described
Cd, Cr (IV), Hg	0.2	no method described
Ni	as low as technically achievable	no method described

aromatic amines that are not allowed in tattoo and PMU products are benzidine, 4-chloroaniline, 6-methoxy-m-toluidine or 2-naphthylamine. In addition, a negative list, or list of forbidden colorants, is also included in this resolution. The limit for polycyclic aromatic hydrocarbons (PAHs) is set at 0.5 ppm, and the limit for benzene-a-pyrene is 5 ppb. Table 2 shows an overview of the limits for aromatic amines, PAHs and heavy metals.

Table 2 also shows that the current resolution is obviously still not sufficient to accurately maintain the toxicological safety of pigments in tattoo and PMU products. For nickel, no specific limits exist, and it is not clear what 'technically achievable limit' really means. Furthermore, an analysis method has only been suggested for the detection of aromatic amines. For PAHs or heavy metals, how to analyze the pigments, so that their safety can be evaluated correctly, has not been recommended, yet. Confusion and misunderstandings between manufacturers and authorities happens, if both are analyzing the products in different ways, because this leads to different results which cannot be compared. In the future, it will be necessary to harmonize the analytical methods for tattoo and PMU products and their related limits; otherwise, it will be impossible for manufacturers to perform and maintain suitable quality controls.

Impurities and Toxicological Aspects

Recent toxicological analysis of high performance pigments found that there is no expected ecotoxicological threat to human health and the environment [5]. These pigments are usually inert and insoluble, which results in minimal ecotoxicological properties. However, the permanent contact of the pigments with human cells or their effects on cells due to cleavage were never considered in any study. Therefore, the several toxicological assessments that have been performed on pigments don't reflect the real environment that they are placed in and are not sufficient to evaluate the toxicological properties of the pigments for long-term stay in the skin. Actually, nearly every existing legislation have referred to the use of possible ingredients in cosmetics; however, none of the substances are intended to be implanted into the skin, especially for years or decades. Furthermore, none of the substances are intended to be spread systemically, as it is known that pigments not only remain in the area where the tattoo has been applied, but are also transported to nearby lymph nodes [6] through the lymphatic system. Therefore, pigments can remain in the region of the tattoo or may travel relatively long distances through our body, as shown in a study published in 2009 [7]. This is why pigment manufacturers have to minimize or remove all unwelcome impurities or by-products in pigments [5]. It was reported that carbon black ink can contain up to 716.94 µg/g of harmful impurities like benzophenone, hexamethylenetetramine or hexachlorobutadiene, which are known to be genotoxic and carcinogenic [8]. These impurities were found after extraction with benzene/acetone using gas chromatography-mass spectrometry analysis. This shows that these compounds can adsorb onto the carbon black pigment surface and can't be determined if the extraction is carried out in a hydrophilic medium [8]. Carbon black is not suspected to cause allergic or irritant skin reactions, but reported cases of tattoos with black ink can potentially be connected to these impurities [1]. Whether the reported toxicological reactions are caused by the pigment itself or by side products has to be investigated. Common cytotoxicity tests analyze extracts and are therefore not suitable for insoluble particles. There is currently no available alternative, validated method to determine the harmful effects caused by applied pigments. Solubilizing pigment particles is also an arguable way to analyze pigments because this would transform an inert and nonbioavailable substance into a bioavailable dyestuff, but this does not represent the reality and can produce 'false-positive' test results [5]. It is mandatory that a standardized and validated method for the safety assessment of tattoo pigments will be available to evaluate the cytotoxicity of pigments according to their long-term stay in the dermis. Heavy metal impurities are often found, especially in inorganic pigments. Jacobsen et al. [9] evaluated the acute or systemic toxicity of heavy metals in tattoo inks in the human body. It is well known that nickel and chromium can cause sensitization issues, but the opinion of the authors is that these elements seem to have less impact on sensitization issues based on allergy test results. Sensitization can also be caused by aromatic amines. Additionally, other heavy metals, like aluminum, can cause granulomas, and barium impacts the cardiovascular system.

Beside the assessment of pigments and their well-known impurities, it is also important to consider that almost every pigment manufacturer uses surface treatments in order to improve the dispersibility or achieve other specific properties of pigments [10]. Inorganic treatments (precipitation of aluminum silicates) of titanium dioxide, for example, can also decrease the photoactivity of the pigment, which is important for tattoo pigments because this reactivity is suspected to induce skin reactions after sun exposure. Another possibility for modifying the surface of pigments is to use organic compounds and to achieve precipitation by spraying combined with intensive milling. Typical compounds for organic surface treatments are polyethylenoxide, Tinuvin® 1130, dioctylphtalate, 3-isobutoxypropylamine or polydimethylsiloxane. Most tattoo ink producers don't know about the surface treatments of their pigments because pigment manufacturers are often not cooperative in exchanging this information. In conclusion, no ink producer is able to evaluate whether there are any potentially harmful impurities in their pigments, and the bioavailability of these coatings during long-term stay in the dermis and their contact with human fluids is unknown. It is possible that these impurities can cause serious reactions, like allergies or granulomas [9]. Toxicity studies of pigments in tattoo inks should consider the pure pigment itself as well as the impurities in the pigments and coatings. However, pure pigments are currently unavailable and are only achievable with high effort and cost [2].

Quality Control of Pigments in the Manufacturing of Tattoo Inks

Because pigments are produced for different applications (table 1), a tattoo ink manufacturer can't act on the assumption that the purchased pigment fulfills all limits prescribed in ResAP(2008) (table 2). Therefore, every new batch of pigment has to go through strict quality controls.

Almost every ink producer does not have the capacity to perform quality control analysis in-

house, so contract analysis is common in this industry. For the determination of aromatic amines, heavy metals and PAHs, the pigment sample is extracted in a buffered solution of 0.1 HCl for 2 h, like is prescribed for the analysis of impurities in textiles [2]. Hence, only extractable impurities can be determined. Subsequently, aromatic amines and PAHs can be determined using gas chromatography-mass spectrometry or liquid chromatography-mass spectrometry, and heavy metals can be determined using inductively coupled plasma-mass spectrometry. Microwave extraction in strong acids is not carried out because this simulates the complete destruction of the pigment, which usually does not happen in the skin. Laser treatment can cleave the pigment into smaller particles, which can release a higher amount of impurities. However, microwave extraction is not comparable to laser treatment because it completely solubilizes the pigment, which doesn't happen during laser treatment. In order to evaluate the safety of pigments according to the impurities, it might be necessary to have two different validated sample preparation methods: (1) simulation of their long-term stay in the bodily fluid of the dermis and (2) simulation of cleavage due to laser removal or ultraviolet exposure. This could help to evaluate the safety of pigments and make the maintenance of their safety during production easier.

Conclusion

Since the EU Resolution on tattoo inks was released, the safety of these products has increased measurably due to the improved quality control of pigment raw materials in ink production and the defined impurity limits that manufacturers are able to refer to. This can be demonstrated by comparing the randomized tests of tattoo inks in Switzerland before and after the adoption of this resolution [8]. However, there are still several tattoo inks on the market that contain forbidden pigments or high levels of impurities. In the past 2 years, the industry has faced problems due to differences between their methods of quality control and those of the authorities. These problems were caused by missing descriptions of the methods that should be used to quantify the impurities in tattoo pigments. High-performance pigments are mostly used in tattoo inks and are very stable and chemically inert. It can be assumed that specific skin reactions after tattooing can often be the result of harmful impurities. However, the needles of tattoo devices should also be investigated because they could be a source of harmful substances, nonsterile particles or microbiological contamination, thus potentially causing serious skin reactions. The development of standardized, validated and well-adapted methods for this application has to be part of prospective efforts. In addition to this, it seems to be important to consider other harmful substances that can be present due to special pigment coatings. Most pigments that are used in tattoo inks were basically developed for other applications, like automotive coatings or plastics, and these pigments are often surface treated in this industry. Only a few pigments that are cosmetic grade are available, but none of these pigments can be purchased in pharmaceutical grade. Even a pharmaceutical-grade pigment might not be sufficient, as these pigments are not intended to be present in the skin and lymph nodes for decades. This underlines that the safety assessment of tattoo pigments has to take into account that the raw materials for these products are often technical grade. Unfortunately, this won't change in the future because tattoo inks belong to a niche market, and no pigment producer will concentrate on this business because it is not profitable enough. Concerning legislation, it might be appropriate that the first regulative approaches are based on those of cosmetics because this would be an improvement to the market, and because cosmetics and tattooing seem to be related applications. But in fact (nearly) none of these raw materials have been tested for intradermal applications and long-term exposure in the human body. Therefore, completely different risk assessments and different approaches are needed to determine their safety for that special kind of use.

References

1 Lehner K: Analysis of Black Tattoo Inks; dissertation, University of Regensburg, Regensburg, Germany, 2012.
2 BFR – German Federal Institute for Risk Assessment: Anforderungen für eine Sicherheitsbewertung von Tätowiermitteln, 2009.
3 Engel E: Tattoo Pigments in Skin; dissertation, University of Regensburg, Regensburg, Germany, 2007, pp 27–30.
4 Council of Europe, Committee of Ministers: Resolution ResAP(2008)1 on requirements and criteria for the safety of tattoos and permanent make-up. Council of Europe, 2008.
5 Faulkner E, Schwartz RJ: High Performance Pigments. Weinheim, Wiley-VCH, 2009.
6 Gopee NV, Cui Y, Olson G, Warbritton AR, Miller BJ, Couch LH, Wamer WG, Howard PC: Response of mouse skin to tattooing. Toxicol Appl Pharmacol. 2005;209:145–158.
7 Kürle S, Schulte KW, Homey B: Accumulation of tattoo pigment in sentinel lymph nodes. Hautarzt 2009;60:781–783.
8 Hauri U: Pigments, preservatives and impurities in tattoo inks (presentation). First International Conference on Tattoo Safety, BFR-Symposium, Berlin, June 2013.
9 Jacobsen E, et al: Chemical Substances in Tattoo Ink. Danmark, Miljøstyrelsen, 2012.
10 Winkler J: Dispergieren von Pigmenten und Füllstoffen, Farbe und Lack ed. Hannover, Vincentz Network, 2010.
11 Cuyper C, Pérez-Cotapos M-L: Dermatologic Complications with Body Art. Berlin, Springer, 2010.

Dr. Henrik Petersen
MT.DERM GmbH
Gustav-Krone-Strasse 3
DE–14167 Berlin (Germany)
E-Mail h.petersen@mtderm.de

Serup J, Kluger N, Bäumler W (eds): Tattooed Skin and Health.
Curr Probl Dermatol. Basel, Karger, 2015, vol 48, pp 142–151 (DOI: 10.1159/000369197)

Survey on European Studies of the Chemical Characterisation of Tattoo Ink Products and the Measurement of Potentially Harmful Ingredients

Manuela Agnello · Marco Fontana

ARPA Piemonte, Regional Agency of Environmental Protection, Igiene Industriale, Grugliasco, Italy

Abstract

The results of the detection of carcinogenic aromatic amines in about 300 ink samples are discussed. All analysed inks contained at least one or more azo compound pigments, and the presence of aromatic amines could only have originated from these compounds through a chemical process named 'reductive cleavage'. Sometimes, aromatic amines were also present as impurities derived from the processing of the pigments. A systematic surveillance programme in Italy, promoted by the Italian Ministry of Health with the involvement of Italian regions, local public health authorities and Agenzia Regionale per la Protezione Ambiente del Piemonte (Environmental Protection Agency), has shown that about 40% of the monitored inks are not regular according to European Resolution ResAP(2008):1. The method utilised for the detection of aromatic amines has allowed the identification of other substances that are not carcinogenic but are toxic or have sensitisation properties that are derived from reductive cleavage or that are present as impurities.

© 2015 S. Karger AG, Basel

Introduction

Since the end of the 1990s, the tattoo fashion has spread widely all over the world. Due to this growth and the lack of information about the substances contained in tattoo inks, in 2006, Regione Piemonte, with the cooperation of Agenzia Regionale per la Protezione Ambiente del Piemonte (ARPA Piemonte), which is an Environmental Protection Agency, and some local public health authorities, promoted a programme for the surveillance of chemicals to ensure the safety of tattoos and permanent make-up.

Local public health authorities and ARPA Piemonte defined a protocol for the inspection of tattoo parlours in Piemonte and included sampling criteria for the products used for tattooing. After a monitoring period, this team found out that the information available for the ingredients contained in tattoo inks was very poor and confusing. A significant number of safety data sheets or technical data sheets that were available at the monitored tattoo parlours were not updated with the current Italian legislations or did not correspond to the products present in the parlours. Analytical studies performed on 30 samples of tattoo inks in 2006–2007 showed that about 40% of the samples were not regular according to European resolution ResAP(2003):2 [1] on tattoos and permanent make-up.

Due to these analytical results, the Italian Ministry of Health has promoted Regione, a national, systematic surveillance programme that samples tattoo inks, since 2009. Surveillance is also conducted by other authorities, such as Nucleo Anti Sofisticazioni – Carabinieri Force, custom agencies and local public health authorities. The analysis of samples is performed by a network of laboratories comprising the Istituto Superiore di Sanità (National Institute of Health) and specialised regional public laboratories according to different analytical methods and chemical matrices.

The legislative instrument utilised in Italy is EU Directive 2001/95/CEE [2], with application of the update for consumer protection (D. Lgs 'Codice del Consumo') n°206 of 2005. This legislation guarantees the safety of all products placed in the Italian market and allows for the application of Resolution ResAP(2008):1 [1] (which supersedes Resolution ResAP(2003):2 on tattoos and permanent make-up) and the development of a surveillance system coordinated by the Ministry of Health. In addition, the Registration, Evaluation, Authorisation and Restriction of Chemicals regulation n°1907/2006 and the Classification, Labelling and Packaging regulation n°1272/2008 provide some restrictions for dangerous substances as well as specific rules for the classification and labelling of substances, mixtures and articles.

The notification system Rapid Information System for Non-food Products is the instrument used in the EU for sharing information about the irregularity of products among local authorities, consumers, producers and users. This system is currently used in Italy.

Ink Characterisation

Tattoo inks consist of pigments combined with a carrier.

Tattoo inks are available in a range of colours that can be thinned or mixed to produce other colours and shades. Most professional tattoo artists purchase pre-made inks (known as pre-dispersed inks), while some tattooists mix their own ink using a dry pigment and a carrier.

Pigments are chemically derived from three main groups of vegetal, inorganic or organic origin.

Vegetal pigments are often derived from root plants or logwood, which is a heartwood extract from 'Haematoxylon campechisnum' that is found in Central America and the West Indies. The most-used black inks are made of Carbon Black (CI 77266), but it is sometimes possible to find black inks made of dried vegetal algae dispersed in a carrier.

Inorganic pigments are made from minerals such as magnetite (Fe_3O_4 or FeO) and are often associated with brown and dark colours. Cinnabar (HgS) is used for red colours, and other kinds of inorganic compounds, such as various metal oxides or sulphides, are used for a wide range of colours. Titanium oxides (TiO_2) are commonly used as white pigments.

The organic pigments are the most variable group and include some different chemical classes that are dependent on characteristic functional groups:

- Nitro dye, associated with yellow colours.
- Xanthenic dye, associated with various colours, mainly various shades of yellow.
- Phtalocyanine compounds, associated with blue and green colours.
- Antraquinone dyes, associated with red and brown colours.
- Mono-azo and di-azo dyes, commonly known as azo dyes. These pigments are used for various colours such as yellow, red or orange.

The colorants (both dyes and pigments) are listed by their colour index numbers. The colour

Table 1. Colour index numbers

Structure	Colour index range
Nitroso	10000–10299
Nitro	10300–10999
Monoazo	11000–19999
Diazo	20000–39999
Stilbene	40000–41999
Diarylmethane	41000–41999
Triarylmethane	42000–44999
Xanthene	45000–45999
Acridine	46000–46999
Quinoline	47000–47999
Methine	48000–48999
Thiazole	49000–49399
Indamine	49400–49699
Indophenol	49700–49999
Azine	50000–50999
Oxazine	51000–51999
Thiazine	52000–52999
Aminoketone	56000–56999
Anthraquinone	57000–72999
Indigoid	73000–73999
Phtalocyanine	74000–74999
Natural dyes	75000–76999
Inorganic pigments	77000–77999

index numbers are grouped into ranges according to their chemical structure, as shown in table 1.

Aromatic Amines in Azo Dyes

Azo compounds are by far the most widely used synthetic organic colorants. The colour index lists more than 2,000 azo compounds. Azo dyes are generally synthesised starting from primary aromatic amines that are diazotisated and coupled with phenols or secondary aromatic amines. In fact, the main chromophore group of the azo compounds is the diarylazo group (Ar-N = N-Ar'), which is derived from simpler molecules known as aromatic amines.

Commercial products often contain high levels of other components that are especially relevant from a toxicological point of view: the aromatic amines, which are chemically characterised by a NH_2 group and are often found in inks as contaminants or reduction (cleavage) products.

According to some studies [3–6], aromatic amines can be formed by the reductive cleavage of azo compounds by human enzymes over a varying range of time beginning from the introduction of the pigments under the skin. Figure 1 shows a hypothetical example: pigment red 5 could be cleaved into three aromatic amines, two of which, p-cresidine and o-toluidine, are carcinogenic.

The chemical analysis discussed in this work focuses on inks containing at least one azo compound and on the determination of certain carcinogenic aromatic amines that could derived from pigment decomposition by means of reductive cleavage.

The aromatic amines that were detected, with their classifications assigned according to regulations by Classification, Labelling and Packaging [7] and other institutions, such as the International Agency for Research on Cancer and the American Conference of Governmental Industrial Hygienists [8, 9], are listed in table 2.

According to Resolution ReSAP(2008):1, these aromatic amines '...*particularly with regard to their carcinogenic, mutagenic, reprotoxic and sensitising properties, ...should neither be present in tattoos and PMU products nor released from azocolorants*'.

The limit of quantification of the method used for the determination of the aromatic amines is 1 mg/kg for each substance listed in table 2. Traces of aromatic amines below this limit of quantification are not considered.

Methodology

The chemical analysis carried out by Arpa Piemonte mainly focused on synthetic pigments specially derived from azo compounds. About

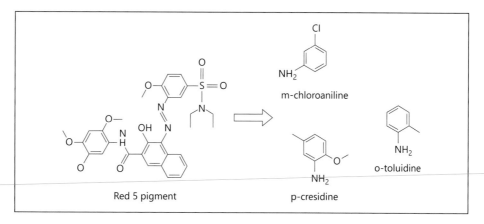

Fig. 1. Cleavage reduction of red 5.

Table 2. List of detected aromatic amines

Substances [CAS number]	Carcinogenic classifications		
	IARC	ACGIH	CLP
o-Toluidine [95–53–4]	2A	A3	Carc. 1B – H350
o-Anisidine [90–04–0]	2B	A3	Carc. 1B – H350
4-Chloroaniline [106–47–8]	2B	–	Carc. 1B – H350
6-Methoxy-m-toluidine [120–71–8]	2B	–	Carc. 1B – H350
2,4,5-Trimethylaniline [137–17–7]	3	–	Carc. 1B – H350
4-Chloro-o-toluidine [95–69–2]	2A	–	Carc. 1B – H350
			Muta. 2 – H341
4-Methyl-m-phenylenediamine [95–80–7]	2B	–	Carc. 1B – H350
			Muta. 2 – H341
			Repr. 2 – H361f
4-Methoxy-m-phenylenediamine [615–05–4]	2B	–	Carc. 1B – H350
			Muta. 2 – H341
2-Naphthylamine [91–59–8]	1	A1	Carc. 1B – H350
Biphenyl-4-ylamine [92–67–1]	1	A1	Carc. 1B – H350
4,4'-Oxydianiline [101–80–4]	2B	–	Carc. 1B – H350
			Muta. 2 – H341
			Repr. 2 – H361f
Benzidine [92–87–5]	1	A1	Carc. 1B – H350
4,4'-Methylenedianiline [101–77–9]	2B	A3	Carc. 1B – H350
			Muta. 2 – H341
4,4'-Methylenedi-o-toluidine [838–88–0]	2B	–	Carc. 1B – H350
3,3'-Dimethylbenzidine [119–93–7]	2B	A3	Carc. 1B – H350
4,4'-Thiodianiline [139–65–1]	2B	–	Carc. 1B – H350
3,3'-Dichlorobenzidine [91–94–1]	2B	A3	Carc. 1B – H350
4,4'-Methylenebis(2-chloroaniline) [101–14–4]	2A	A2	Carc. 1B – H350
3,3'-Dimethoxybenzidine [119–90–4]	2B	–	Carc. 1B – H350
5-Nitro-o-toluidine [99–55–8]	3	A3	Carc. 1B – H351
o-Aminoazotoluene [97–56–3]	2B	–	Carc. 1B – H351
4-Aminoazobenzene [60–09–3]	2B	–	Carc. 1B – H351

Table 3. Comparison of two methods

Inks	O-anisidine with ISO 17234 mg/kg	O-anisidine with ISO 14362 mg/kg
Yellow 1	318	46
Yellow 2	177	11
Yellow 3	242	78
Yellow 4	113	18
Yellow 5	69	32

300 ink samples of various colours were analysed for the determination of aromatic amines.

The analytical method was derived from EN ISO 17234 [10], which is normally used for the determination of aromatic amines in leather samples. The method consists of three stages:

(1) Chemical reduction of pigments with sodium dithionite as a reduction agent.

(2) Extraction of aromatic amines that could be formed by sodium dithionite by means of methyl tert butyl ether.

(3) Quantitative analysis by gas chromatography followed by mass spectrometry.

The method used for leather samples was adapted to ink samples and then compared to the method described in ResAP, which was derived from the determination of aromatic amines in textiles (ISO 14362 – Textiles. Methods for the determination of certain aromatic amines derived from azo colorants. Detection of certain azo colorants that are accessible with and without extracting the fibres) [11].

These two methods are rather similar, except for the first step, the pigment reduction. The concentration of sodium dithionite in ISO 17234 is about 200 mg/ml; 3 ml of this solution is added to the samples, and the samples are pre-heated for 20 min at 70°C in 17 ml of citrate buffer at pH 6 for other 20 min.

In the model method derived from ISO 14362, 5 ml of dithionite solution (5%) in phosphate buffer is added to the sample. Then, the reduction continues at 70°C for 90 min.

The leather method is more effective when compared to this method, but its application is in agreement with the directives of the Ministry of Heath, which are based on a 'precaution principle'.

Table 3 shows the concentrations of o-anisidine in a group of samples, compared to the above-described methods. The classification of these samples does not conform to Resolution ResAP(2008):1 when both methods are considered.

Data Evaluation

The analytical results of the detection of carcinogenic aromatic amines in about 300 samples showed the presence of carcinogenic compounds in more than 40% of the inks that were considered [12].

Higher irregularities were found in yellow and red colours and related shades, such as orange, flesh and green (green colour is sometimes derived from blue pigment mixed with yellow pigment).

The aromatic amines that were frequently determined were o-toluidine, which was found in 24 samples; o-anisidine, which was found in 64 samples; 4-chloroaniline (also known as p-chloroaniline), which was found in 5 samples; 3,3'-dichlorobenzidine, which was found in 6 samples; 5-nitro-o-toluidine (also known as 2-methyl-5-nitroaniline), which was found in 5 samples; and 4-methyl-m-phenylenediamine (also known as 2,4-diaminotoluene), which was found in 4 samples. Often, the reduction split the pigments into more than one aromatic amine; therefore, two or more aromatic amines were detected in a significant number of irregular samples. In a red sample, 5 different carcinogenic aromatic amines were found.

The aromatic amines that were most frequently detected were o-toluidine, which is generally related to red colours, and o-anisidine, which is generally related to yellow colours.

The amounts of the aromatic amines that were found were quite variable, and a graphical representation is shown in figure 2.

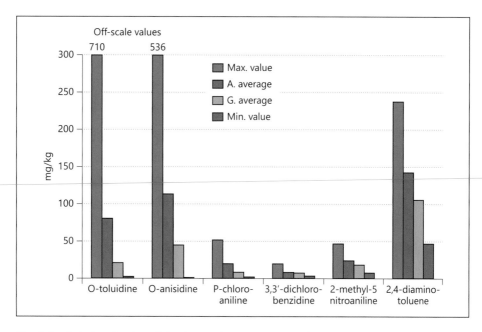

Fig. 2. Statistical evaluation of the detected concentrations of aromatic amines.

A very large number of irregular samples contained a considerable amount of aromatic amines, and in about 44% of the irregular samples, these quantities exceeded 100 mg/kg (see fig. 3). The highest concentration was found in a shade of red: up to 700 mg/kg of o-toluidine. Furthermore, a shade of yellow had about 550 mg/kg of o-anisidine (see fig. 2).

Despite the strong reduction of the azo compound pigments, a significant percentage didn't show the presence of carcinogenic aromatic amines. This fact shows that it is possible to produce safe inks containing azo compound pigments.

Considerations

Our results led us to affirm that the determination of aromatic amines mostly depends on the specific lot number. In fact, some inks of the same brand and colour showed different results.

Table 4 shows some examples: the green, orange and yellow inks that were analysed could be either regular or irregular, based on the lot number.

The origin of the pigments is probably the key. Even though producers always use chemically equal pigments during the production of the various ink lots, the country of origin and the quality of the pigments could differ from one to the other.

One more test was carried out on two equal orange samples that had the same lot number. The analysis showed different results: one sample was regular, and the other one wasn't (see table 4, first row).

When investigating this peculiar case, the irregular sample that had a remarkable amount of o-toluidine was identified as a fake. The label was counterfeit and didn't correspond to the real product. It had been falsified. This situation represents a further danger in the production of tattoo inks and in the safety of customers.

Moreover, qualitative screening performed with the same method used for the determination

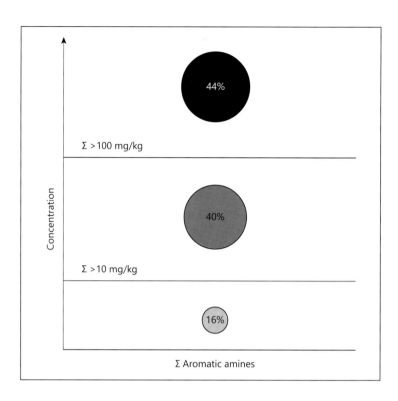

Fig. 3. Distribution of amounts of aromatic amines in different ranges of concentrations.

Table 4. Conformity by lot number

Orange ink – Brand A (Lot N° ABXXX10) Irregular 3,3'-dichlorobenzidine	Orange ink – Brand A (Lot N° ABXXX09) Irregular O-toluidine	Orange ink – Brand A (Lot N° ABXXX09) Regular
Green ink – Brand B (Lot N° CDXXX42) Irregular O-toluidine, O-anisidine	Green ink – Brand B (Lot N° CEXXX04) Regular	
Yellow ink – Brand C (Lot N° FGXXX88) Irregular O-anisidne	Yellow ink – Brand C (no lot number) Regular	

of carcinogenic aromatic amines revealed that other compounds, including aromatic amines that were not carcinogenic but were toxic (see table 5), were found in about 30% of the samples, both regular and irregular.

Future Developments

The evaluation of risks associated with the use of inks for tattoos carried out in recent years has allowed a frequent exchange of experiences at the Italian and European levels.

Agnello · Fontana

Table 5. H phrases about chemical substances found in the qualitative analyses

Substances [CAS number]	H phrases and notes from the American Conference of Governmental and Industrial Hygienists and the International Agency for Research on Cancer
Aniline [62–53–3]	H351 Suspected of causing cancer H341 Suspected of causing genetic defects H331 Toxic if inhaled H311 Toxic when in contact with skin H301 Toxic if swallowed H372 Causes damage to organs through prolonged or repeated exposure H318 Causes serious eye damage H317 May cause an allergic skin reaction H400 Very toxic to aquatic life ACGIH: Skin, A3
2-Ethoxyaniline [94–70–2]	H331 Toxic if inhaled H311 Toxic when in contact with skin H301 Toxic if swallowed H372 Causes damage to organs through prolonged or repeated exposure
3,4-Dichlorobenzenamine [95–76–1]	H331 Toxic if inhaled H311 Toxic when in contact with skin H301 Toxic if swallowed H317 May cause an allergic skin reaction H318 Causes serious eye damage H400 Very toxic to aquatic life H410 Very toxic to aquatic life with long-lasting effects
4-Ethoxyaniline [156–43–4]	H341 Suspected of causing genetic defects H322 May be harmful if inhaled H312 Harmful when in contact with skin H302 Harmful if swallowed H319 Causes serious eye irritation H317 May cause an allergic skin reaction
N-Isopropyl-N'-phenyl-p-phenylendiamine (IPPD) [101–72–4]	H302 Harmful if swallowed H317 May cause an allergic skin reaction H400 Very toxic to aquatic life H410 Very toxic to aquatic life with long-lasting effects
Styrene [100–42–5]	H226 Flammable liquid and vapour H332 May be harmful if inhaled H319 Causes serious eye irritation H315 Causes skin irritation IARC NOTE: 2B (possibly carcinogenic)
3-Butenylbenzene [768–56–9]	H315 Causes skin irritation H411 Toxic to aquatic life with long-lasting effects
Biphenyl [92–52–4]	H319 Causes serious eye irritation H335 May cause respiratory irritation H315 Causes skin irritation H400 Very toxic to aquatic life H410 Very toxic to aquatic life with long-lasting effects

Table 5. Continued

Substances [CAS number]	H phrases and notes from the American Conference of Governmental and Industrial Hygienists and the International Agency for Research on Cancer
Thymol [89–83–8]	H302 Harmful if swallowed H314 Causes severe skin burns and eye damage H411 Toxic to aquatic life with long-lasting effects
1,2-Dichlorobenzene [95–50–1]	H302 Harmful if swallowed H319 Causes serious eye irritation H335 May cause respiratory irritation H315 Causes skin irritation H400 Very toxic to aquatic life H410 Very toxic to aquatic life with long-lasting effects
3,4-Dichlorobenzene [95–76–1]	H331 Toxic if inhaled H311 Toxic in contact with skin H301 Toxic if swallowed H318 Causes serious eye damage H317 May cause an allergic skin reaction H400 Very toxic to aquatic life H410 Very toxic to aquatic life with long-lasting effects
2,4,5-Trichlorophenol [95–95–4]	H302 Harmful if swallowed H319 Causes serious eye irritation H315 Causes skin irritation H400 Very toxic to aquatic life H410 Very toxic to aquatic life with long-lasting effects
1-Naphthol [90–15–3]	H312 Harmful in contact with skin H302 Harmful if swallowed H335 May cause respiratory irritation H315 Causes skin irritation H318 Causes serious eye damage

The goals of these collaborative efforts between institutions and laboratories in different countries are the more effective coordination of supervisory actions as well as the adoption of criteria that are as homogeneous as possible.

The purpose of the European Society of Tattoo and Pigment Research, in collaboration with producers and tattoo parlours, is the sharing of methods and objectives for improving the safety of these products.

The activities planned in Italy in the next few years will be oriented according to the following main guidelines:

a. Proposal of a single method, which is in accordance with guidelines of the national authorities, for the determination of different hazardous substances, among which are first-stage aromatic amines, polycyclic aromatic hydrocarbons and heavy metals.

b. Consideration of the adoption of limits for the concentrations of the aromatic amines listed in ResAP.

c. The extension of measures to restrict the levels of other hazardous aromatic amines, as a consequence of their high percentage of occurrence in the analysed samples, such as for the example substances listed in table 5.

References

1 Council of Europe: Resolution ResAP(2008)1 on requirements and criteria for the safety of tattoos and permanent make-up (superseding Resolution ResAP(2003)2 on tattoos and permanent make-up), Adopted by the Committee of Ministers on 20 February 2008 at the 1018th meeting of the Ministers' Deputies.

2 European Commission: Directive 2001/95/EC of the European Parliament and of the Council of 3 December 2001 on General Product Safety.

3 Gregory AR: The carcinogenic potential of benzidine-based dyes. J Environ Pathol Toxicol Oncol 1984;5:243–259.

4 Kennelly JC, Hertzog PJ, Martin CN: The release of 4,4'-diaminobiphenyls from azodyes in the rat. Carcinogenesis 1982; 3:947–951.

5 Cerniglia CE, Freeman JP, Franklin W, Pack LD: Metabolism of azo dyes derived from benzidine, 3,3'-dimethylbenzidine, and 3,3'-dimethoxybenzidine to potentially carcinogenic aromatic amines by intestinal bacteria. Carcinogenesis 1982;3:1255–1260.

6 Dewan A, Jani JP, Patel JS, Gandhi DN, Variya MR, Ghodasara NB: Benzidine and its acetylated metabolites in the urine of workers exposed to Direct Black 38. Arch Environ Health 1988;43:269–272.

7 European Union: Regulation (EC) No 1272/2008 of the European Parliament and of the Council of 16 December 2008 on classification, labelling and packaging of substances and mixtures, amending and repealing Directives 67/548/EEC and 1999/45/EC, and amending Regulation (EC) No 1907/2006.

8 IARC Monographs Working Group on the Evaluation of Carcinogenic Risks to Humans: IARC Monographs on the Evaluation of Carcinogenic Risks to Humans: Volume 99: Some Aromatic Amines, Organic Dyes, and Related Exposures. Lyon, International Agency for Research on Cancer, 2010.

9 AGCIH – American Conference of Governmental Industrial Hygienists, www.acgih.org (accessed August 2012).

10 ISO: ISO 17234–1:2010: Leather – Chemical tests for the determination of certain azo colorants in dyed leathers – Part 1: Determination of certain aromatic amines derived from azo colorants. Geneva, ISO.

11 ISO: EN 14362–1:2012: Textiles – Methods for determination of certain aromatic amines derived from azo colorants – Part 1: Detection of the use of certain azo colorants accessible with and without extracting the fibres. Geneva, ISO.

12 Agnello M, Fontana M, Mulatero G: Aromatic amines in tattoo inks: surveillance activities in Italy, 1st European Congress of Tattoo and Pigment Research, Copenhagen, 2013.

Marco Fontana
ARPA Piemonte, Regional Agency of Environmental Protection, Igiene Industriale
Via Sabaudia, 164
IT–10095 Grugliasco (Italy)
E-Mail m.fontana@arpa.piemonte.it

Serup J, Kluger N, Bäumler W (eds): Tattooed Skin and Health.
Curr Probl Dermatol. Basel, Karger, 2015, vol 48, pp 152–157 (DOI: 10.1159/000369196)

Tattoo Inks: Legislation, Pigments, Metals and Chemical Analysis

Gerald Prior

CTL Bielefeld GmbH, Bielefeld, Germany

Abstract

Legal limits for chemical substances require that they are linked to clearly defined analytical methods. Present limits for certain chemicals in tattoo and permanent make-up inks do not mention analytical methods for the detection of metals, polycyclic aromatic hydrocarbons or forbidden colourants. There is, therefore, no established method for the determination of the quantities of these chemicals in tattoo and permanent make-up inks. Failing to provide an appropriate method may lead to unqualified and questionable results which often cause legal disputes that are ultimately resolved by a judge with regard to the method that should have been applied. Analytical methods are tuned to exactly what is to be found and what causes the health problems. They are extremely specific. Irrespective of which is the correct method for detecting metals in tattoo inks, the focus should be on the actual amounts of ink in the skin. CTL® has conducted experiments to determine these amounts and these experiments are crucial for toxicological evaluations and for setting legal limits. When setting legal limits, it is essential to also incorporate factors such as daily consumption, total uptake and frequency of use. A tattoo lasts for several decades; therefore, the limits that have been established for heavy metals used in drinking water or soap are not relevant. Drinking water is consumed on a daily basis and soap is used several times per week, while tattooing only occurs once.

© 2015 S. Karger AG, Basel

Introduction

CTL® Bielefeld GmbH is the leading commercial laboratory for the investigation of tattoo and permanent make-up (PMU) inks. This laboratory has been conducting tests in this field for over a decade and has customers based in locations ranging from Europe to the US, Asia and Australia. CTL® not only tests products but also helps manufacturers to improve quality and meet legislative requirements. The managing director of CTL®, Dr. Gerald Prior, has recently published a book [1] containing more in-depth details on many more issues than are mentioned here.

The key question when evaluating the potential risks of tattoo inks is how much ink is in the skin as a result of the tattooing. A test was conducted by CTL® using a marker in a tattoo ink. A tattoo was performed by a professional tattoo artist, which left an average amount of 0.4 mg/cm^2 of ink in the skin [1]. The size of the tattoo was 910 cm^2. These results can be used to determine the actual quantities of contaminants in the skin.

An example using the data from the above-mentioned experiment demonstrates basic calculations for determining ink amounts in skin. A product has been banned from the EU market because it contains 12.2 mg/kg of nickel (Germany, Rapex Reference 24 A12/1380/12). If the above-mentioned large tattoo of 910 cm^2 in size had been tattooed on the back of a person using this banned ink, they would have had a total of 0.0057 mg of nickel in their skin. The average content of nickel per cm^2 would have been 0.000006 mg. Whether it is reasonable to ban a tattoo ink containing 12.2 mg/kg of nickel is questionable.

The basis for the ban of inks are limits contained in two resolutions published by the Council of Europe (CoE), ResAP(2003)2 [2] and ResAP(2008)1 [3]. The limit defined for nickel is 'as low as technically achievable'. This value is not only dependent on the method used for the analysis but also on the product used. For certain pigments, values of zero can be achieved, but this is not true for all pigments. Iron oxide pigments always contain minor amounts of nickel as impurities. The nickel in these products is not soluble and therefore, it is unclear whether it causes allergic reactions.

Resolutions ResAP(2003)2 and ResAP(2008)1 of the CoE

The resolutions published by the CoE contain limits for contaminants, bans for several chemicals and instructions for labelling products. The most important requirement is that inks must not endanger the health or safety of persons or the environment. Further, inks must not contain carcinogenic, mutagenic or reproduction-toxic substances of categories 1, 2 and 3 as classified in the EU Directive 67/548/EEC. Limits have also been set for polycyclic aromatic hydrocarbons (PAHs) and metals. Certain aromatic amines that may be released from colourants and certain colourants themselves are forbidden.

Most interesting is the fact that the limits for metals in these resolutions are exceedingly lower than those for food colourants, according to the Directive 95/45/EEC. For example, the amount of chromium allowed in food colourants is 100 mg/kg, while for tattoo inks it is 0.2 mg/kg according to ResAP(2008)1. This means that food colourants may contain 500 times more chromium than tattoo ink. In addition, 25 times more cadmium is allowed in food colourants than in tattoo ink. The reasoning for the set limits for tattoo and PMU inks is hard to understand.

The resolutions of the CoE also do not mention any methods for the analysis of metals, PAHs or the forbidden colourants. This is a sincere drawback and is discussed later in detail.

Pigments

Pigments used in the tattoo and PMU industries are both organic and inorganic. Organic pigments are mainly synthetically made and contain carbon. Inorganic pigments are minerals that are also often found in nature. The main inorganic pigments are titanium dioxide, barium sulphate and iron oxides. Titanium dioxide and barium sulphate are used for white colours or to brighten darker shades. Iron oxides are used to achieve the colours red, brown and black and are often used for colours similar to the shade of the skin. These pigments are all insoluble in aqueous solutions and precipitate in the skin.

A major issue is the purity of the barium sulphate used. Impurities of soluble barium salts, e.g.

barium carbonate, can cause respiratory paralysis, cardiac arrest or death [4–6]. It is therefore of utmost importance that barium sulphate is analysed for soluble barium salts as described for medical (barium meal) or cosmetic products [7, 8]. Failing to do so may cause death. The severe problem arising from impure barium sulphate is not at all addressed in the resolutions. For some, this could be a deadly omission.

Iron oxide pigments are found in nature and all contain nickel as an impurity. They are refined before use to achieve a high degree of purity and to obtain a defined colour. The nickel contained in iron oxides is not soluble and is seemingly part of the crystal structure [1]. Therefore, it is questionable whether the contained nickel can cause allergic reactions.

Several different classes of organic pigments are used in tattoo and PMU inks, including azo pigments, polycyclic pigments, and phthalocyanine pigments. The frequently used black pigment is the main source of carcinogenic PAHs. Its purity is dependent on the source and manufacturing process. Although there is only one colour index (CI) number for black pigment, CI 77266, it has many physical variations that are all listed under the same CI number. Therefore, the CI number gives only limited information about a product and its quality. The purity and structure of a black pigment and whether it contains problematic PAHs can in no way be derived from the CI number. This information would require detailed chemical analysis, but again, no methods are mentioned in the resolutions of the CoE.

Azo pigments are mainly used to achieve bright and vibrant colours and can be a source of carcinogenic amines if the azo bond is cleaved to produce such amines. Azo colourants pose a smaller health risk than the amines that they produce. Cancer-causing amines were documented in the colour and textile dyeing industry more than a century ago [9]. There are indications that only soluble azo colourants are cleaved to form carcinogenic amines in the human body. Insoluble pigments, such as those used in tattoo and PMU inks, appear to be stable [10]; therefore, they should not lead to health problems. The question remains as to whether solubility is generally equivalent to bioavailability.

Phthalocyanine pigments have a base structure similar to several pigments found in nature, including haem, which gives the red colour to blood, and green chlorophyll in plants. The pigments used in tattoo inks contain copper as a central atom in their structures and the copper ion is firmly bonded to the base structure, similar to haem, which contains iron, and chlorophyll, which contains magnesium as a central atom. Microwave analysis of these copper-based pigments have shown copper levels of more than 1,000 mg/kg but have not revealed the amounts of soluble copper in products. Because the copper is firmly bound to the base structure, it is unclear whether it causes health problems. On the other hand, soluble copper should be limited. Here again, the microwave digestion method has not produced any useful results or information.

Analysis of Metals in Tattoo Inks

There are two methods being used on the market for the analysis of metals in tattoo and PMU inks. They differ considerably with regard to the first part of the procedure, which is called the work-up. The procedures for the final analysis of the metals themselves are identical. Authorities use a method commonly known as microwave digestion. The work-up of this method uses strong acids and a microwave oven to digest the sample. Due to the strong acids and high temperature and pressure, nearly everything can be digested and broken down into their elements. Even high-quality steels and jewellery can be dissolved using this fierce method. The form of a metal cannot be established using this method. It may have been soluble in water or insoluble and part of a crystal structure of a pigment or it may even have been in an organic or a mineral form. In 2009, CTL® devised an

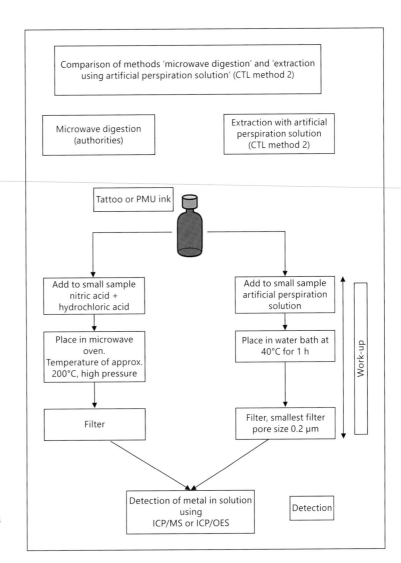

Fig. 1. Different work-up methods for the analysis of metals in tattoo and PMU inks.

alternative work-up method for microwave digestion for analysing metals in tattoo and PMU inks
which only detects soluble metals. This method involves extraction with an artificial perspiration solution and microfiltration [1]. It is quite similar to
the legal method used for the release of nickel in
jewellery [11]. For nickel in jewellery, only the
nickel that is soluble in an artificial perspiration
solution is detected. Figure 1 demonstrates the different work-up methods for microwave digestion
and extraction with artificial perspiration.

Limitations and Weaknesses of the Resolutions

The resolutions ResAP(2003)2 and ResAP(2008)1
are only recommendations and are not legally
binding. Nevertheless, several manufacturers use
the limits mentioned in ResAP(2008)1 as a minimum standard for their inks.

A major drawback of the resolutions are the
missing analytical methods. Due to this lack of
information, it is unclear what the limits mean

and what they refer to; for example, whether they pertain to soluble metals or insoluble metals and other chemicals. If soluble chemicals are of concern, then the solvent in which they are to be solubilised must be defined, e.g. artificial perspiration or hydrochloric acid, such as that in the stomach. The legal methods for detecting metal in toys [12] and in jewellery [11] are specific in this respect. The method for toys only detects metals that are soluble in the hydrochloric acid of the stomach, and for jewellery, only released soluble nickel is detected.

A previous publication [13] has described the limits for allergic reactions to metals in products which are based on soluble nickel, not insoluble nickel. The dose-response tests conducted used soluble nickel salts, such as nickel sulphate and nickel chloride, applied directly on the skin [14]. Furthermore, the missing analytical methods in the resolutions are responsible for much confusion on the market, many unjust and illegal market recalls and arbitrary decisions by authorities. The resolutions have not been implemented into national law in any of the EU member states and they are therefore not binding. As previously mentioned, the amounts of contaminants found in inks are highly dependent on the analytical method used. Furthermore, when the amount of ink in the skin is taken into consideration, the amount of contaminants in the skin becomes extremely small. The microwave digestion method has failed in the evaluation of barium and copper, and the results achieved for nickel are questionable.

The limit for nickel in the resolution ResAP(2008)1 is 'as low as technically achievable'. Of course, products containing no nickel can be found on the market, e.g. a simple black pigment, but this cannot be the reason for the use of a general limit of zero. Whether zero nickel is achievable also depends upon whether an ink contains organic or inorganic pigments. For inorganic iron oxides, a limit of zero is not 'technically achievable'.

The limits for some metals in ResAP(2008)1 are similar to those for drinking water. The level for nickel according to the drinking water regulation in Germany is 0.02 mg/l, which is approximately 0.02 mg/kg [15]. As previously mentioned, the large tattoo performed at CTL® with the banned ink containing 12.2 mg/kg of nickel contained as little as 0.0057 mg of nickel. This is well below the set limits for drinking water in Germany. It should be further considered that the intake of water is at least 1 kg every day for 365 days a year. A tattoo, on the other hand, should have a lifetime of 20 years, and ink is therefore only applied once every 20 years. Considering the legal limits for jewellery [11] and comparing them to those of tattoos reveals the following:

- the legal limit for nickel release in jewellery is $0.2 \ \mu g/cm^2/week$; and
- the average content of nickel in large tattoos using the values from the above-mentioned banned ink is $0.006 \ \mu g/cm^2$.

This comparison shows that the amount of nickel in the skin is substantially (approximately 33 times) lower than the legal limit for nickel in jewellery.

Irrespective of whether ResAP(2008)1 refers to soluble or insoluble metals, it is questionable whether these limits are realistic. Quite obviously, factors such as the amount of ink in the skin, daily uptake or daily consumption, total uptake and frequency of use have not been taken into consideration. Comparisons with several food products consumed on a daily basis by many people have shown that these foods contain as much nickel as the above-mentioned $910\text{-}cm^2$ tattoo, which will only be performed once in a span of 20 years.

It must be mentioned that iron oxide-based inks are also used in hospitals for areola tattooing after breast reconstruction or breast cancer. In addition, these inks are used following the development of alopecia after chemotherapy or for cosmetic corrections after burns. This cosmetic tattooing improves the quality of life for many people. In particular, iron oxide pigments allow for the imitation of skin colour. If the limits for nickel in ResAP(2008)1 are enforced and the use of the microwave digestion method is required, then practically all iron oxide-based inks would become illegal.

The analysed amount of ink in the skin resulting from tattooing has been used here only for calculations of the resulting quantities of metal impurities in the skin. This fundamental data can also be used to calculate the actual amounts of other contaminants in the skin, which are listed in the resolutions of the CoE.

References

1 Prior G: Tattoo Inks: Analysis, Pigments, Legislation. Berlin, epubli, 2014.
2 Council of Europe, Committee of Ministers: Resolution ResAP(2003)2 on Tattoos and Permanent Make-Up. Strasbourg, France, Council of Europe, 2003.
3 Council of Europe, Committee of Ministers: Resolution ResAP(2008)1 on Tattoos and Permanent Make-Up. Strasbourg, France, Council of Europe, 2008.
4 Radiology dye kills six. The Age, Fairfax Digital, 2003. http://www.theage.com.au/articles/2003/07/23/1058853117047.html (accessed February 10, 2014).
5 Johnson CH, VanTassell VJ: Acute barium poisoning with respiratory failure and rhabdomyolysis. Ann Emerg Med 1991;20:1138–1142.
6 Ghose A, Sayeed AA, Hossain A, Rahman R, Faiz A, Haque G: Mass barium carbonate poisoning with fatal outcome, lessons learned: a case series. Cases J 2009;2:9327.

7 Commission of the European Communities: Fifth Commission Directive 93/73/EEC of 9 September 1993 on the methods of analysis necessary for checking composition of cosmetic products. Official Journal of the European Communities 1993;L 231:34–53.
8 Eurpopäisches Arzneibuch (European Pharmacopoeia). Stuttgart, Deutscher Apotheker Verlag, 1997.
9 Rehn L: Blasengeschwülste bei fuchsinarbeitern. Arch Klein Chir 1895;50:588–600.
10 Golka K, Kopps S, Myslak ZW: Carcinogenicity of azo colorants: influence of solubility and bioavailability. Toxicol Lett 2004;151:203–210.

11 DIN EN 1811:2012-10, Reference test method for release of nickel from all post assemblies which are inserted into pierced parts of the human body and articles intended to come into direct and prolonged contact with the skin. Berlin, Beuth Verlag, 2012.
12 CEN EN 71–3:2013 Safety of toys – Part 3: Migration of certain elements. European Committee for Standardisation, Brussels, 2013.
13 Basketer DA, Angelini G, Ingber A, Kern PS, Menné T: Nickel, chromium and cobalt in consumer products: revisiting safe levels in the new millenium. Contact Dermatitis 2003;49:1–7.
14 Fischer LA, Menné T, Johansen JD: Experimental nickel elicitation thresholds – a review focusing on occluded nickel exposure. Contact Dermatitis 2005;52:57–64.
15 Bundesgesetzblatt Teil 1, BGBl. I 2013, 2993 – 2995, Anlage 2 zu § 6 Absatz 2), Chemische Parameter.

Gerald Prior
CTL Bielefeld GmbH
Krackserstrasse 12
DE–33659 Bielefeld (Germany)
E-Mail info@ctl-bielefeld.de

Serup J, Kluger N, Bäumler W (eds): Tattooed Skin and Health.
Curr Probl Dermatol. Basel, Karger, 2015, vol 48, pp 158–163 (DOI: 10.1159/000369221)

The Challenges and Limitations of Chemical Analysis of Particulate Pigments of Very Low Solubility

Ole Olsen

Medico Chemical Lab ApS, Vedbaek, Denmark

Abstract

When performing a chemical analysis of colorants in tattoo products, specific degradation products as well as impurity patterns can be predicted. Mislabeling or false declarations can also be avoided using this test. It is notable that pigment identification in tattoo products may serve as a precursory technique to recognize the colorants contained in a patient's tattoo prior to laser removal therapy. In contrast to the analysis of banned pigments, positive identification of pigments will normally require few reference substances. Given the fact that tattoo pigments are nearly insoluble in water and many organic solvents, different chemical pigment analyses are outlined and evaluated. Related publications from the study of art are also mentioned. It is recommended that access to comprehensive pigment standards and spectroscopic databanks should be offered to laboratories dealing with tattoo product analysis in the future.

Introduction

Tattoo products consist of colorants dispersed in a suitable matrix, which is normally a solution of water, glycerin, alcohol, resins, surfactants, and witch hazel. Different types of colorants are responsible for the final motif of the tattoo. The concentrations of the colorants in tattoo products are often above 50% (w/w) [1]. As tattoos are meant to last for a lifetime, the colorants have to be very stable after placement in the dermis. This means that the colorants have to be insoluble in water. If not, they will be washed away during contact with the tissue. When a colorant is insoluble in its own matrix, it is called a pigment. Today, approximately 80% of the pigments in tattoo products are synthetic organic molecules, mostly azo pigments and polycyclic compounds [2]. The most frequently used inorganic pigments are titanium dioxide, barium sulfate, and iron oxides [3].

Organic pigments are favored for tattooing because of their high tinting strengths, light fastness, enzymatic resistance, dispersion, and relatively inexpensive production [4]. In order to secure the safety and quality of tattoo products for the consumer, different regulatory guidelines have been developed during the last 20 years. The European guideline from Council of Europe, 2008, Resolution ResAP(2008)2 on tattoos and permanent make-up [5] is the most significant example to be mentioned. According to this guideline, the only identification required to verify the pigments in tattoo products is the color index (CI) number printed on the label. No chemical identification of the pigment is needed. As some pigments (mostly azo pigments) are known to degrade into potentially harmful substances, such as primary amines, the guideline contains a list of 35 banned pigments suspected of being potential precursors of degradation products, such as the carcinogenic primary amines o-anisidine, 5-nitro-o-toluidine, 4-chloro-o-toluidine, and 3,3-dichlorobenzidine [1]. To fulfill this requirement, a reference sample of all 35 different pigments is needed for the chemical analysis of pigments. Engel et al. [6] and Vasold et al. [7] conducted in vitro experiments to show that potentially toxic/carcinogenic decomposition products form when using a typical Q-switched Nd:YAG (532 nm) laser on two common red tattoo inks.

As the market for tattoo products is huge and nontransparent, it could be desirable for positive identification of the pigments in tattoo products to be established as a standard safety test. This would also avoid mislabeling or false declarations. In contrast to the analysis of the banned pigments, positive identification of pigments will normally require few reference pigments, depending of the type of tattoo product.

Another important reason to know the identity of the pigments in tattoo products is related to tattoo removal. Here, it is necessary to know the absorption wavelengths of the actual pigments so that the laser light can be matched to the absorption spectra of the tattooed compounds. In other words, the identification of pigments in tattoo products might serve as an important precursory technique prior to laser removal therapy [4]. As some impurities are related to specific pigments [8], positive pigment identification could predict the impurity pattern of the actual tattoo product. As noted by Bäumler et al. [9], the analysis of pigments using standard methods has turned out to be very troublesome because of their extremely low solubility. This is a general problem in all analytical quantification methods in which sample preparations are included. If the solubility is less than 1 mg/ml at 22°C, the compound is generally characterized as insoluble [1]. It has been observed that pigments are generally considered as insoluble in water and also partially insoluble in most organic solvents. In many of the chemical methods described below, the pigment concentration is very low and close to the insoluble limit.

When setting up an analytical standard method for the analysis of pigments in tattoo products, one also has to take into account the variable solubility of the pigments. In other words, the pigments with the lowest solubility will be responsible for the final setting of the pigment concentration in the analytical standard. If quantification of the pigment is needed, one has to ensure that all pigments are totally dissolved when making the calibration curve.

As reference pigments are necessary for the performance of analytical procedures, it should be noted that access to a suitable selection of reference pigments seems to be a serious problem for routine laboratories.

Chemical Analyses of Tattoo Pigments

During the last 20 years, several investigations of the pigment content of tattoo products have been performed, and a survey of the many pigments used in tattoo inks is given in [1, 10, 11]. Inorganic pigments can be analyzed relatively straightforwardly with techniques such as energy-dispersive spectrometry, X-ray fluorescence, or X-ray diffraction [4, 12]. In the following sections, different published analytical methods are listed and discussed. The analytical methods are arranged according to their analyzing principle.

Fourier Transform Infrared Spectroscopy
Poon et al. [4] carried out an analytical procedure in which organic pigments were identified in situ and post-tattoo procedure by Fourier transform infrared spectroscopy (FTIR). The pigments were filtrated from the tattoo ink, finely ground with analytical-grade KBr, and pressed into pellets. Peak wave numbers and spectra were visually compared and cross-referenced against the active reference material and existing databases. The method was used as a complementary technique to Raman spectroscopy to confirm the identity of the pigments.

Bäumler et al. [9] analyzed 41 tattoo inks and identified 16 different pigments using FTIR. The pigments were placed in a KBr disc (pigment concentration 0.1% w/w) and identified by computer-assisted pattern comparison with original pigment spectra from databanks. According to the authors, the analysis of the pigments by using standard methods turned out to be very troublesome because of the pigments' extremely low solubility or volatility. Using this method, 16 different pigments were determined.

Vila and Garcia [13] investigated the composition of red pigments and inks for the characterization and differentiation of prints. They used a combination of FTIR and an energy-dispersive X-ray-analyzing system (scanning electron microscopy-energy-dispersive X-ray (SEM-EDX)), which are common techniques available in museums and at centers related to the study of artwork. FTIR provides information about the organic and some inorganic components of pigments and inks, whereas SEM-EDX provides the elemental composition of the material. The mid-IR range is

very useful for detecting the fingerprint of organic materials, although it does not allow the identification of inorganic pigments with absorptions below 400 cm^{-1}, such as vermilion, titanium, and cadmium pigments. In the study, the inks were spread on top of a pure KBr pellet. The authors concluded that due to the complexity of the synthetic organic pigments, a combination of the two methods (FTIR and SEM-EDX) was needed for the identification of all components in the actual inks.

Schaening et al. [14], from the Academy of Fine Arts, used FTIR for the identification and classification of synthetic organic pigments in a collection from the 19th and 20th centuries. Different organic pigments could be detected by FTIR in combination with a diamond sample cell. The identification was based on reference material taken from a large pigment database. In another study [15], the authors used a multivariate data analysis of FTIR spectra to support the classification of synthetic organic pigments. FTIR seems to be a very useful method for the examination of pigments in old paintings. Learner [16], from the Tate Gallery, used FTIR to analyze pigments in paintings, and FTIR has proven to be a very useful method for rapid differentiation between the main types of 20th-century paint media. In forensic paint examinations, FTIR analysis seems to be the routine choice. The FBI Laboratory for Paints and Polymers [17] has developed a standard operating procedure regarding the identification of pigments in paints. The paint is placed between two inactive IR windows or in a diamond cell.

High-Pressure Liquid Chromatography
Using high-pressure liquid chromatography (HPLC) and diode array detection (DAD), Bhakti and Petigara [18] identified the two major classes of organic pigments, along with benzimidazolone-based organic pigments for orange and brown ink colors. The retention times and spectral data for the pigments in the examined tattoo inks were correlated with those of reference

standards. The complexity of the ink mixtures did complicate the correlation with the specific pigments.

Investigating the photodecomposition of Pigment Yellow 74 (PY74), Cui et al. [19] analyzed seven yellow tattoo inks. The inks were mixed with water and extracted with methylene chloride. The samples were analyzed using HPLC equipped with a diode array detector. PY74 was identified in six of the seven inks by comparing the HPLC retention times and absorbance spectra of the eluting components with those of authentic PY74.

Engel et al. [20] have established a protocol to analyze tattoo pigments in situ by HPLC and DAD. Using a rather complicated extraction method, nearly complete recovery from aqueous suspension was achieved. This is an interesting study because quantification of the pigments was included.

Vasold et al. [7] used the same instrumentation when looking at degradation products after laser light cleavage of the two pigments CI 12315 and CI 12460. The pigments were identified by their retention times and spectral data in comparison with those of reference pigments.

A well-known method to identify and quantify organic pigments in textiles is described in Textilien-Nachweis von Dispersionsfarbstoffen [21]. Some laboratories are using this method for the identification of the 35 banned pigments, as stated in the Council of Europe, 2008, Resolution ResAP(2008)2 on tattoos and permanent make-up. The method uses HPLC and DAD, with methanol as the extraction solvent. The retention times and spectral data for the pigments in the examined tattoo inks are correlated with those of reference standards. The detection limit is approximately 1–2 mg/l. As the method was developed for the analysis of textiles, modifications have to be implemented for the analysis of tattoo inks.

Raman Spectroscopy

Poon et al. [4] carried out an analytical procedure in which organic pigments were identified in situ and post-tattoo procedure by Raman spectroscopy. During the sample preparation, separation from the carrier solution was necessary, as overwhelming fluorescence was observed when the tattoo inks were simply smeared onto glass slides and analyzed by Raman spectroscopy. Using this method, TiO_2 was identified separately. Raman analysis was performed on reference material and tattoo pigments separated from the pre-mixed ink by focusing the laser on the sample mounted onto the glass slides. Beyond the rather comprehensive sample preparation, the method seems suitable for routine purposes. Vandenabeele et al. [12] investigated the pigments in different paintings using a fiber-optic probe combined with a Raman spectrophotometer. In this direct analysis, the probe was placed approximately 1 cm above the object (which could be tattoo ink evaporated on a glass plate). Several pigments in the painting could be identified using reference samples. The method seems interesting, as it is a direct and fast analysis.

Different Time-of-Flight-Based Analytical Methods

Hauri [8] analyzed 167 tattoo ink samples for their content of pigments; aromatic amines; carcinogenic, mutagenic, and reprotoxic substances; and preservatives. The method used for qualitative analysis of organic pigments was matrix-assisted laser desorption ionization time-of-flight (TOF) mass spectrometry (MS). This allowed most of the pigments that were used to be analyzed directly from the dyes themselves, without adding a matrix. Along with the poor solubility, the biggest problem in the analysis lay in obtaining reference substances.

The Mass Spectrometry Application Group at JEOL Ltd. [22] has described a method in which Pigment Yellow 83 and Pigment Red 144 are identified using a direct exposure probe (DEP) and a TOF gas chromatography mass spectrometer (AccuTOF GCv 4G). Regarding the DEP, the analyte solution (or suspension) is placed on a coiled platinum filament at the end of the probe. The probe is introduced into the ion source, and the analyte is rapidly heated and vaporized by passing an electric current through the filament. Since the analyte is vaporized by rapid heating with the DEP, this method is efficient and suitable for the analysis of high-boiling-point and thermally labile compounds. As the method has only been tested on two different pigments, it is unknown whether it is suitable for analyses of pigment mixtures.

Oxidative degradation of the azo pigment CI 13020 was studied by Djelal et al. [23] using direct analysis in real time TOF MS. The method is similar to the method described above, and again, only data based on experiments on one pigment are available. Fang et al. [24] have developed a highly advanced method for the low-level detection of organic pigments. The method is based on a combination of HPLC and mass-selective detector (MSD) TOF. The liquid chromatography (LC) system will separate the different pigments before the identification/quantification takes place. The high mass accuracy of the LC/MSD TOF allows the user to confirm the identity as well as the quantity of each compound analyzed. Due to the better precision and accuracy of the mass measurement, LC/MSD TOF appears to represent a very precise analytical method, especially for the identification of unknown pigments.

Conclusion

As indicated in this chapter, several analytical methods are used in the identification of pigments in tattoo products, paint, and paintings. The choice of method will depend on the purpose, e.g. pigment identification/quantification or identification only. As mentioned in the introduction, the chemical identification of pigments in tattoo products is important to establish a pig-

ment-related safety profile, which has been the main focus of this chapter. When characterizing pigment degradation products and impurities, quantification methods will be necessary. For the routine laboratory, several analytical methods seem to be possible.

For the world of art, where the identification of pigments is a very important issue, the scientific literature points out FTIR to be the best choice. Forensic laboratories also use this method as standard option. The sample preparation is minor, as the tattoo ink can be placed directly on the IR transparent window and evaporated, or the pigments can be filtrated and pressed in the KBr disc. As reference spectral data are necessary in the identification procedure, it is notable that several FTIR pigment reference databases are available (http://www.ir-spectra.com/2012/indexes/index_p.htm).

HPLC has been used by several scientists and routine laboratories when separation of pigments is necessary. For example, the identification of the 35 banned pigments requires proper separation before final identification. The identification is based on comparison of retention times and spectral data from reference samples. Raman spectroscopy has been performed on paintings and tattoo ink as well. In the analysis of tattoo ink, the sample preparation seems to be rather comprehensive to avoid interfering fluorescence signals from TiO_2. It should be mentioned that several Raman pigment reference databases exist [6]. All of the above-mentioned methods are suitable for routine laboratories. Once again, it should be noted that access to relevant pigment reference samples as well as spectral databases is crucial.

For the research laboratories with access to more advanced equipment, LC/MSD TOF, direct analysis in real time TOF MS, or matrix-assisted laser desorption ionization TOF with a DEP seem to be the state-of-the-art methods. Access to research laboratories is important in situations in which the routine methods are insufficient.

References

1 Baeumler W, Vasold R, Lundsgaard J, Talberg HJ: Chemicals used in tattooing and permanent make up products; in Papameletiou D, Schwela D, Zenie A, Baeumler W (eds): Workshop on the technical/scientific and regulatory issues on the safety of tattoos, body piercing and related practices. Ispra, European Commission, 2003, pp 21–48.

2 De Cuyper C, D'hollander D: Materials Used in Body Art; in De Cuyper C, Pérez-Cotapos S ML (eds): Dermatologic Complications with Body Art. Dordrecht, Springer-Verlag Berlin/Heidelberg, 2010, pp 13–28.

3 Prior G: Tattoo Inks: Analysis, Pigments, Legislation. Berlin, epubli, 2014.

4 Poon KWC, Dadour IR, McKibley J: In situ chemical analysis of modern organic tattooing inks and pigments by micro-Raman spectroscopy. J Raman Spectrosc 2008;39:1227–1237.

5 Council of Europe: Resolution ResAP(2008)1, on Requirements and criteria for the safety of tattoos and permanent make-up.

6 Engel E, Vasold R, Bäumler W: Tätowierungspigmente im Focus der Forschung. Nachr Chem 2007;55:847–851.

7 Vasold R, Naarmann N, Ulrich H, Fisher D, König B, Landthaler M, Bäumler W: tattoo pigments are cleaved by laser light- the chemical analysis in vitro provide evidence for hazardous compounds. Photochem Photobiol 2004;80:185–190.

8 Hauri U: Inks for tattoos and PMU (permanent make-up)/organic pigments, preservatives and impurities such as primary aromatic amines and nitrosamines. State Laboratory of the Canton Basel City. 2011. Available from: www.kantonslabor-bs.ch/files/berichte/6729_111012_JB_Tattoo_PMU_2011_EN.pdf.

9 Bäumler W, Eibler ET, Hohenleutner U, Sens B, Sauer J, Landthaler M: Q-Switch laser and tattoo pigments: first results of the chemical and photophysical analysis of 41 compounds. Lasers Surg Med 2000;26:13–21.

10 Timko AL, Miller CH, Johnson FB: In vitro quantitative chemical analysis of tattoo pigments. Arch Dermatol 2001; 137:143–147.

11 Danish Environmental Protection Agency: Chemical Substances in Tattoo Ink. Survey of chemical substances in consumer products (Kortlægning af kemiske stoffer i forbrugerprodukter) No. 116, 2012.

12 Vandenabeele P, Verpoort F, Moens L: Non-destructive analysis of paintings using Fourier transform Raman spectroscopy with fibre optics. J Raman Spectrosc 2001;32:263–269.

13 Vila A, Garcia FJ: Analysis of the chemical composition of red pigments and inks for the characterization and differentiation of contemporary prints. Anal Lett 2012;45:1274–1285.

14 Schaening A, Schreiner M, Jembrih-Simburger: Identification and classification of synthetic organic pigments of a collection of the 19th and 20th century by FTIR; in Picollo M (ed): The Sixth Infrared and Raman Users Group Conference (IRUG6), 29.3.–1.4., Florence, Italy, 2004, pp 302–305.

15 Schäning A, Varmuza K, Schreiner M: Pigment classification of synthetic organic pigments by multivariate data analysis of FTIR spectra. e-PS 2009;6: 75–80.

16 Learner T: The use of a diamond cell for the FTIR characterization of paints and varnishes available to twentieth century artists. Postprints: IRUG2 Meeting, pp. 7-20. Available at http://www.getty.edu/conservation/our_projects/science/modpaints/1Learner.pdf.

17 FBI Laboratory Chemistry Unit: FTIR Analysis of Paints, Tapes, and Polymers. FBI Laboratory Chemistry Unit SOP Manual PPSU 200–0.doc, 2006, pp 1–12.

18 Bhakti R, Petigara B: Separation and identification of pigments found in permanent cosmetic/tattoo inks using reversed-phase high performance liquid chromatography and photodiode array detection. Abstracts of the 230th ACS National Meeting, August 28–September 1, Washington, DC, 2005.

19 Cui Y, Spann AP, Couch LH, Gopee NV, Evans FE, Churchwell MI, Williams LD, Doerge DR, Howard PC: Photodecomposition of Pigment Yellow 74, a pigment used in tattoo inks. Photochem Photobiol 2004;80:175–184.

20 Engel E, Santarelli F, et al: Establishment of an extraction method for the recovery of tattoo pigments from human skin using HPLC diode array detector technology. Anal Chem 2006;15:78: 6440–6470.

21 Deutsches Institut für Normung: Textilien-Nachweis von Dispersionsfarbstoffen. DIN 54231, 2005. Available at: http://www.din.de/cmd%3Bjsessionid=JD9UB2Z2AKIJVC2RHGRWHYZX.1?workflowname=infoInstantdownload&docname=9642857&contextid=din&servicerefname=dino&ixos=toc.

22 Analysis of organic pigments using a direct exposure probe on JMS-T100GC 'AccuTOF GC' Jeol MS Data Sheet no 085, 2006.

23 Djelal H, Cornée C, Tartivel R, Lavastre O, Abdeltif A: The use of HPTLC and Direct Analysis in Real Time-Of-Flight Mass Spectrometry (DART-TOF-MS) for rapid analysis of degradation by oxidation and sonication of an azo dye. Arabian J Chem 2013. http://dx.doi.org/10.1016/j.arabjc.2013.06.003

24 Fang Y, Li P, Zumwalt M: Determination of EU-Banned Disperse Dyes by LC/MSD TOF. Agilent Technologies, 2005. Available at: http://www.chem.agilent.com/Library/applications/5989-3859EN.pdf.

Ms. Sci. Chem. Ole Olsen
Medico Chemical Lab ApS
Skelstedet 5
DK–2950 Vedbaek (Denmark)
E-Mail OO@medico.dk

Serup J, Kluger N, Bäumler W (eds): Tattooed Skin and Health.
Curr Probl Dermatol. Basel, Karger, 2015, vol 48, pp 164–169 (DOI: 10.1159/000369225)

Photostability and Breakdown Products of Pigments Currently Used in Tattoo Inks

Urs Hauri · Christopher Hohl

State Laboratory of Basel-City, Analytical Department, Basel, Switzerland

Abstract

Tattoos fade with time. Part of this fading can be attributed to the photodegradation of pigments. When people get tired of their tattoos, removal by laser irradiation is the method of choice. In vivo laser irradiation of tattoos on mice has shown that the degradation of pigments can result in toxic compounds. Various in vitro studies on photodegradation by sunlight or laser have shown similar degradation products for both irradiations. Even visible light was shown to be able to decompose some pigments to toxic degradation products in vitro. Whereas the investigated phthalocyanins (C.I. 74160, 74260), quinacridones (C.I. 73915) or dioxazines (C.I. 51319) were fairly photostable in vitro, all azo pigments exposed to sunlight or laser were degraded into a variety of products, some of which were toxic or even carcinogenic, such as 2-amino-4-nitrotoluene, 3,3′-dichlorobenzidine and o-toluidine. Up to now, the absence of specific toxicological data is the reason why legal restrictions for tattoo inks are derived from those for cosmetics, toys and textiles. Photodegradation has not been considered. In light of the present analytical findings, even with their possible shortcomings, the evidence weighs heavily enough to consider banning azo pigments containing carcinogenic aromatic amines or allergens in their structure from use in tattoo inks.

Introduction

Organic pigments are the main components of coloured tattoo inks. Appropriate toxicological data being unavailable, the legal restrictions for tattoo inks in Europe still lean on restrictions for cosmetics, toys and textiles [1]. Specific toxicological data are desperately needed to establish a list of pigments safe for tattooing. From today's perspective, however, it is unlikely that such data will be available in the near future. At the moment, it seems more promising to improve consumer safety using chemical analysis to sort out those pigments which potentially can degrade to allergens or carcinogenic, mutagenic or reprotoxic compounds in the human body.

Tattoos fade with time. Several mechanisms are thought to play a part in this. Some fading can be attributed to the transport of the injected pigments away from the skin into the regional lymph nodes and other parts of the body [2, 3], where their fate remains unknown. Pigments may also be metabolised by enzymes [4], as was discussed for azo reductases, which are able to split azo colourants into hazardous aromatic amines [5]. If this also happens in the dermis, where metabolic activity is low [6], seems questionable. Pigments, however, are transported to other parts of the body where they might be metabolised.

As pigments remain in the skin for the rest of life, lightfastness is an important criterion for them. Colourants used for cars and plastic materials for outdoor purposes must withstand solar radiation and have therefore been deemed suitable for tattoo inks, regardless of the possible toxicological consequences. While their lightfastness is tested under outdoor conditions, screening for photodegradation products is not performed.

If people get tired of their tattoos, removal by laser irradiation is the method of choice. Upon absorbing laser light energy, pigment crystals are superheated to several hundred degrees Celsius and break into fragments which are washed away by lymphatic transport [7]. Thermic decomposition of the pigments is also to be expected.

Irradiation with Sunlight

Up to now, only a few studies have investigated the photodegradation of pigments used in tattoos. C.I. 11741, a yellow mono-azo pigment, was subjected to simulated solar light in a solution of tetrahydrofuran [8]. Three of the major fragments (table 1) were identified, suggesting cleavage at the hydrazine and amide groups. Photodegradation was also studied for the red mono-azo pigment C.I. 12315, which was dissolved in organic solvents and subjected to ultraviolet B (UVB) radiation (2.5–8 h; 14–43 J/cm^2) and natural sunlight (10–110 days) [9]. Depending on the solvent and light source, a slight discolouration up to the complete mineralisation of C.I. 12315 was observed. The nature of degradation products (table 1) suggests a reductive cleavage of the azo bridge as well as cleavage at the site of the azo bond under loss of nitrogen. The fate of this pigment was also studied in vivo using tattooed mice as a model [10]. Irradiation with simulated solar radiation for 32 days caused a pigment reduction of about 60% in the skin. The decomposition products identified in vitro, however, were not observed in vivo. The authors reckoned that these substances were formed temporarily but disappeared either by on-site metabolism, additional photochemistry or dissemination throughout the body. This would not be surprising, as the expected decomposition products are much more soluble than the pigment itself. While the in vitro studies investigated pigments dissolved in strong solvents, in the dermis, pigments occur as little crystals that are mostly surrounded by body fluids [7]. We therefore designed a study [11], where ready-to-use tattoo inks containing often-used pigments [12] were suspended in water or squeezed between glass plates as a thin layer. The samples were then exposed to natural sunlight for at least 35 days in late spring, with the UVB part of the spectrum being partly blocked by the glass plates. Liquid chromatography with ultraviolet/visible (UV/VIS) and mass spectrometric detection were used as methods. The irradiated samples were also screened for bioactive substances using thin layer chromatography followed by *Vibrio fisheri* detection. Irradiation between glass plates resulted in a stronger photodegradation. With the exception of a violet ink, all exposed samples produced bioactive fragments. Examination of the data revealed that for the pigments C.I. 51319, C.I. 73915, C.I. 74160 and C.I. 74260, no bioactive substances were detected. A highly bioactive substance that was present in all samples containing the pigments C.I. 21095, C.I. 21110 and C.I. 21115 was identified to be 3,3′-dichlorobenzidine (3,3′-DCB), a structural element of all these

Table 1. Degradation products of pigments under sunlight and laser irradiation

Pigment	Irradiation with different light sources	Laser irradiation products
C.I. 11741	o-acetoacetanisidide, 2-(hydroxyimine)-N-(2-methoxyphenyl)-3-oxobutanamide, N,N0-bis(2-methoxyphenyl)urea [8]; 2-methoxyacetanilide [13]	none identified [13]
C.I. 11767	none identified [13]	aniline [13]
C.I. 12315	2-amino-4-nitrotoluene, 4-nitrotoluene [9]	2-amino-4-nitrotoluene, 4-nitrotoluene, naphthol AS [14]
C.I. 12370	2-toluidin, 2,4,5-trichloroaniline, 2-methylformanilide, 2-methylacetanilide [13]	2-toluidin, 2,4,5-trichloroaniline [13]
C.I. 12460	not investigated	2,5-dichloroaniline, 1,4-dichlorobenzene, methoxy-naphthol AS [14]
C.I. 12475	benzamide [11, 13]; 4-hydroxybenzamide, 4-aminobenzamide [11]	not investigated
C.I. 21095	2-methylformanilide, 2-methyl-acetanilide, 3,3'-dichlorodiphenyl [13]; 3,3'-dichlorobenzidine [11]	3,3'-dichlorobenzidine [13]
C.I. 21108	not investigated	3,3'-dichlorobenzidine [13]
C.I. 21110	3,3'-dichlorobenzidine [11, 13]; 3,3'-dichlorodiphenyl [13]	3,3'-dichlorobenzidine [13]; aniline [13]
C.I. 21115	3,3'-dichlorobenzidine [11]	not investigated
C.I. 21160	formanilide, acetanilide, 3,3'-dimethoxydiphenyl [13]	none identified [13]
C.I. 51319	none identified [11, 13]	none identified [13]
C.I. 56110	none identified [13]	none identified [13]
C.I. 73907	4-chloroaniline [13]	none identified [13]
C.I. 73915	none identified [11, 13]	none identified [13]
C.I. 74160	none identified [11, 13]	none identified [13]
C.I. 74260	none identified [11, 13]	none identified [13]

pigments that was released by reductive cleavage of the azo bonds. A list of several other identified degradation products is shown in table 1. In a second study [13], pure pigments were submitted to the glass-plate experiment. In general, irradiation by artificial sunlight, which is commonly used for determining the photostability of sunscreens, gave similar results as irradiation with natural sunlight. Comparison of the degradation of pigments in inks with that of the pure pigments showed a much faster reaction in the inks. We assume that the finer pigment particles in tattoo inks have a higher specific surface than the agglomerated particles of pure pigments, thus leading to higher reaction rates. In most cases, degradation of inks led to the same compounds as were found in irradiated pigments. Especially, azo pigments in tattoo inks were easily degraded under artificial sunlight, whereas other important pigments, like quinacridones (C.I. 73915,

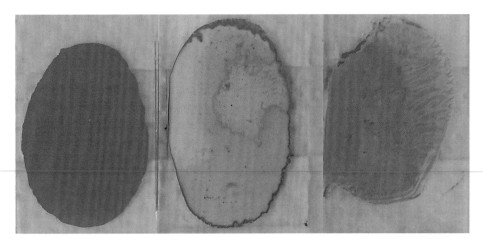

Fig. 1. Orange tattoo ink containing C.I. 21110 and titanium dioxide. From left to right: dark control sample, sample irradiated for 7 days with artificial sunlight, and sample irradiated for 7 days with visible (VIS) light only.

73907), phthalocyanins (C.I. 74160, 74260, 74265) or dioxazines (C.I. 51319, 51345), seemed fairly stable. Chromatographic runs revealed many peaks but only a few of them were identified (table 1). The main problem with in vitro assays lies in the elimination of photolabile products due to further reactions when under continued irradiation. In vivo, soluble ink components and degradation products are washed away by body fluids. In an attempt to preserve these photolabile degradation products, artificial irradiation with only the visible part of the spectrum was used, thus as a further benefit, simulating the situation of pigments in the dermis where only UVA and visible radiation can penetrate; UVB irradiation being mostly blocked by the epidermis. Figure 1 shows aliquots of orange tattoo ink, containing C.I. 21110 and titanium dioxide, that were subjected to 7 days of either artificial sun irradiation or visible light irradiation [13]. Exposure to visible light led to an obvious degradation of the inks. Full-spectrum light not only promoted degradation but also led to a variety of new degradation products when compared to aliquots exposed only to the visible spectrum. Inter-

estingly, the expected degradation product 3,3′-DCB was only found in the full-spectrum-irradiated sample, whereas on the other hand 3,3′-dichlorobiphenyl (PCB-11) was only found in the VIS-irradiated sample.

Laser Irradiation

In the first study investigating breakdown products after laser irradiation [14], the authors chose two red mono-azo pigments (C.I. 12315 and C.I. 12460) because red tattoos are the cause of most allergic reactions to tattooing. Laser irradiation performed on suspensions of the pigments in acetonitrile resulted in several fragments, of which three were identified (table 1). In the case of C.I. 12315, two of the identified products (4-nitrotoluene and 2-amino-4-nitrotoluene) were also found after irradiation with sunlight. In a second study [13], commercial tattoo inks instead of pure pigments were diluted with water and irradiated as in the first study [14]. For the azo pigments C.I. 11767, C.I. 12370, C.I. 21095, C.I. 21108 and C.I. 21110 similar degradation products as those observed in the first study [14] were detected. In the case of C.I. 11741, the expected reduction of the azo bridge could not be confirmed due to the presence of o-anisidine as an impurity in high concentration levels. The results of the tests are summarised in table 1.

Discussion

Identifying the photodegradation products of pigments is a difficult task. Even for pure pigments only few studies are available, and all have downsides. Photodegradation of C.I. 12315 was shown in vivo with mice [10], but the postulated decomposition products were not detected, presumably because they were eliminated during the period of irradiation. In vitro tests, besides their obvious shortcomings, have another flaw: In contrast to the in vivo situation, where decomposition products are constantly washed away from the dermis, they remain at their site of reaction and are prone to decay and react with other fragments. Subsequent screening would then reveal fragments unrelated to in vivo conditions. More lightfast pigments take longer to degrade, making it more difficult to detect photolabile degradation products. Some samples can even be completely mineralised under prolonged irradiation. Several potential azo pigment degradation products, like naphthol AS-type compounds or acetoacetarylamides (e.g., o-acetoacetanisidide), are not only formed after irradiation [13], they also occur as impurities in pigments, thus complicating the interpretation of irradiation experiments. Upon first view, inks do not appear suitable for in vitro experiments. Their ingredients, e.g. surfactants, thickeners or preservatives, form a reaction environment which is not relevant in vivo. Still, the investigation of inks has certain advantages. Presumably because of their very fine pigment dispersions, photodegradation is accelerated, and degradation products may be easier to detect. Further-more, effects on photostability by the specific pigment combination used have to be taken into account. When new inks containing C.I. 21110 were irradiated [13], the previously found degradation product 3,3′-DCB [11] was only found in traces. We suppose that the much higher content of titanium dioxide present in the older sample had a catalysing effect on C.I. 21110 degradation. Titanium dioxide is very often used in tattoo inks.

Laser irradiation experiments seem to better simulate in vivo conditions; it was even possible to detect the same degradation products in vivo and in vitro for the pigment C.I. 12315 [10]. Two mono-azo pigments (C.I. 12315 and C.I. 12460) showed the same degradation patterns. Bonds were cleaved at the junctions of the azo bridges, and interestingly, a reduction of the azo bridge yielding free amines also occured. Experiments with laser irradiation of similar mono-azo pigments suspended in water, however, only partly revealed analogous degradation products [13]. The presence of a relatively high amount of impurities certainly complicated any verification of photolysis. The choice of solvent or energy dose, however, could be another reason for these discrepancies. In the case of the 3,3′-DCB-based pigments C.I. 21095, C.I. 21108 and C.I. 21110, laser treatment led to the expected reduction of the azo bridge, resulting in the formation of 3,3′-DCB, but not of 3,3′-dichlorodiphenyl.

Regardless of any shortcomings of the described in vitro assays, some reaction pathways are very likely to happen in vivo and sometimes result in the same degradation products, regardless of the irradiation source. Whereas sunlight irradiation leads to continuous, low-level production of degradation compounds, comparable to degradation by enzymes, laser irradiation releases a momentary, high-level spike comparable to concentration spikes of pigment impurities when a tattoo ink is injected into the body. For the carcinogenic aromatic amines identified, toxicological data are available; therefore, worst-case toxicological evaluations using published pigment concentrations in the skin should be possible.

Conclusion

All organic pigments undergo photodegradation. In vitro experiments show that even the visible range of the sun spectrum degrades them to potentially hazardous compounds. It is reasonable to relate this process to in vivo conditions where this range of light penetrates into the dermis. Laser irradiation may also degrade pigments. For some pigments, toxic or carcinogenic degradation substances have been identified. In vitro analytical screenings, even with their inherent shortcomings, have provided evidence that certain azo pigments release carcinogenic aromatic amines like o-toluidine, 2-amino-4-nitrotoluene and 3,3'-dichlorobenzidine under sunlight or laser irradiation. In light of these findings, it is time to consider banning tattoo inks with azo pigments containing carcinogenic aromatic amines or strong allergens in their structure.

References

1 Council of Europe (CoE): Resolution ResAP(2008)1 on requirements and criteria for the safety of tattoos and permanent make-up. Adopted by the Committee of Ministers on 20 February 2008 at the 1018th meeting of the Ministers' Deputies.

2 Lehner K, Santarelli F, Penning R, et al: The decrease of pigment concentration in red tattooed skin years after tattooing. J Eur Acad Dermatol Venereol 2011; 25:1340–1345.

3 Moehrle M, Blaheta HJ, Ruck P: Tattoo pigment mimics positive sentinel lymph node in melanoma. Dermatology 2001; 203:342–344.

4 Cui Y, Churchwell MI, Couch LH, et al: Metabolism of pigment yellow 74 by rat and human microsomal proteins. Drug Metabolism Disposition 2005;33:1459–1465.

5 Platzek T, Lang C, Grohmann G, et al: Formation of a carcinogenic aromatic amine from an azo dye by human skin bacteria in vitro. Hum Exp Toxicol 1999; 18:552–559.

6 Serup J: News and challenges. European Congress on Tattoo and Pigment Research, Copenhagen, November 13–14, 2013. http://www.iss.it/binary/ondi/cont/SERUP.pdf (accessed September 3, 2014).

7 Ferguson JE, Andrew SM, Jones CJ, et al: The Q-switched neodymium:YAG laser and tattoos: A microscopic analysis of laser-tattoo interactions. Br J Dermatol 1997;137:405–410.

8 Cui Y, Spann AP, Couch LH, et al: Photodecomposition of pigment yellow 74, a pigment used in tattoo inks. Photochem Photobiol 2004;80:175–184.

9 Engel E, Spannberger A, Vasold R, et al: Photochemical cleavage of a tattoo pigment by UV-B radiation or natural sunlight. J Dtsch Dermatol Ges 2007;5:583–589.

10 Engel E, Vasold R, Santarelli F, et al: Tattooing of skin results in transportation and light-induced decomposition of tattoo pigments – a first quantification in vivo using a mouse model. Exp Dermatol 2010;19:54–60.

11 Gaugler S: Analysis of Bioactive Compounds in Tattoo Inks Before and After Irradiation with Sunlight Using HPTLC and In Situ Detection with Vibrio fischeri; thesis, University of Hohenheim, Stuttgart, 2011.

12 Hauri U: Pigments, preservatives and impurities in tattoo inks. Presentation at the First International Conference on Tattoo Safety BfR-Symposium, Berlin, June 6–7, 2013.

13 Wezel K: Untersuchung des Verhaltens von Tätowiertinten und Pigmenten unter Lichteinfluss; thesis, University of Giessen, Giessen, 2013.

14 Vasold R, Naarmann N, Ulirch H, et al: Tattoo pigments are cleaved by laser light – the chemical analysis in vitro evidence for hazardous compounds. Photochem Photobiol 2004;80:185–190.

Urs Hauri, PhD
State Laboratory of Basel-City, Analytical Department
PO Box
CH–4012 Basel (Switzerland)
E-Mail urs.hauri@bs.ch

Serup J, Kluger N, Bäumler W (eds): Tattooed Skin and Health.
Curr Probl Dermatol. Basel, Karger, 2015, vol 48, pp 170–175 (DOI: 10.1159/000369319)

Carbon Black Nanoparticles and Other Problematic Constituents of Black Ink and Their Potential to Harm Tattooed Humans

Nicklas Raun Jacobsen · Per Axel Clausen

The National Research Centre for the Working Environment, Copenhagen, Denmark

Abstract

Black is the most common tattoo color, but only a few studies have shed light on the multitude of functional and contaminating chemicals present in black inks. These studies have generally shown that black inks are a diverse group, containing anything from 5 to 50+ organic components. Little is known about the possible effects on humans of internalizing these chemicals. Analysis has shown that the production of the main component, carbon black, can lead to the formation of pigments with polycyclic aromatic hydrocarbon (PAH) contents that range from very high to almost completely absent. Similar variations in PAH concentrations are observed in black inks. PAHs are known carcinogens and thus, low recommended levels have been suggested by the Council of Europe. Reactive oxygen species (ROS) have recently been a topic in scientific literature related to tattoo ink. Again, it has been shown that some inks produce deleterious ROS (e.g. singlet oxygen or peroxyl radicals), presumably via either adhered organic compounds or particle surface defects. It has been shown that black tattoo inks may contain a multitude of chemicals, including car- cinogens and allergens, and some have unknown toxicologies. However, it has additionally been demonstrated that some black inks already on the market do not produce ROS and also contain PAHs at levels that are below those recommended by the Council of Europe and very few additional contaminants.

© 2015 S. Karger AG, Basel

Tattoos have become increasingly popular in the Western world. Surveys have shown that 15% of the whole population is tattooed, and this proportion is almost doubled for young to middle aged people. The numbers are relatively similar for surveyed countries, such as Denmark [1], the United States [2] and Australia [3]. In spite of the recent increase in tattooed individuals and the wide popularity of tattooing amongst young people of both sexes, little is known about chemicals and contaminants in tattoo ink. Black is by far the most common color used in tattoos. However, so far, only a couple of research projects in which the content of black ink was thoroughly character-ized have reached the literature. The main sub-stance in black inks is carbon black (CB). One project has shown that the average CB content in 4 inks is 0.3 g/g [1], whereas another has reported ultra-centrifuged dry weight percentages of be-tween 31 and 67% for 11 black inks [4]. CB is one of the major chemicals used in the world with an annual global production of 5–10 million tons per year. By far, the majority (70%) is used for the re-inforcement of rubber in the production of auto-mobile tires, and 20% is used for the production of black plastic [5, 6]. Nine percent is used for inks and paints, which includes tattoo inks. CB is very diverse, being produced by many different manu-facturers from different types of highly controlled incomplete combustion of hydrocarbons (gases or liquids). Thus, there is a wide variety of particle sizes, surface areas, structures, purities and ad-hered chemicals, such as polycyclic aromatic hy-drocarbons (PAHs). An illustration of the latter has been demonstrated by a characterization of 5 commercial CB products, in which a 3,000-fold difference (0.123–330 µg/g) in PAH content was detected between the highest and lowest extract-able PAH contents. For a strong carcinogen and the most frequently examined PAH (benzo[a]py-rene), this difference was 0 versus 6.8 µg/g [1]. The latter of these two products contained even higher amounts of PAHs than those found in standard diesel exhaust particles from a forklift engine (NIST SRM 2975).

A wide variety of chemicals with different functions may be added to tattoo ink, including dispersed pigment particles, dispersants (poly-mers and surfactants), solvents (water and/or or-ganic solvents), polymeric resins for binding, an-tifoaming agents (e.g. fatty oils), wetting agents (surfactants), rheological modifiers to control viscosity, pH modifiers, and biocides to prevent microbiological growth. In addition to the inten-tionally added chemicals, inks contain contami-nants that are associated with the added chemi-cals, e.g. PAHs in CB. However, it must also be mentioned that some inks used in tattoo shops are commonly used for paper printing and are thus not manufactured for the purpose of tattoo-ing and being injected into the human body.

We have previously shown in a study of 11 black tattoo inks that they contain a wide variety of at least 50 different organic compounds in amounts (excluding low boiling solvents) of about 1% (w/w) or below [4]. All of the investi-gated tattoo inks contained CB and 2–3 other main components in addition to surfactants and contaminants. The main components constituted 65–100% of the organic compounds and were all oxygenated compounds, such as butanediol, glyc-erol and phenol, but in some cases, more exotic compounds were observed, such as Texanol, which is usually used in waterborne paints. In 6 of the 11 inks, surfactants were found, including nonylphenol ethoxylates (Surfonic N-X), octyl-phenol ethoxylates (Triton X), heptylphenol pro-poxylates, alkenyl ethoxylates, a mixture of poly-ethylene glycol, isosorbide oligomers and sorbi-tan ethoxylates (Tween), alcohol ethoxylates and 2,4,7,9-tetramethyl-5-decyne-4,7-diol ethoxylate (Surfynol 4XX). However, their contents were not quantified. Most of the tentatively identified minor organic compounds were derivatives of PAHs, with a few exceptions, such as trichloro-benzene, and were all considered contaminants. The inks were screened for dimethyl phthalate, diethyl phthalate, butyl benzyl phthalate and di-octyl phthalate, but only dibutyl phthalate in con-centrations of up to 5 µg/g and di-(2-ethylhexyl) phthalate in concentrations of up to 19 µg/g ink were found. One of the interesting findings of this study was that the total content of PAHs varied by up to a factor of 63 among the 11 black inks (0.46–29 µg/g), showing that there are commercial inks with PAH contents that are below the Council of Europe recommendation of <0.5 µg/g. This find-ing was also supported by Regensburger et al. [7], who showed that 19 commercial black tattoo inks contained total PAHs at concentrations ranging from 0.14 to 201 µg/g ink. A third study showed similar results, in which 8 black inks were found to contain from 0.8 to 118 µg/g, and two inks were shown to contain no PAHs (i.e. under the detection limit) [1]. All of these results clearly show that it is possible to produce black tattoo inks with very low levels of carcinogenic PAHs and that such products already exist on the market. PAHs represent a large group of organic chemicals with more than two fused aromatic rings, which are often formed as a result of incomplete combustion. Within inks, these chemicals have received special attention due to their possible toxicities. Although only one PAH has been classified by the International Agency for Research on Cancer (IARC) as a group 1 human carcinogen (benzo[a]pyrene), numerous others have been classified as group 2b (probably) and group 2a (possibly) human carcinogens [8]. Several metabolized PAH intermediates (via the cytochrome P-450 subfamily) are able to interact with DNA, forming bulky adducts with known carcinogenic effects. Skin cells are able to metabolize and activate PAHs, although this occurs at a much lower rate compared with other cell types e.g. liver and lung cells [9]. Human skin cells may be less sensitive to the genotoxicity of PAHs. However, it should be considered that the dermis is not the only and final destination of inks. Local lymph nodes are also recipients [10], and it is likely that systemic exposure occurs as well. Circulating particles above the size of glomerular filtration of <10 nm (a small subset of 2% of renal pores are 15–20 nm) [11] will likely be largely taken up by the liver. However, removing PAHs from particle surfaces requires harsh chemical treatments. Borm et al. [12] did not find any leakage of PAHs when CB particles were shaken in a water bath (24 h at 37°C in the dark) in a range of saline/dipalmitoylphosphatidylcholine concentrations. Thus, the bioavailability of particle-adhered PAHs in inks can be questioned. Because metabolized PAHs are excreted in the feces or urine, and such excretion has been demonstrated, for example, for PAHs taken up through the skin [13, 14], it

should be possible to determine whether PAHs in deposited ink are systemically bioavailable after tattooing. Although mutations and cancers are the main events in PAH carcinogenesis, some *in vitro* studies have indicated that nongenotoxic mechanisms may influence this process. For example, PAHs have been linked to promoter hypermethylation and increased cell proliferation [15, 16]. In addition to carcinogenesis, PAHs have been linked to several other toxicological end points, such as skin sensitization, skin photosensitivity, and immunotoxicity (see discussion in [17]).

The production of chemically highly reactive oxygen species (ROS) by tattoo inks has so far only been shown and discussed in two publications. It has previously been shown that PAHs are able to generate singlet oxygen ($O_2^{\cdot}$) under ultraviolet A (UVA) radiation [18]. Importantly, UVA is able to penetrate the skin to a depth of 1.5 mm. This includes the entire dermis with tattooed particles and PAHs. Regensburger et al. [7] tested the production of singlet oxygen by all PAHs present in a wide selection of black inks. Then, they exposed primary normal human dermal keratinocytes to PAH extracts of inks and UVA light. A good correlation between the generation of singlet oxygen by PAHs (the PAH composition of the extract) and decreased mitochondrial activity in the keratinocytes was observed [7]. Høgsberg et al. [4] used a broad indicator of ROS when they analyzed the production of 11 black inks. Surprisingly, they found huge differences in the ability to produce ROS, identifying 2 inks that produced very high amounts and 9 that produced relatively low amounts. Experiments with different specific ROS scavengers were performed to specify which ROS were produced by the two inks. For the first ink, it was shown that the peroxyl radical accounted for 44–69% of the ROS, whereas hydrogen peroxide and hydroxyl radicals accounted for less than 10%, depending on the tested concentration. The second ink showed relatively similar results, with the peroxyl radical accounting for

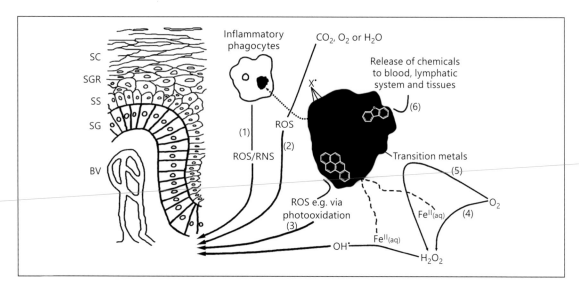

Fig. 1. Tattoo inks may cause the formation of highly reactive molecules via a number of mechanisms. (1) Inflammatory cells, such as macrophages or neutrophils, are activated during phagocytosis, leading to the formation of reactive oxygen species (ROS) and reactive nitrogen species (RNS). (2) Surface defects on particles may be involved in the catalysis of ROS. (3) Adsorbed organic chemicals, such as polyaromatic hydrocarbons and quinones, are depicted. Quinones can, in the presence of biological reductants, be involved in redox cycles that form the semiquinone radical (SQ') and also can yield O_2^{-}, H_2O_2 and 'OH [20]. (4) The release of redox-active metal ions from tattoo particles can lead to the formation of O_2^{-}, H_2O_2 and 'OH via the Haber-Weiss and Fenton reactions. (5) Same as (4) but occurring on the surfaces of tattoo particles. BV = Blood vessel; SG = stratum germinativum; SS = stratum spinosum; SGR = stratum granulosum; SC = stratum corneum.

45–72% of the ROS, and hydrogen peroxide and hydroxyl radicals accounting for less than 16%. Additionally, these results were somewhat similar to those detected for a highly pure (>99.9% C; 75 ng PAH/g [19]), high ROS-producing CB product (Printex 90), with peroxyl radicals, hydrogen peroxide and hydroxyl radicals accounting for 26–57, 1–20 and 0–10%, respectively [4].

The production of ROS by inks is an important finding that indicates the possibility of new mechanisms that may lead to mild or even more severe toxicological symptoms in tattooed individuals. Possible mechanisms underlying ROS production by inks are illustrated in figure 1. Toxicological symptoms could be anything from membrane destabilization, over reduced skin integrity to genotoxicity and cancer; proximal or even distal to the site of deposition. In this regard, it should be mentioned that Printex 90 has previously been shown to be able to both oxidize DNA and induce DNA strand breaks in a pulmonary cell line and *in vivo* in rodent lungs following pulmonary exposure [21–23]. Prolonged *in vitro* exposure caused mutations to form in the damaged DNA [21]. Mutation spectrum analysis has revealed that the mutations possess the same genetic fingerprint as that of high ROS production [24]. It is therefore important that both of the abovementioned studies have shown that there are several commercial black inks without or with very limited ROS production. Based on these findings, one could expect that long-term exposure to some black inks may cause genotoxicity, mutations and cancer. On the other hand, a recent literature survey has indicated that cancer in tattoos is rare and coincidental [25]. However, these cases have not been linked to specific ink products, and as mentioned above, it appears that only some samples produce high amounts of ROS. Additionally, no one has examined whether a correlation exists for other possible target sites, such as the lymph nodes or liver.

Regensburger et al. [7] also measured phenol and found concentrations of up to 385 µg/g. Phenol is thus far unclassifiable as a human carcinogen (IARC group 3). However, in addition to causing cutaneous burns, it has been shown in mice that the external skin application of 3 mg of phenol twice a week for up to 20 weeks promotes papilloma formation with the risk of malignant conversion [26]. However, the implication of the detected concentrations in inks is unknown.

Lehner et al. [27] investigated 14 black tattoo inks and found that they all contained dibutyl phthalate in concentrations ranging from 0.12 to 691.2 µg/g. Some of the inks also contained the contaminants hexachloro-1,3-butadiene (0.08–4.52 µg/g), methenamine (0.08–21.64 µg/g), dibenzofuran (0.02–1.62 µg/g), benzophenone (0.26–556.66 µg/g), and 9-fluorenone (0.04–3.04 µg/g) [27]. Some of these compounds have been suspected of causing irritant skin reactions or allergies.

The Danish Environmental Protection Agency measured metals and other elements, primary aromatic amines and phenylene diamine in 61 tattoo inks, including 11 black inks. The only problematic metals/elements found in the black inks were (in µg/g ink) the following: Cr, 8.9 and Ni, 2.5 [1]. The council of Europe recommends that hexavalent Cr should be present at <0.2 µg/g, whereas the level of Ni should be as low as possible due to the possibility of allergies. Additionally, these elements have been linked to genotoxicity via direct DNA-Cr adducts or the inhibition of DNA repair enzymes [28]. One black ink was screened for 23 different primary aromatic amines, and only o-anisidine was detected, at a concentration of 4.9 µg/g. O-anisidine is possibly carcinogenic to humans (IARC group 2b) based on sufficient evidence of carcinogenicity in animals [29].

Some black tattoo inks have been shown to contain a multitude of chemicals, including known allergens and carcinogens. This might well be connected to the fact that a large fraction of the tattooed population appears to suffer from persistent skin reactions, including sunlight sensitivity [30, 31]. It is therefore important to mention that all of the abovementioned studies of ink composition have shown that there are products that are presently on the market that contain very low amounts or the complete absence of PAHs, ROS production and other associated chemicals.

References

1 Danish EPA: Chemical Substances in Tattoo Ink. Mapping of Chemical Substances in Consumer Products 2012 nr. 115. København, Miljøstyrelsen, 2012.

2 Laumann A-E, Derick AJ: Tattoos and body piercings in the United States: a national data set. J Am Acad Dermatol 2006;55:413–421.

3 Makkai T, McAllister I: Prevalence of tattooing and body piercing in the Australian community. Commun Dis Intell Q Rep 2001;25:67–72.

4 Høgsberg T, Jacobsen NR, Clausen PA, Serup J: Black tattoo inks induce reactive oxygen species production correlating with aggregation of pigment nanoparticles and product brand but not with the polycyclic aromatic hydrocarbon content. Exp Dermatol 2013;22:464–469.

5 IARC: Carbon Black, Titanium Dioxide and Talc. Monograph vol. 93. Lyon, International Agency for Research on Cancer, 2010.

6 ICBA: Carbon Black User's Guide: Safety, Health and Environmental Information. The International Carbon Black Association, 2004.

7 Regensburger J, Lehner K, Maisch T, Vasold R, Santarelli F, Engel E, Gollmer A, König B, Landthaler M, Bäumler W: Tattoo inks contain polycyclic aromatic hydrocarbons that additionally generate deleterious singlet oxygen. Exp Dermatol 2010;19:e275–e281.

8 IARC: Some Non-Heterocyclic Polycyclic Aromatic Hydrocarbons and Some Related Exposures. Monograph vol. 92. Lyon, International Agency for Research on Cancer, 2010.

9 WHO: Polycyclic aromatic hydrocarbons; in Air Quality Guidelines for Europe, ed 2. Copenhagen, World Health Organization, 2000, pp 92–97.

10 Lehner K, Santarelli F, Vasold R, Penning R, Sidoroff A, Konig B, Landthaler M, Baumler W: Black tattoos entail substantial uptake of genotoxicpolycyclic aromatic hydrocarbons (PAH) in human skin and regional lymph nodes. PLoS One 2014;9:e92787.

11 Haraldsson B, Sorensson J: Why do we not all have proteinuria? An update of our current understanding of the glomerular barrier. News Physiol Sci 2004; 19:7–10.

12 Borm PJ, Cakmak G, Jermann E, Weishaupt C, Kempers P, van Schooten FJ, Oberdörster G, Schins RP: Formation of PAH-DNA adducts after in vivo and in vitro exposure of rats and lung cells to different commercial carbon blacks. Toxicol Appl Pharmacol 2005;205:157–167.

13 Sanders CL, Skinner C, Gelman RA: Percutaneous absorption of [7.10–14C] benzo[a]pyrene and [7, 12–14C] dimethylbenz[a]anthracene in mice. Environ Res 1984;33:353–360.

14 Yang JJ, Roy TA, Mackerer CR: Percutaneous absorption of benzo[a]pyrene in the rat: comparison of in vivo and in vitro results. Toxicol Ind Health 1986;2: 409–416.

15 Damiani LA, Yingling CM, Leng S, Romo PE, Nakamura J, Belinsky SA: Carcinogen-induced gene promoter hypermethylation is mediated by DNMT1 and causal for transformation of immortalized bronchial epithelial cells. Cancer Res 2008;68:9005–9014.

16 Oguri T, Singh SV, Nemoto K, Lazo JS: The carcinogen (7R,8S)-dihydroxy-(9S,10R)-epoxy-7,8,9,10-tetrahydrobenzo[a]pyrene induces Cdc25B expression in human bronchial and lung cancer cells. Cancer Res 2003; 63:771–775.

17 WHO: Guidelines for Indoor Air Quality: Selected Pollutants. Copenhagen, World Health Organization, 2010.

18 Bao L, Xu A, Tong L, Chen S, Zhu L, Zhao Y, Zhao G, Jiang E, Wang J, Wu L: Activated toxicity of diesel particulate extract by ultraviolet a radiation in mammalian cells: role of singlet oxygen. Environ Health Perspect 2009;117:436–441.

19 Jacobsen NR, Pojana G, White P, Møller P, Cohn CA, Korsholm KS, Vogel U, Marcomini A, Loft S, Wallin H: Genotoxicity, cytotoxicity, and reactive oxygen species induced by single-walled carbon nanotubes and C60 fullerenes in the FE1-Muta™ Mouse lung epithelial cells. Environ Mol Mutagen 2008;49: 476–487.

20 Bolton JL, Trush MA, Penning TM, Dryhurst G, Monks TJ: Role of quinones in toxicology. Chem Res Toxicol 2000;13: 135–160.

21 Jacobsen NR, Saber AT, White P, Møller P, Pojana G, Vogel U, Loft S, Gingerich J, Soper L, Douglas GR, Wallin H: Increased mutant frequency by carbon black, but not quartz, in the *lacZ* and *cII* transgenes of muta™mouse lung epithelial cells. Environ Mol Mutagen 2007;48: 451–461.

22 Jacobsen NR, Møller P, Jensen KA, Vogel U, Ladefoged O, Loft S, Wallin H: Lung inflammation and genotoxicity following pulmonary exposure to nanoparticles in ApoE–/– mice. Part Fibre Toxicol 2009;6:2.

23 Bourdon JA, Saber AT, Jacobsen NR, Jensen KA, Madsen AM, Lamson JS, Wallin H, Møller P, Loft S, Yauk CL, Vogel UB: Carbon black nanoparticle instillation induces sustained inflammation and genotoxicity in mouse lung and liver. Part Fibre Toxicol 2012;9:5.

24 Jacobsen NR, White PA, Gingerich J, Møller P, Saber AT, Douglas GR, Vogel U, Wallin H: Mutation spectrum in FE1-muta™ mouse lung epithelial cells exposed to nanoparticulate carbon black. Environ Mol Mutagen 2011;52:331–337.

25 Kluger N, Koljonen V: Tattoos, inks, and cancer. Lancet Oncol 2012;13:e161–e168.

26 Spalding JW, Momma J, Elwell MR, Tennant RW: Chemically induced skin carcinogenesis in a transgenic mouse line (TG.AC) carrying a v-Ha-ras gene. Carcinogenesis 1993;14:1335–1341.

27 Lehner K, Santarelli F, Vasold R, König B, Landthaler M, Bäumler W: Black tattoo inks are a source of problematic substances such as dibutyl phthalate. Contact Dermatitis 2011;65:231–238.

28 Beyersmann D, Hartwig A: Carcinogenic metal compounds: recent insight into molecular and cellular mechanisms. Arch Toxicol 2008;82:493–512.

29 IARC: Some Chemicals that Cause Tumours of the Kidney or Urinary Bladder in Rodents and Some Other Substances. Monograph vol. 73. Lyon, International Agency for Research on Cancer, 1999.

30 Klugl I, Hiller KA, Landthaler M, Bäumler W: Incidence of health problems associated with tattooed skin: a nationwide survey in German-speaking countries. Dermatology 2010;221:43–50.

31 Høgsberg T, Hutton Carlsen K, Serup J: High prevalence of minor symptoms in tattoos among a young population tattooed with carbon black and organic pigments. J Eur Acad Dermatol Venereol 2013;27:846–852.

Nicklas Raun Jacobsen
The National Research Centre for the Working Environment
105 Lerso Parkallé
DK–2100 Copenhagen (Denmark)
E-Mail nrj@nrcwe.dk

Serup J, Kluger N, Bäumler W (eds): Tattooed Skin and Health.
Curr Probl Dermatol. Basel, Karger, 2015, vol 48, pp 176–184 (DOI: 10.1159/000369222)

Absorption, Distribution, Metabolism and Excretion of Tattoo Colorants and Ingredients in Mouse and Man: The Known and the Unknown

Wolfgang Bäumler

Department of Dermatology, University of Regensburg, Regensburg, Germany

Abstract

During tattooing, high amounts of tattoo colorants, which usually contain various substances, are injected into skin. The major ingredient in tattoo colorants is the coloring component, which can be assigned to two different groups. First, amorphous carbon particles (Carbon Black) are found almost exclusively in black tattoos. Second, tattooists use azo and polycyclic pigments to create nearly all colors of the visible spectrum. Due to their different chemistries, those tattoo colorants usually contain various compounds, such as by-products and impurities. Professional tattooists inject the colorant mixture into skin using the solid needles of tattoo machines, and studies have shown that about 2.5 mg of tattoo pigment is injected to stain about 1 cm^2 of skin. Animal experiments revealed that about one-third of that amount disappeared from skin within weeks after tattooing, and this finding was confirmed by pigment extraction from long-existing tattoos. It is assumed that some of the tattoo colorants stay in the skin because the pigment particles are insoluble and too large to be transported. The other part of the tattoo colorants shows up at least in the lymph nodes located next to the tattoo. To date, no investigations determining whether and to what extent tattoo colorants can be found in any other organs of the human body have been performed. Thus, tattooing of colorants into skin entails a complex reaction of the skin that triggers the immune system and launches manifold transport processes, which might pose additional health risks not only to skin but also to other organs of humans.

© 2015 S. Karger AG, Basel

Introduction

Tattooing is an ancient technique used to stain the skin of humans. Tattoos have been identified in human beings dating back to the Stone Age [1]. In some cultures, like Polynesian tribes, tattooing was an important tool in religion and hierarchy. However, the meaning of tattoos in the western world became ambiguous during the past centuries and was consistently associated with low social status.

Nowadays, tattooing has become very popular worldwide. The current tattoos are black or multicolored and can be found on almost all parts of the human body. Many tattooed role models, like football, pop or movie stars, have led to a broader cultural acceptance of tattoos. A special category of tattoos is the so-called permanent make-up, in which colorants are placed in the skin to mimic normal make-up [2].

Tattooists usually inject colorants as a suspension into the skin using solid needles, which are actuated by tattoo machines. Tattooists purchase black colorants from tattoo suppliers or through the internet. A fraction of the injected colorant stays in the dermis as particles, and their light absorption within a specific spectral range results in the color of the tattoo. Another fraction of the injected colorant is removed from the skin via the lymphatic or blood vessel systems. As a result, tattoo colorants can be found in the lymph nodes located next to the tattoo [3–6]. An internet-based survey showed that about 60% of tattoos are either completely or partly black [7].

Chemistry of Tattoo Colorants and the Related Health Concerns

From a chemical point of view, colorants are classified as either pigments or dyes; however, the chemical structures of pigment and dye molecules are frequently the same. In contrast to dyes, pigments are practically insoluble in the medium in which they are incorporated, and this insolubility is achieved by avoiding solubilizing groups in the molecules, yielding small particles, the so-called pigments. Pigments may be inorganic or organic, colored, white or black materials.

Thus, making a persistent tattoo in skin requires the use of water-insoluble colorants in the form of pigments. In the past, tattooists used inorganic pigments that contained heavy metals such as mercury, chromium or cadmium, resulting in the typical colors yellow (cadmium sulfide), mercury sulfide (red), or chromium oxide (green). Two important inorganic pigments are still in use: Carbon Black for black tattoos and titanium dioxide to reduce the color strength of colored pigments.

Nowadays, colored tattoo colorants mainly consist of organic pigments like azo or polycyclic pigments, which are usually obtained from the chemical industry [8]. These pigments comprise two features perfect for use in tattoos: the pigments exhibit brilliant colors, and they are insoluble in aqueous tissue. The chemistry of black inks, which predominantly contain Carbon Black, has not changed over time. Carbon Black is a powder that mainly comprises amorphous particles of carbon with diameters of a few tenths of nanometers (fig. 1).

Although they are injected into the human body, tattoo colorants usually have no pharmaceutical requirements. Beside the coloring compound (black, red, green, blue, etc.), the colorants may contain other various substances depending on the production methods. The colorants comprise educts, products, and by-products of the respective coloring compound [9]. Different solvents (water, isopropanol, etc.) are used to dissolve the pigment powder, other substances are applied as preservatives, and titanium dioxide is frequently added to change the color strength [8, 10]. Tattoo colorants might also contain various impurities that accidentally got into colorants for unknown reasons. Thus, tattoo colorants usually exhibit a complex mixture of various chemical compounds [11–13]. At present, the list of identified admixtures and impurities is rather incomplete, and further chemical analysis of the tattoo colorants that are present in the market is required. It is known that the chemistries for colored and black tattoo colorants are rather different, and hence, the colorants may contain different by-products and impurities [8, 11].

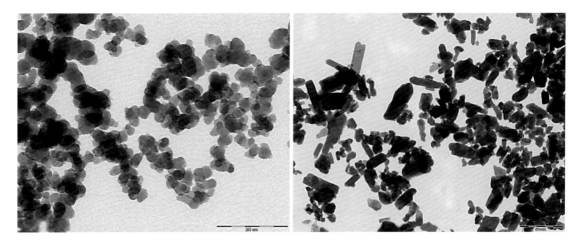

Fig. 1. Electron microscopy images showing the details of commercially available tattoo colorants. The black colorant is comprised of rounded particles (left), whereas red azo pigments (PR22) have a more elongated shape (right). The mean diameter of the particles is in the range of several tenths of nanometers.

Colored Pigments

Colored pigments are classified by their chemical constitution and can be roughly assigned to azo or polycyclic pigments. Pigments are identified either by their chemical index number or by the pigment shortcut. The azo pigments are subdivided in mono-azo (greenish to medium yellow, reddish yellow to orange), dis-azo (greenish, reddish to orange red), β-naphtol (orange to medium red), naphtol AS (medium red to violet) and metal complex pigments containing nickel, copper or cobalt. The polycyclic pigments are generally condensed aromatic or heterocyclic ring systems. Two important examples are the phthalocyanines (green, blue) and the quinacridone pigments (bluish red, red, violet) [8]. The production of such pigments requires complex chemical synthesis, and the resulting colorant may contain different educts, products and by-products as well as titanium dioxide, to lighten the colorant, and different concentrations of other non-specified compounds.

Colored tattoo pigments like PR.22 can be decomposed by solar radiation [14, 15] or by laser light [16], yielding decomposition products such as 2-methyl-5-nitroaniline (2,5-MNA), 4-nitrotoluene (4-NT), 2,5-dichloroaniline (2,5-DCA) and 1,4-dichlorobenzene (1,4-DCB) (fig. 1). 4-NT was genotoxic in a human lymphocyte assay [17], and 2,5-MNA, also referred to as 5-nitro-*o*-toluidine, was shown to cause liver dysfunction in workers from a hair dye factory [18]. Additionally, Sayama et al. [19] showed that 2,5-MNA and some dinitrotoluenes are mutagenic to *Salmonella typhimurium* YG. Furthermore, 1,4-DCB induced kidney tumors in male rats and liver tumors in male and female mice [20], whereas 2,5-DCA was nephrotoxic in rats [21].

Black Colorants

Black colorants are usually produced by the imperfect combustion of hydrocarbons, yielding soot with polycyclic aromatic hydrocarbons (PAHs). The major constituent of black tattoo colorants is Carbon Black, which has been listed by the International Agency of Research in Cancer (IARC) as possibly carcinogenic to humans (group 2B) [22]. High amounts of hazardous PAHs, up to 201 μg/g, were found when analyzing different commercially available black tattoo colorants [11]. PAH molecules are either unbound in the colorant suspension or are attached to the surface of Carbon Black particles. PAHs such as benzo[a]pyrene belong to a large class of well-studied chemical pollutants that ubiquitously occur in the environment. They consist of two or more fused benzene rings and are generated naturally or are found as a result of incomplete combustion of organic materials, fossil fuels, vehicular emissions or even tobacco smoke. Some PAHs are classified by the IARC as human carcinogens (e.g., benzo[a]pyrene), and several others are classified as probably or possibly carcinogenic to humans [23]. The active metabolite benzo[a]pyrene-7,8-diol-9,10-epoxide probably represents the ultimate carcinogen [24].

It is well known that human exposure to complex mixtures of PAHs occurs primarily through three routes: the respiratory tract through the smoking of tobacco products and the inhalation of polluted air, the gastrointestinal tract through the ingestion of contaminated drinking water and food, and skin contact, which usually occurs from occupational exposure [25].

In contrast to topical coal tar application and possible penetration into skin, black colorants are injected into skin during the making of a black tattoo, resulting in an almost complete penetration of PAHs into the skin, after which the substances can distribute throughout the entire body. In addition to their carcinogenic properties, PAHs exert a wide range of deleterious effects towards tissue and cells, including the mutagenesis of oncogenes in skin [26]. PAHs are thus potent immunotoxic agents that impair the functional activation of lymphocytes [27] and inhibit macrophage differentiation [28]. Other analytical investigations revealed the presence of additional hazard substances, such as the softener di-buthyl-phthalate [29]. Another problem may arise from the fact that the particles have small diameters of tenths of nanometers [30]. Thus, the potential of the particles for nanotoxicology should be investigated [31].

Consequently, the skin might react to either colored or black ink suspensions in different manners. Many side effects of tattoos, such as granulomatous, lichenoid or hypersensitive allergic reactions, infections, and malignant skin tumors, have been described in the medical literature [2, 12, 13, 32]; however, the latter might be coincidental [33].

Tattoo Colorants in Skin

In the western world, most tattooists inject tattoo colorants into skin using the rapidly vibrating needles of a tattoo machine to transport a certain amount of colorant suspension into the skin. The needles thereby leave punctures in the skin that pierce the thin epidermis and may reach the middle of the dermis (fig. 2, left). Experiments with pig and human skin revealed the concentration of, e.g., red pigment, that is placed in skin by such tattoo machines. As tattooing is an archaic procedure, the experiments yielded a concentration range of about 0.60–9.42 mg of pigment per cm^2 of tattooed skin [34]. The concentrations depended on the size of the pigment crystals, the concentration of pigment applied to the skin surface, the desired color strength of the tattoo, and the tattooing procedure using needles of different sizes and shapes. The mean value was estimated to be about 2.5 mg/cm^2.

Tattooing damages the skin, causing pain and superficial bleeding. In an internet-based survey, tattooed people reported crust formation, itching, swelling and even superficial infections during the healing process [7]. Being a superficial injury to the skin, the tattooed area should heal within a couple of days. However, the survey also revealed that 8% of the participants still had health problems 4 weeks after tattooing, and 6% had persistent skin problems in the tattooed area. Additionally, 3% stated other health problems such as psychiatric problems and light sensitivity of the tattooed skin. These problems were significantly related to the color of the tattoo, which obviously meant that they were related to the specific chemistry of the colorant. This finding was confirmed by comparing the data of that survey with medical case reports

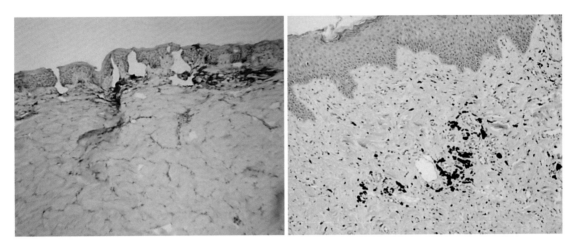

Fig. 2. Pig skin tattooed with a red-colored pigment (left). The histology shows the color in the superficial dermis and that the tattooing needles left holes in the skin. A punch biopsy was taken from black-tattooed skin (right). The histological slice shows black particles in the dermis. Only large agglomerates of pigments can be detected in the histology using light microscopy at a spatial resolution of about 0.5 μm. Regardless of the place of injection, the pigment particles move to different sites within the dermis by carriers such as macrophages.

on the location and color of tattoos. The results clearly showed that colored tattoo pigments, in particular red pigments, are mainly responsible for adverse skin reactions and that these reactions occur more often on the extremities [12, 13].

After tattooing skin, pigment particles are exclusively found in the cytoplasm of cells in membrane-bound structures identified as secondary lysosomes [35]. Also, macrophages may contain pigment particles. At first view, the injected tattoo colorants seem to stay in skin forever. However, three major mechanisms may reduce the concentration of colorants that is initially placed in the skin. First, part of the colorant may leave the skin with the bleeding during or directly after tattooing. Second, part of the colorant may be transported away from the skin via the lymphatic or blood vessel system. Third, part of the colorant is decomposed months or years after tattooing because the pigments in the dermis are repeatedly exposed to different light sources, in particular, solar radiation, including UV radiation. Azo pigments are chemically unstable when exposed to UV radiation [14, 15].

Recent investigations provided evidence that the major part of tattoo colorants, such as red pigments (87–99%), disappears from skin months or years after tattooing [36], which could cause a fading of the colored skin. However, when asking tattooed people, almost nobody perceives a change in the tattoo color [7]. The change in the color concentration can be overlooked because of the very high color strength of azo pigments. The decrease in the pigment concentration appears to be very high; however, an in vivo animal model showed that about 30% of intradermally injected PR22 disappeared from skin within 6 weeks after tattooing [37], and up to 60% of tattooed PR22 disappeared when applying excess solar radiation to the animal skin [37]. Thus, the disappearance of such a high fraction of the tattooed pigments is a result of either light-induced decomposition in tattooed skin or pigment transport to other anatomical locations in the body via the lymphatic system.

For example, black tattoo colorants frequently contain substantial amounts of PAHs [11], and enzymatic and non-enzymatic pathways can convert PAHs into hazardous diol-epoxides, such as benz[a]pyrene-7,8-diol-9,10-epoxide [38]. Both pathways might also occur in tattooed skin. First, cytochrome P450-dependent enzymes can be triggered by injecting foreign material, such as tattoo ink, into skin [39]. Second, PAHs in tattooed skin generate singlet oxygen when exposed to UV radiation, leading to oxidation of the PAHs. Akintobi et al. showed the induction of cytochrome P450 1B1 (CYP1B1) expression in human dermal fibroblasts when exposed to xenobiotic substances like 2,3,7,8-tetrachlorodibenzo-p-dioxin [40]. Recent studies have shown that CYP1B1, a newly identified member of the CYP1 family, plays a very important role in the metabolic activation of PAHs [41, 42]. Whether such cytochrome P450-dependent enzymes also play a role in tattooed skin has not been investigated.

Thus, educts, by-products, impurities, and admixtures can be punctured into skin to an unknown extent during tattooing. These compounds may cause various adverse skin reactions, which have been consistently published in the literature [12, 43]. Also, case reports about skin tumors from tattoos have been published and summarized in a recent review article [33]. However, it is still under discussion whether the malignancies, including basal cell carcinoma [44] or malignant melanoma, were coincident.

Transport of Tattoo Colorants to Other Anatomical Sites

Tattoo colorants are a rather complex mixture of various compounds that exhibit different chemical and physical structures. The colorants contain pigment particles of different sizes and molecules, and many of the molecules are in the form of monomers, dimers, or polymers with different solubilities, which influences the extent and the route of transport inside the dermis and to other organs. In addition to transport, some constituents of the colorants can be metabolized in skin or

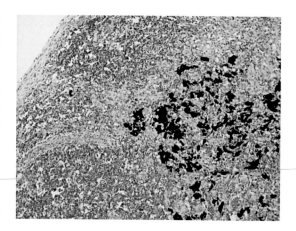

Fig. 3. A histological slice showing black colorant particles in a lymph node located in the axilla.

in the organs to which the compounds were transported. Thus, tattooing of colorants into skin entails a complex reaction of the skin that triggers the immune system and launches manifold transport processes.

After injection into skin, some of the tattoo pigment particles are encapsulated in the dermis. As mentioned above, the colorants can be transported to other anatomical locations in the body via the blood vessel and lymphatic systems directly after tattooing or via the lymphatic system years or months after tattooing. In particular, a portion of the small particles, admixtures, impurities, as well as educts and products of the pigment molecules may leave the skin directly or during the weeks after tattooing. These transportable compounds have the potential to reach other anatomical locations and might be stored in other organs or may leave the human body via the urinary system or defecation. Thus, organs such as liver, spleen and kidney could be destinations of constituents of tattoo colorants, depending on the route of transport via the lymphatic or blood vessel systems. Consequently, after tattooing the skin, the injected colorants may pose a risk to other organs in the human body. However, except for the transport of tattoo colorants to the lymph nodes (fig. 3) [3, 4, 45–48], all other transport processes and routes in a human body have been unexplored.

It is assumed that especially large particles, which cannot pass the lymph nodes, stay in the dermis. Thus, any process that reduces the size of the particles will assist in reducing the concentration of pigment particles in skin. A major mechanism for disintegration of the particles is the light-induced decomposition of pigment molecules that may continuously occur whenever tattooed skin is exposed to light sources [14]. Other mechanisms, like enzymatic activities or the recurring activation of macrophages, might contribute to pigment particle transport. However, the contribution of other mechanisms is unknown.

There are currently no indications regarding the systemic effects of tattoo colorants and of their decomposition products because scientific investigations or epidemiologic data are lacking. Millions of people have many and large tattoos [7], with sizes of 600 cm^2 and more. In cases of such tattoos, about 1,500 mg of, e.g., azo pigments are injected into the human body. In light of the 80% decrease, one should deliberate about whether 1,200 mg of azo pigments and their possible decomposition products could cause health problems in the skin or in the rest of the human body.

In the case of black colorants, substantial amounts of PAHs are injected into skin and hence should be partially transported to other organs.

This is of great importance because those PAHs might cause deleterious effects elsewhere in the human body. Recently, placental concentrations of PAHs were analyzed by gas chromatography-mass spectrometry. PAH concentrations above the median, as detected in some cases, were associated with a 4.52-fold increased risk for neural tube defects, a 5.84-fold increased risk for anencephaly, and a 3.71-fold increased risk for spina bifida [49]. PAHs are an important class of environmentally prevalent xenobiotics that can activate oxidative and electrophilic signaling pathways in lymphoid and non-lymphoid cells, including myeloid, epithelial, and other cells [50]. Beside toxicity and mutagenicity [23, 51], PAHs, including the non-classified PAHs such as phenanthrene, are also known to cause immunotoxic effects, particularly IgE regulation [52].

In conclusion, millions of people worldwide have tattoos, for which high amounts of tattoo colorants are injected into the human body. A recent survey revealed that 28% of tattooed individuals have more than four tattoos and that 36% have tattoos that are larger than 900 cm^2, implying that several grams of tattoo colorants have been injected into skin. Any systemic effects of tattoo colorants, which are administered via tattooing, have not been investigated; thus, we highly recommend performing pharmacological, toxicological and epidemiological studies to clarify the possible impact of tattooing on human health.

References

1 Dorfer L, Moser M, Bahr F, Spindler K, Egarter-Vigl E, Giullen S, Dohr G, Kenner T: A medical report from the stone age? Lancet 1999;354:1023–1025.
2 Ortiz AE, Alster TS: Rising concern over cosmetic tattoos. Dermatol Surg 2012; 38:424–429.
3 Soran A, Kanbour-Shakir A, Bas O, Bonaventura M: A tattoo pigmented node and breast cancer. Bratisl Lek Listy 2014;115:311–312.
4 Balasubramanian I, Burke JP, Condon E: Painful, pigmented lymphadenopathy secondary to decorative tattooing. Am J Emerg Med 2013;31:1001.e1–e2.
5 Yactor AR, Michell MN, Koch MS, Leete TG, Shah ZA, Carter BW: Percutaneous tattoo pigment simulating calcific deposits in axillary lymph nodes. Proc (Bayl Univ Med Cent) 2013;26:28–29.
6 Peterson SL, Lee LA, Ozer K, Fitzpatrick JE: Tattoo pigment interpreted as lymph node metastasis in a case of subungual melanoma. Hand (N Y) 2008;3:282–285.
7 Klugl I, Hiller KA, Landthaler M, Bäumler W: Incidence of health problems associated with tattooed skin: a nationwide survey in German-speaking countries. Dermatology 2010;221:43–50.

8 Baumler W, Eibler ET, Hohenleutner U, Sens B, Sauer J, Landthaler M: Q-switch laser and tattoo pigments: first results of the chemical and photophysical analysis of 41 compounds. Lasers Surg Med 2000;26:13–21.

9 Timko AL, Miller CH, Johnson FB, Ross E: In vitro quantitative chemical analysis of tattoo pigments. Arch Dermatol 2001; 137:143–147.

10 Papameletiou D, Zenie A, Schwela D, Bäumler W: Risks and health effects from tattoos, body piercing and related practices. http://gesundheit-nds.de/downloads/risksandhealth.pdf, 2003 (accessed January 14, 2015).

11 Regensburger J, Lehner K, Maisch T, Vasold R, Santarelli F, Engel E, Gollmer A, Konig B, Landthaler M, Bäumler W: Tattoo inks contain polycyclic aromatic hydrocarbons that additionally generate deleterious singlet oxygen. Exp Dermatol 2010;19:e275–e281.

12 Wenzel SM, Rittmann I, Landthaler M, Bäumler W: Adverse reactions after tattooing: review of the literature and comparison to results of a survey. Dermatology 2013;226:138–147.

13 Serup J, Hutton Carlsen K: Patch test study of 90 patients with tattoo reactions: negative outcome of allergy patch test to baseline batteries and culprit inks suggests allergen(s) are generated in the skin through haptenization. Contact Dermatitis 2014;71:255–263.

14 Engel E, Spannberger A, Vasold R, Konig B, Landthaler M, Bäumler W: Photochemical cleavage of a tattoo pigment by UVB radiation or natural sunlight. J Dtsch Dermatol Ges 2007;5:583–589.

15 Cui Y, Spann AP, Couch LH, Gopee NV, Evans FE, Churchwell MI, Williams LD, Doerge DR, Howard PC: Photodecomposition of pigment yellow 74, a pigment used in tattoo inks. Photochem Photobiol 2004;80:175–184.

16 Vasold R, Naarmann N, Ulirch H, Fischer D, König B, Landthaler M, Bäumler W: Tattoo pigments are cleaved by laser light – the chemical analysis in vitro evidence for hazardous compounds. Photochem Photobiol 2004;80:185–190.

17 Huang QG, Kong LR, Liu YB, Wang LS: Relationships between molecular structure and chromosomal aberrations in in vitro human lymphocytes induced by substituted nitrobenzenes. Bull Environ Contam Toxicol 1996;57:349–353.

18 Shimizu H, Kumada T, Nakano S, Kiriyama S, Sone Y, Honda T, Watanabe K, Nakano I, Fukuda Y, Hayakawa T: Liver dysfunction among workers handling 5-nitro-o-toluidine. Gut 2002;50:266–270.

19 Sayama M, Mori M, Shoji M, Uda S, Kakikawa M, Kondo T, Kodaira KI: Mutagenicities of 2,4- and 2,6-dinitrotoluenes and their reduced products in salmonella typhimurium nitroreductase- and o-acetyltransferase-overproducing ames test strains. Mutat Res 1998;420:27–32.

20 National Toxicology Program: Toxicology and carcinogenesis studies of 1,4-dichlorobenzene (cas no. 106–46–7) in f344/n rats and b6c3f1 mice (gavage studies). Natl Toxicol Program Tech Rep Ser 1987;319:1–198.

21 Lo HH, Brown PI, Rankin GO: Acute nephrotoxicity induced by isomeric dichloroanilines in Fischer 344 rats. Toxicology 1990;63:215–231.

22 IARC: Carbon Black; in IARC Monographs on the Evaluation of Carcinogenic Risks to Humans. Volume 93: Carbon Black, Titanium Dioxide, and Talc. Lyon, International Agency for Research on Cancer, 2010. http://monographs.iarc.fr/ENG/Monographs/vol93/mono93.pdf (accessed January 14, 2015).

23 IARC: IARC Monographs on the Evaluation of Carcinogenic Risks to Humans. Volume 92: Some Non-Heterocyclic Polycyclic Aromatic Hydrocarbons and Some Related Exposures. Lyon, International Agency for Research on Cancer, 2010. http://monographs.iarc.fr/ENG/Monographs/vol92/mono92.pdf (accessed January 14, 2015).

24 Koreeda M, Moore PD, Wislocki PG, Levin W, Yagi H, Jerina DM: Binding of benzo[a]pyrene 7,8-diol-9,10-epoxides to DNA, RNA, and protein of mouse skin occurs with high stereoselectivity. Science 1978;199:778–781.

25 Newman MJ, Light BA, Weston A, Tollurud D, Clark JL, Mann DL, Blackmon JP, Harris CC: Detection and characterization of human serum antibodies to polycyclic aromatic hydrocarbon diol-epoxide DNA adducts. J Clin Invest 1988;82:145–153.

26 Bizub D, Wood AW, Skalka AM: Mutagenesis of the ha-ras oncogene in mouse skin tumors induced by polycyclic aromatic hydrocarbons. Proc Natl Acad Sci U S A 1986;83:6048–6052.

27 Davila DR, Romero DL, Burchiel SW: Human t cells are highly sensitive to suppression of mitogenesis by polycyclic aromatic hydrocarbons and this effect is differentially reversed by alpha-naphthoflavone. Toxicol Appl Pharmacol 1996;139:333–341.

28 van Grevenynghe J, Rion S, Le Ferrec E, Le Vee M, Amiot L, Fauchet R, Fardel O: Polycyclic aromatic hydrocarbons inhibit differentiation of human monocytes into macrophages. J Immunol 2003;170:2374–2381.

29 Lehner K, Santarelli F, Vasold R, Konig B, Landthaler M, Baumler W: Black tattoo inks are a source of problematic substances such as dibutyl phthalate. Contact Dermatitis 2011;65:231–238.

30 Hogsberg T, Loeschner K, Lof D, Serup J: Tattoo inks in general usage contain nanoparticles. Br J Dermatol 2011;165:1210–1218.

31 Zhang M, Jin J, Chang YN, Chang X, Xing G: Toxicological properties of nanomaterials. J Nanosci Nanotechnol 2014;14:717–729.

32 Varga E, Korom I, Varga J, Kohan J, Kemeny L, Olah J: Melanoma and melanocytic nevi in decorative tattoos: three case reports. J Cutan Pathol 2011;38:994–998.

33 Kluger N, Koljonen V: Tattoos, inks, and cancer. Lancet Oncol 2012;13:e161–e168.

34 Engel E, Santarelli F, Vasold R, Maisch T, Ulrich H, Prantl L, Konig B, Landthaler M, Baumler W: Modern tattoos cause high concentrations of hazardous pigments in skin. Contact Dermatitis 2008; 58:228–233.

35 Ferguson JE, Andrew SM, Jones CJ, August PJ: The q-switched neodymium:Yag laser and tattoos: a microscopic analysis of laser-tattoo interactions. Br J Dermatol 1997;137:405–410.

36 Lehner K, Santarelli F, Penning R, Vasold R, Engel E, Maisch T, Gastl K, Konig B, Landthaler M, Bäumler W: The decrease of pigment concentration in red tattooed skin years after tattooing. J Eur Acad Dermatol Venereol 2011;25:1340–1345.

37 Engel E, Vasold R, Santarelli F, Maisch T, Gopee NV, Howard PC, Landthaler M, Bäumler W: Tattooing of skin results in transportation and light-induced decomposition of tattoo pigments – a first quantification in vivo using a mouse model. Exp Dermatol 2010;19:54–60.

38 Gelboin HV: Benzo[alpha]pyrene metabolism, activation and carcinogenesis: role and regulation of mixed-function oxidases and related enzymes. Physiol Rev 1980;60:1107–1166.

39 Moraitis AG, Hewison M, Collins M, Anaya C, Holick MF: Hypercalcemia associated with mineral oil-induced sclerosing paraffinomas. Endocr Pract 2013;19:e50–e56.

40 Akintobi AM, Villano CM, White LA: 2,3,7,8-tetrachlorodibenzo-p-dioxin (tcdd) exposure of normal human dermal fibroblasts results in ahr-dependent and -independent changes in gene expression. Toxicol Appl Pharmacol 2007; 220:9–17.

41 Shimada T, Fujii-Kuriyama Y: Metabolic activation of polycyclic aromatic hydrocarbons to carcinogens by cytochromes p450 1a1 and 1b1. Cancer Sci 2004;95: 1–6.

42 Buters JT, Sakai S, Richter T, Pineau T, Alexander DL, Savas U, Doehmer J, Ward JM, Jefcoate CR, Gonzalez FJ: Cytochrome p450 cyp1b1 determines susceptibility to 7, 12-dimethylbenz[a]anthracene-induced lymphomas. Proc Natl Acad Sci U S A 1999;96:1977–1982.

43 Kaur RR, Kirby W, Maibach H: Cutaneous allergic reactions to tattoo ink. J Cosmet Dermatol 2009;8:295–300.

44 Engel E, Ulrich H, Vasold R, Konig B, Landthaler M, Suttinger R, Baumler W: Azo pigments and a basal cell carcinoma at the thumb. Dermatology 2008;216: 76–80.

45 Jaigirdar AA, Yeh MW, Sharifi E, Browne LW, Leong SP: Coexisting tattoo pigment and metastatic melanoma in the same sentinel lymph node. J Cutan Med Surg 2009;13:321–325.

46 Dominguez E, Alegre V, Garcia-Melgares ML, Laguna C, Martin B, Sanchez JL, Oliver V: Tattoo pigment in two lymph nodes in a patient with melanoma. J Eur Acad Dermatol Venereol 2008;22:101–102.

47 Honegger MM, Hesseltine SM, Gross JD, Singer C, Cohen JM: Tattoo pigment mimicking axillary lymph node calcifications on mammography. AJR Am J Roentgenol 2004;183:831–832.

48 Schlager A, Laser A, Melamed J, Guth AA: A tattoo-pigmented node masquerading as the sentinel node in a case of breast cancer. Breast J 2008;14:299–300.

49 Ren A, Qiu X, Jin L, Ma J, Li Z, Zhang L, Zhu H, Finnell RH, Zhu T: Association of selected persistent organic pollutants in the placenta with the risk of neural tube defects. Proc Natl Acad Sci U S A 2011;108:12770–12775.

50 Burchiel SW, Luster MI: Signaling by environmental polycyclic aromatic hydrocarbons in human lymphocytes. Clin Immunol 2001;98:2–10.

51 EC-SCF: Polycyclic aromatic hydrocarbons – occurrence in foods, dietary exposure and health effects. SCF/CS/CNTM/PAH/29 ADD1. 2002. http://ec.europa.eu/food/fs/sc/scf/out154_en.pdf (accessed January 14, 2015).

52 Tsien A, Diaz-Sanchez D, Ma J, Saxon A: The organic component of diesel exhaust particles and phenanthrene, a major polyaromatic hydrocarbon constituent, enhances ige production by ige-secreting ebv-transformed human b cells in vitro. Toxicol Appl Pharmacol 1997;142:256–263.

Prof. Dr. Wolfgang Bäumler
Department of Dermatology, University of Regensburg
DE–93042 Regensburg (Germany)
E-Mail baeumler.wolfgang@klinik.uni-regensburg.de

Serup J, Kluger N, Bäumler W (eds): Tattooed Skin and Health.
Curr Probl Dermatol. Basel, Karger, 2015, vol 48, pp 185–189 (DOI: 10.1159/000369224)

Towards the Limiting of Health Risks Associated with Tattooing: Whitelists for Tattoo Pigments and Preservatives

Annegret Blume · Thomas Platzek · Bärbel Vieth ·
Christoph Hutzler · Andreas Luch

German Federal Institute for Risk Assessment (BfR), Department of Chemicals and Product Safety,
Berlin, Germany

Abstract

The number of pigments that could potentially be used in tattoo inks is vast. However, pigments are generally not manufactured for the purpose of being injected into subepidermal layers of the skin. Assuming 100% bioavailability after injection means that pigments can be imminently hazardous to human health. Given the ever-increasing number of pigments being circulated on the market or through the internet, a 'negative list' ('black' list) containing pigments with known adverse effects will never be finalised. If incriminated, substances could easily be replaced by structurally similar pigments that might be even more deleterious to human health. Therefore, we and others suggest the establishment of a whitelist ('positive list') that would only contain pigments that had undergone a risk assessment specifically for their application into the dermis. Some of the problems associated with such a 'positive list' are discussed. Another important issue with regard to tattoo safety is related to the preservatives used in ink preparations. Notwithstanding the demand for sterile tattoo inks, a whitelist for these compounds would be beneficial. At present, many technical preservatives are being used, despite their known detrimental effects to human health. Criteria for the inclusion of preservatives in a 'positive list' are also discussed.

© 2015 S. Karger AG, Basel

Pigments

According to Colour Index International, which is jointly published by the British Society of Dyers and Colourists (UK) and the American Association of Textile Chemists and Colorists (US) and which serves as standard library for the identification of pigments, about 27,000 products residing under more than 13,000 generic colour index names are used for the manufacturing of colours [1]. To be suitable for tattoo inks, a pigment must display light-fastness, a certain degree of resistance to ultraviolet light, brilliance and equal distribution in suspension. These requirements are met only by a subset of all pigments, but the number of pigments that might be applicable for tattoo inks is still large. Pigments are not specifically manufactured for use in tattoo inks. Instead, pigments initially manufactured for use in paints, plastics, glazes or other applications are being included in viscous ink formulations for insertion into the skin, more specifically, into the upper layer of the dermis right beneath the epidermis. To do so, pricking needles that penetrate the natural (epidermal) skin barrier are used.

The pigments being discussed are not specifically manufactured for any kind of application in the human body. Hence, the raw materials used for their production are not controlled with regard to contamination or other chemical hazards. Consequently, carcinogenic polycyclic aromatic hydrocarbons or nitrosamines and allergenic substances like nickel are frequently reported to be present in tattoo inks [2]. In particular, the 'modern practice' of applying organic pigments in tattoo inks is not usually backed-up by minimal toxicity testing. Yet, toxicity data for certain pigments are available and thus can be utilised for health risk assessment purposes. Some of these data have previously been compiled into a list of colours that should not be used in tattoo inks ('negative list') [3].

Currently, there is no authoritative European regulation on tattoo inks; however, some member states of the European Union have set up their own national legislations that are mostly based on resolution ResAP(2008)1 of the Council of Europe in Strasbourg [3]. ResAP(2008)1 includes a list of pigments that should not be included in tattoo inks ('negative list') as well as provisions stating that pigments that are prohibited or restricted from cosmetic products and that are listed in Annexes II and IV of the European Regulation (EC) No. 1223/2009 on Cosmetic Products should not be contained in tattoo inks [4]. Usually, these annexes are compiled based on existing toxicological data that have been fed into the corresponding risk assessments by expert groups. As a prerequisite for the risk assessment of cosmetic ingredients, a dossier summarising the related toxicological data has to be provided by the industry. However, it should be noted that the majority of substances on the list of cosmetic colourants (Annex IV of Regulation 1223/2009) have not undergone a recent safety assessment.

Given the great number of pigments on the market, 'negative lists' and restrictions cannot and do not cover all potentially problematic pigments; furthermore, effectively regulating hazardous colourants based on 'negative lists' is not feasible. First, the inclusion of a pigment in a 'negative list' would require further substantiation, usually via assessing toxicological data. However, it currently remains unclear who would be in charge of delivering such data. Industry certainly would have no interest in delivering the data due to the lack of any additional benefit from the prohibited compounds and pigments that would fill such black lists. On the other hand, it seems equally questionable to address the taxpayer when it comes to the funding of research that, after all, would ultimately back-up the commercialisation of non-listed alternatives by private companies. Second, the prohibition of one pigment might easily pave the way for structurally similar pigments of equally questionable toxicology. An example of this is provided by phthalocyanine 'Pigment Green 7' (CI 74260; see fig. 1). According to ResAP(2008)1, this pigment should not be a part of tattoo inks because its use is restricted in EU Regulation (EC) No. 1223/2009 (Annex IV, no. 107, 'not to be used in eye products'). The very similar substance 'Pigment Green 36' (CI 74265; see fig. 1), however, is not present in any of the above-mentioned lists and therefore remains currently unrestricted with regard to tattoo inks. Accordingly, 'Pigment Green 7' is currently being substituted by 'Pigment Green 36' on the market. When analysing the structures of both compounds, it becomes evident that the chlorine substituents of Pigment Green 7 have just been replaced by bromine in Pigment Green 36 (6 of 16). Since there was only an exchange from one halogen to another, it seems reasonable to expect that

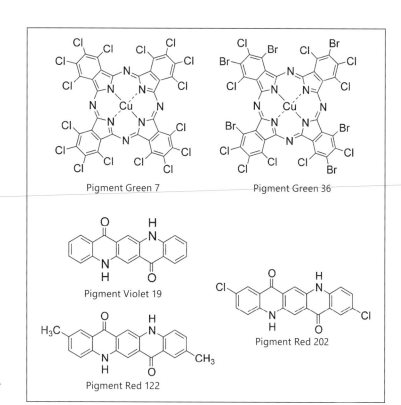

Fig. 1. Comparison between structurally similar phthalocyanine and quinacridone pigments.

Pigment Green 7

Pigment Green 36

Pigment Violet 19

Pigment Red 202

Pigment Red 122

both compounds would not differ much in terms of their toxicological properties. It might even be possible that the latter compound would actually show increased potential as a health hazard. Another example is provided by the quinacridones 'Pigment Violet 19' (CI 73900) and 'Pigment Red 122' (CI 73915), both of which are restricted from use according to EU Regulation (EC) No. 1223/2009 (Annex IV, no. 102, 103 'rinse-off products'). These compounds have been replaced by 'Pigment Red 202' (CI 73907), which carries two chlorine substituents instead of hydrogen or methyl groups (fig. 1).

Although 'negative lists' of pigments and other compounds prohibiting their use in tattoo inks might be helpful to some extent, 'positive lists' are now clearly favoured by experts in light of the issues described above. The establishment of whitelists would require submission of dossiers

compiling toxicological data, which could then be assessed regarding the potential health risks of the pigments by expert committees. Pigments that pass the risk assessment procedure with no or only little concern could then be included in such a list. This course of action has been generally followed in the cosmetics sector in the EU. Interested companies or, in some cases, industry consortia supply the required toxicological data, and the Scientific Committee on Consumer Safety (SCCS) of the EU commission takes the task of evaluating the dossiers for health issues. It is expected that 'positive lists' would provide higher levels of safety when compared to 'negative lists'. However, different from the situation in the cosmetics sector, manufacturers of tattoo inks are mostly small companies that presumably would have difficulties paying for all of the requested toxicological and analytical data, especially if new experiments have to be conducted to fill knowledge gaps. On the other hand, the manufacturers of pigments are mostly large, often international companies that are likely to be in a (financial) position to afford the research. For these companies, however, the market dealing with tattoo pigments simply represents a 'much-too-small segment' of their portfolio; therefore, they usually refuse to get involved in the safety discussion and evaluation process. Even existing data might not be disclosed because pigment manufacturers, in principal, do not endorse the use of their pigments for the purpose of tattooing. The questions of how to overcome these difficulties and of how to ensure that the pigments used in tattoo inks do not pose a risk to consumers still exist.

According to tattoo ink manufacturers, about 15–20 pigments would be sufficient to satisfy the demands on the market for preparing all shades of tattoo inks imaginable (personal communication, Ralf Michel, Tattoo Ink Manufacturers of Europe). A pragmatic approach would be for tattoo ink manufacturers to form a consortium that would focus on drafting a comprehensive list of indispensable pigments to be assessed for possible health issues. The costs of data compilation – which certainly should be manageable for 15–20 substances – could be shared among all members of the consortium. Subsequently, all prepared dossiers could then be evaluated by a committee of experts similar to the SCCS. Data specific for application of the pigments into skin would have to be included, and in most cases, newly generated data, such as studies on biokinetics (e.g. distribution of pigments or tattoo ink ingredients throughout the body), will probably have to be included. Therefore, another important aspect has to be considered: although tattoo inks are not by any means comparable to cosmetic products, the prohibition of animal experiments for the testing of cosmetic ingredients has begun to cast a shadow over the necessary research on the biokinetics of tattoo ink ingredients in the living body. At present, it is difficult to predict how this will affect and

interfere with research on tattoo inks. However, tattooed individuals are not a minority anymore, and these data have to be provided somehow to ensure the safety of consumers.

Preservatives

According to ResAP(2008)1, inks used for tattoos and permanent make-up should be 'sterile and supplied in a container which maintains the sterility of the product until application, preferably in a packaging size appropriate for single use. In case multi-use containers are used, their design should ensure that the contents will not be contaminated during the period of use'. The resolution also specifies that 'preservatives should only be used to ensure the preservation of the product after opening and by no means as a correction of insufficient microbiologic purity in the course of manufacture and of inadequate hygiene in tattooing and PMU (permanent make-up) practice' and that they 'should only be used after a safety assessment and in the lowest effective concentration' [3]. Based on market surveillance, e.g. in Switzerland and Germany, it is known that tattoo inks usually contain preservatives [5, 6]. These compounds belong to two categories: (1) preservatives that are included in a 'positive list' for use in cosmetics (Annex V of EU-Regulation 1223/2009) and that have been approved after a risk assessment by the SCCS or its predecessor committees for use on the skin; and (2) technical preservatives that have not been approved for safe use on skin and/or have never been intended for use in tattoo inks. Examples of this second category include substances like benzisothiazolinone or octylisothiazolinone, both of which are strong sensitisers, or the corrosive phenol. Again, candidate preservatives are numerous, and a 'negative list' would hardly be adequate to ensure that the health of the consumer would not be adversely affected by tattoo inks.

However, even preservatives in category 1, which, as ingredients of cosmetic products, have been approved for use on the skin, are not necessarily safe for injection into the skin. The latter would occur once they become ingredients of tattoo inks. Yet, at least some toxicological data for these substances that can provide some kind of grounding for the compilation of a whitelist of preservatives to be used in tattoo inks exist. Still, some substances listed in Annex V of the EU cosmetics regulation (i.e. preservatives allowed in cosmetic products) are certainly not suitable for the purpose of tattooing, including:

- mercury-containing preservatives (e.g. thiomersal, phenylmercury and phenylmercury salts)
- substances with a high sensitization potency (e.g. Kathon CG, formaldehyde, glutaraldehyde)
- formaldehyde-releasing substances
- substances for which specific limits are effective or for which a warning must be included on the label according to cosmetics regulations
- corrosive or irritating substances
- triclosan

- iodopropinylbutyl carbamate.

The remaining substances listed in Annex V would still need to undergo a systematic risk assessment for the application route 'injection into the skin' in order to be eligible to become part of a 'positive list' of preservatives for tattoo inks. With Annex V as the basis, the number of potential candidates is still limited, thus enabling risk assessment based on the data that are already available in conjunction with the supplementary toxicokinetics data.

In conclusion, although it is useful in the short term to ban some of the most harmful substances, 'negative lists' will always be incomplete. Although the compilation of 'positive lists' requires a huge effort by both industry and authorities and might not be possible within a short time frame, these lists seem indispensable for providing the highest level of safety possible. This also holds true for the safety of tattoo inks and for the protection of consumers against any adverse health effects that might occur immediately after the process of tattooing or over the long term.

References

1 Society of Dyers and Colorists (SDC) and American Association of Textile Chemists and Colorists (AATCC), Color Index, 1924, 4th edition online, last accessed Jan 9, 2015. http://www.sdc.org.uk/technical-services/colour-index/.

2 Gesundheitsdepartement des Kantons Basel-Stadt, Bereich Gesundheitsschutz, Kantonales Laboratorium, Jahresbericht (annual report) 2009. 2009, p. 75, last accessed Jan 9, 2015. http://www.gesundheitsschutz.bs.ch/konsum-umwelt/berichte/jahresberichte.html.

3 Council of Europe, Committee of Ministers, Resolution ResAP(2008)1 on requirements and criteria for the safety of tattoos and permanent make-up, adopted on 20 Feb 2008, last accessed Jan 9, 2015. http://www.coe.int/t/e/social_cohesion/soc-sp/ResAP_2008_1%20E.pdf.

4 The European Parliament and the Council of the European Union, Regulation (EC) No 1223/2009 of the European parliament and of the Council of November 30 2009 on cosmetic products, 2009, last accessed Jan 9, 2015. http://eur-lex.europa.eu/LexUriServ/LexUriServ.do?uri=OJ:L:2009:342:0059:0209:EN:PDF.

5 Bundesamt für Verbraucherschutz und Lebensmittel (BVL), Berichte zur Lebensmittelsicherheit 2007, 2007, p.75, last accessed Jan 9, 2015. http://www.bvl.bund.de/SharedDocs/Downloads/01_Lebensmittel/02_BUEp_dokumente/buep_berichte_archiv/BUEp_Bericht_2007.pdf?__blob=publicationFile&v=5.

6 Gesundheitsdepartement des Kantons Basel-Stadt, Bereich Gesundheitsschutz, Kantonales Labor, Urs Hauri, Tinten für Permanent Make Up (PMU) und zur Tätowierung / Organische Pigmente, Konservierungsmittel, Verunreinigungen (Nitrosamine, Polyaromatische Kohlenwasserstoffe (PAK), Aromatische Amine), 2012, last accessed Jan 9, 2015. http://www.gesundheitsschutz.bs.ch/konsum-umwelt/berichte/2012.html#page_section3_section2.

Annegret Blume
German Federal Institute for Risk Assessment (BfR)
Department of Chemicals and Product Safety
Max-Dohrn-Strasse 8–10
DE–10589 Berlin (Germany)
E-Mail annegret.blume@bfr.bund.de

Serup J, Kluger N, Bäumler W (eds): Tattooed Skin and Health.
Curr Probl Dermatol. Basel, Karger, 2015, vol 48, pp 190–195 (DOI: 10.1159/000369226)

Survey of Studies on Microbial Contamination of Marketed Tattoo Inks

Lucia Bonadonna

National Institute of Health, Rome, Italy

Abstract

Tattooing became a popular phenomenon during the late twentieth century. Because the act of tattooing involves repeated injection of ink through the skin, a risk of contracting infections from contaminated tattooing equipment and ink and the surrounding environment exists. Progress has been made in infection control strategies; however, contraction of bacterial and viral infections from tattooing continues to occur. The risk of acquiring a tattoo-related infection largely depends on the hygiene conditions under which the tattoo is applied. Nevertheless, even when adequate hygiene and sanitation measures are taken, the inks themselves may contain infectious microorganisms that are able to survive under hostile conditions, such as in inks. The results of the few studies on the microbiological quality of unopened and opened tattoo inks are reported. Some authors' conclusions demonstrated that the current ink sterilisation systems show a low capability to inactivate microbial contamination in tattoo inks. At the moment, European Resolution ResAP2008–1 recommends that the ink be sterile and supplied in containers that maintain the sterility of the product until application. In light of the outcomes of published studies, at the moment, preservation of the microbial quality and safety of ink seems challenging and still difficult to reach. © 2015 S. Karger AG, Basel

In the last few decades, tattoos have become trendy and socially acceptable, especially among adolescents and young adults, and information regarding the prevalence of tattooing among these categories of people continues to be widespread.

In recent years, infectious diseases transmitted through the practice of tattooing seem to have decreased with the step-up of professional tattoo studios and the adoption of safety measures. However, this technique is not devoid of potential adverse effects, and numerous cases of cutaneous and systemic infectious complications following tattooing are still reported [1, 2].

Infectious disease can be transmitted as the exogenous pigments and/or dyes penetrate the dermis and come into contact with both capillaries and lymph vessels. The risk of acquiring a tattoo-related infection largely depends on the hygiene conditions under which the tattoo is applied, and secondary infections of the tattoo lesions can also occur during the healing process.

Nevertheless, even when adequate hygiene and sanitation measures are taken, the inks themselves may contain infectious microorganisms, which together with the diluents and instruments, are effectively often referred to as the putative agents of tattoo-related infections [3].

Contamination may occur at various points in the ink-production process due to unsanitary manufacturing processes or use of contaminated ingredients and containers.

The actual epidemiology of tattoo-related infections is not known. In fact, it is difficult to determine the true incidence of tattoo-related infections because late, retrospective investigations are commonly conducted. Furthermore, the real incidence of infective complications after tattooing is definitely not known because most subjects choose to return to the tattoo parlour rather than consulting their own physician. In the majority of cases, it is not possible to relate the aetiological agent and the specific cause of infection; namely, it is not possible to demonstrate a cause-effect relationship. That is often due to different factors: (i) analytical investigation of the products (needles, inks, etc.) generally takes place with a delay with respect to the notification of infection; (ii) it is difficult to demonstrate an unequivocal relationship between a product and an infection, and (iii) microbiological cultural analyses of tattoo inks are complex because these products represent a very hostile environment for most microorganisms.

An Internet survey on the possible health risks associated with tattoos reported that people described skin problems (67.5%), systemic reactions (6.6%), fever directly after tattooing (1.1%), and pus-filled tattoo lesions (0.4%), which are health problems that might be associated with bacterial infections [4].

The introduction of tattoo inks into the skin has been associated with the potential entry of a great number of microorganisms, including bacteria, viruses, and fungi. *Streptococcus pyogenes*, methicillin-resistant *Staphylococcus aureus, Pseudomonas aeruginosa*, and non-tuberculous mycobacteria are often reported as bacterial aetiological agents of tattoo-related infections. In addition to local infections, increasing numbers of cases of systemic infections following professional tattoo-ing have been reported, including polymicrobial septicaemia, cases of endocarditis associated with tattooing in patients with congenital heart failure, and mycoses [5–9].

Several outbreaks of non-tuberculous mycobacterial infections in tattoo parlours, especially due to *Mycobacterium chelonae*, have been reported during the past few years. In these cases, the source of infection was presumed to be tap water, and the tattooist was subsequently instructed to use only sterile water for solution and dye preparation [10, 11].

Tattoos also represent a known risk factor for certain viral infections, such as hepatitis B and C and human immunodeficiency virus infections, although, epidemiologically, this risk factor is not considered to be statistically relevant. Both skin infection caused by the human papillomavirus and molluscum contagiosum following tattoo application have also been reported. Fungal infections due to *Trichophyton rubrum* and *Epidermophyton floccosum* have also been associated with tattoos [12–16].

Infection may also occur in the case of severe immunodeficiency, as illustrated by a lethal case of *echtyma gangrenosum* in a young patient with acute leukaemia [17].

As mentioned, in most cases, tattoo-related infections are caused by improper use of hygiene regimens, but sometimes pigments, diluents, and instruments can also be contaminated. Despite claims of sterility, opened and even sealed stock bottles of tattoo ink may contain microorganisms that are pathogenic for humans [18].

In the literature, very few data have been published on microorganisms present in tattoo inks and pigments in opened/unopened containers.

In 2004, a brand of a tattoo ink was removed from the market: *P. aeruginosa* and the mould *Acremonium* sp. were the ink contaminants [19].

A follow-up report after the introduction of the European Resolution ResAP2008–1 verified that 3% of inks from tattoo parlours were microbiologically contaminated [20].

Kluger and colleagues conducted bacteriological analyses on 16 tattoo inks that had previously been opened and were at that moment in use. None of the samples showed microbial or fungal growth, even if the authors did not exclude the possibility of ink contamination during the manufacturing process [21].

In total, 145 tattoo pigments (39 unopened and 106 in use) have been bacteriologically analysed. In most cases, contaminations were in a low concentration range (10^1–10^2 CFU/ml). Higher counts (10^3–10^8 CFU/ml) were recorded in four samples. Among the 31 isolated bacterial species, 64.5% were Gram-positive rods, 25.8% were Gram-positive cocci, and 9.7% were Gram-negative rods. Pathogens were never detected [22].

Similarly, a study conducted in Denmark on 58 original tattoo inks proved microbial contamination of unopened stock bottles in 10% of the examined samples, and only one out of six in-use samples (17%) showed microbial growth. Microbial concentrations ranged from 100 bacteria/ml to 650 bacteria/ml, whilst yeast and moulds were never detected. Environmental bacteria and potentially pathogenic bacteria were also identified: *Pseudomonas* sp., *Aeromonas* sp., *Staphylococcus* sp., *Enterococcus faecium*, *Streptococcus sanguinis*, *Streptococcus salivarius*, and *Acinetobacter* sp. These three last strains were recovered from both opened and unopened ink bottles [23].

In the USA, non-tuberculous mycobacteria have often been detected in both opened and unopened bottles of ink. In most cases, non-sterile water, used as a diluent of the ink, was reported as responsible for the contamination because of the ubiquitous nature of mycobacteria [24].

Analytical controls conducted by the author and colleagues examined the microbial product safety of a total of 34 sealed and opened tattoo inks. Only three inks were not contaminated, whilst 86% of the unopened inks showed microbial growth. Different bacterial species were detected, and the concentration range (from 1 to >1,000 CFU/ml) was very wide. Moulds were detected at lower concentrations than bacteria. Many species had a strictly environmental origin, but some of them were opportunistic pathogens (e.g., *Neosartorya hiratsukae*). As was predicted, most of the identified microbial strains were represented by highly resistant environmental microorganisms. A prevalence of endospore-forming bacteria (e.g., different species of *Bacillus*); anaerobic, spore-forming bacteria; and aerobic, spore-forming bacteria, such as *Alicyclobacillus acidocaldarius*, were cultured from the sealed inks. Most of the strains isolated from the opened tattoo inks belonged instead to the cutaneous human microbiome (e.g., *Staphylococcus* sp.) [25].

The Food and Drug Administration has published advice related to recalling lots of tattoo inks and tattoo needles due to pathogenic bacterial contamination. From the tattoo kits (inks and needles), a variety of potentially pathogenic organisms were isolated and identified, including Gram-negative bacteria and Gram-positive rods and cocci. In particular, *Bacillus* sp., *Sphingomonas paucimobilis*, *Micrococcus luteus*, *Corynebacterium* sp., and species belonging to the genus *Clostridium* were identified [26].

The sterility of manufactured inks has recently been questioned [27]. In national and European frameworks, the lack of specific regulation requiring ink sterility control has disallowed the assessment of the infectious risk to public health. In contrast, in the USA, under the Federal Food, Drug, and Cosmetic Act, tattoo inks are considered to be cosmetics, whereas the pigments used in the inks are colour additives that require pre-marketing approval. This law requires that cosmetics and their ingredients not be adulterated or misbranded, which means that they cannot contain poisonous or deleterious substances or unapproved colour additives, be manufactured or held under unsanitary conditions, or be falsely labelled. Furthermore, cosmetic manufacturers are supposed to ensure the safety of a product before marketing it.

Table 1. Notifications of microbial tattoo ink contamination reported by RAPEX

Year	Notifying country	Risk
2006	France	*Moraxella, Staphylococcus warneri*
2007	The Netherlands	*P. aeruginosa* 1,500 CFU/ml
2007	Germany	Mesophiles, total bacteria 7.71×10^5 CFU/g
2008	Germany	Mesophiles, total bacteria 8.1×10^7 CFU/g, *P. aeruginosa*
		Mesophiles, total bacteria 3.6×10^6 CFU/g, *P. aeruginosa*
		1.1×10^6 CFU/g, yeast 9×10^5 CFU/g
2009	The Netherlands	*Pseudomonas*: 41 contaminated inks
2010	Italy	General microbial risk

In fact, tattooing is subject to little control regarding both ink production/sterilisation and tattooing practices in order to ensure the consumers' health. In table 1, the advice of RAPEX, the European rapid alert system, on the microbial risk associated with tattooing products is reported. The few notifications are probably due to scarce microbiological controls executed by European laboratories [28].

In the last decade, two recommendations have been made by the Council of Europe regarding the safety of tattooing. ResAP2003–2 [29] established that tattoo products had to be manufactured in sterile single-use containers without preservatives, while ResAP2008–1 [30] subsequently legalised the use of preservatives and multi-use containers, without providing appropriate details on sterilisation and preservation modalities. Furthermore, national regulations can greatly vary. According to ResAP2008–1, tattoo inks should be sterilised before marketing. Both beta and gamma radiations are generally suitable for sterilisation. This sterilisation technology is widely used in many countries and enables products, including their packaging, to be sterilised without altering their organoleptic, physical, and chemical characteristics. The main difference between beta and gamma radiations lies in their material penetration and their dose rates (beta rays: high dose rate and limited penetration depth; gamma rays: high penetration capability and relatively low dose

rate). Both types of ionising radiation should destroy the DNA of microorganisms, thus inactivating them. Radiation resistance varies widely among different microorganisms, and this is related to differences in their chemical and physical structures as well as in their ability to recover from radiation injury. The radiation technology is considered safe, reliable, and highly effective. As recommended by the International Organization for Standardization [31], the sterilisation dose must be set for each type of product depending on its bioburden, and the manufacturer has the responsibility of identifying the sterilisation dose.

Nevertheless, it is recognised that the sterility of an individual item in a population of sterilised products cannot be ensured in the absolute sense.

According to the Pharmacopeia [32], for products to be considered sterilised, the sterility assurance level (SAL) is accepted. Since achievement of the absolute state of sterility cannot be demonstrated, the sterility of a product can be defined only in terms of probability. Thus, the SAL is the probability that not more than one viable microorganism is present in an amount of one million sterilised items of the final product (SAL 10^{-6}). The probability of microbial survival is a function of the number and species of microorganisms present in the product (bioburden), the sterilisation process lethality, and the type of product submitted to sterilisation treatment.

The sterility process needs well-planned quality control to ensure that irradiation reaches the inner part of the product, killing microorganisms and preventing their ability to recover from radiation injury. It is evident, therefore, that understanding the specific nature of radiation is important in order to properly use this sterilisation technique in practice.

Most bacterial isolates in the mentioned studies had particular resistance capability (e.g., *Bacillus* sp.), which is also true for moulds able to survive under unfavourable environmental conditions.

In light of the data reported in the literature and in view of a revision of the European principles on tattooing, in order to obtain reliable results, it is important to highlight that microbiological quality control should contemplate the use of appropriate microbial parameters and valid analytical methods.

References

1 Kazandjieva J, Tsankov N: Tattoos: dermatological complications. Clin Dermatol 2007;25:375–382.

2 Kaatz M, Elsner P, Bauer A: Body-modifying concepts and dermatologic problems: tattooing and piercing. Clin Dermatol 2008;26:35–44.

3 Kennedy BS, Bedard B, Younge M, Tuttle D, Ammerman E, Ricci J, Doniger AS, Escuyer VE, Mitchell K, Noble-Wang JA, O'Connell HA, Lanier WA, Katz LM, Betts RF, Mercurio MG, Scott GA, Lewis MA, Goldgeie MH: Outbreak of *Mycobacterium chelonae* infection associated with tattoo ink. N Engl J Med 2012;367:1020–1024.

4 Klügl I, Hiller KA, Landthaler M, Bäumler W: Incidence of health problems associated with tattooed skin: a nationwide survey in German-speaking countries. Dermatology 2010;221:43–50.

5 Korman TM, Grayson ML, Turnidge JD: Polymicrobial septicaemia with *Pseudomonas aeruginosa* and *Streptococcus pyogenes* following traditional tattooing. J Infect 1997;35:203.

6 Mathur DR, Sahoo A: *Pseudomonas* septicaemia following tribal tattoo marks. Trop Geogr Med 1984;36:301–302.

7 Charnack C: Tattooing dyes and pigments contaminated with bacteria. Tidsskr Nor Laegeforen 2004;124:2278.

8 Kluger N, Muller C, Gral N: Atypical mycobacteria infection following tattooing: review of an outbreak in 8 patients in a French tattoo parlor. Arch Dermatol 2008;144:941–942.

9 Wolf R, Wolf DA: Tattooed butterfly as a vector of atypical Mycobacteria. J Am Acad Dermatol 2003;48:S73–S74.

10 Falsey RR, Kinzer MH, Hurst S, Kalus A, Pottinger PS, Duchin JS, Zhang J, Noble-Wang J, Shinohara MM: Cutaneous inoculation of nontuberculous mycobacteria during professional tattooing: a case series and epidemiologic study. Clin Infect Dis 2013;57:e143–e147.

11 Kay MK, Perti TR, Duchin JS: Tattoo-associated *Mycobacterium haemophilum* skin infection in immunocompetent adult, 2009. Emerg Infect Dis 2011; 17:1734–1736.

12 Rosario Pac M, Arnedo A, Montaner MD, Prieto P, García J, Izuel M, León P, López JA, Echevarría JM: Epidemic outbreak of hepatitis B from the tattoo in gypsy families. Rev Esp Salud Publica 1996;70:63–69.

13 Limentani AE, Elliott LM, Noah ND, Lamborn JK: An outbreak of hepatitis B from tattooing. Lancet 1979;2:86–88.

14 Miller DM, Brodell RT: Verruca restricted to the areas of black dye within a tattoo. Arch Dermatol 1994;130:1453–1454.

15 Pérez Gala S, Alonso Pérez A, Ríos Buceta L, Aragüés Montañés M, García Díez A: Molluscum contagiosum on a multicoloured tattoo. J Eur Acad Dermatol Venereol 2006;20:221–222.

16 Salmaso F, Gnecchi L, Gianotti R, Veraldi S: Molluscum contagiosum on a tattoo. Acta Derm Venereol 2001;81:146–147.

17 Tendas A, Niscola P, Barbati R, Abruzzese E, Cuppelli L, Giovannini M, Scaramucci L, Fratoni S, Ales M, Neri B, Morino L, Dentamaro T, De Fabritiis P: Tattoo related pyoderma/ectyma gangrenous as presenting feature of relapsed acute myeloid leukaemia: an exceptionally rare observation. Injury 2011;42:546–547.

18 Le Blanc PM, Hollinger KA, Klontz KC: Tattoo ink – related infections – awareness, diagnosis, reporting, and prevention. N Engl J Med 2012;367:985–987.

19 Harp BP: FDA: tattoos and permanent makeup. 2009. http://learningcenter. nsta.org/products/symposia_seminars/ fall09/fda/files/WS4–12–17–09.ppt (accessed September 29, 2014).

20 Swiss Confederation: Conformity of tattooing- and permanent make-up-colours not satisfied. 2006. http://ctl-tattoo.net/FOPH-Report_tattoo-colours_control-campaign.pdf (accessed September 29, 2014).

21 Kluger N, Terru D, Godreuil S: Bacteriological and fungal survey of commercial tattoo inks used in daily practice in a tattoo parlor. J Eur Acad Dermatol Venereol 2011;25:1230–1231.

22 Baumgartner A, Gautsch S: Hygienic-microbiological quality of tattoo- and permanent make-up colours. J Verbrauch Lebensmitt 2011;6:319–325.

23 Høgsberg T, Saunte DM, Frimodt-Møller N, Serup J: Microbial status and product labelling of 58 original tattoo inks. J Eur Acad Dermatol Venereol 2013;27:73–80.

24 Kennedy BS, Bedard B, Younge M, Tuttle D, Ammerman E, Ricci J, Doniger AS, Escuyer VE, Mitchell K, Noble-Wang JA, O'Connell HA, Lanier WA, Katz LM, Betts RF, Mercurio MG, Scott GA, Lewis MA, Goldgeier MH: Outbreak of *Mycobacterium chelonae* infection associated with tattoo ink. N Engl J Med 2012;367:1020–1024.

25 Bonadonna L, Briancesco R, Coccia A, Fonda A, Meloni P, Semproni M: Microbiological quality and product labelling of tattoo inks. Proceedings 1st European Congress on Tattoo and Pigment Research, Copenhagen, November 13–14, 2013.

26 U.S. Food and Drug Administration: Voluntary nationwide recall of tattoo ink, tattoo needles, tattoo kits due to microbial contamination. 2014. http://www.fda.gov/Safety/Recalls/ucm405474.htm (accessed September 29, 2014).

27 Centers for Disease Control and Prevention (CDC): Tattoo-associated nontuberculous mycobacterial skin infections – multiple states, 2001–2012. Morb Mortal Wkly Rep 2012;61:653–656.

28 European Commission: Health and consumers. RAPEX notification. 2014. http://ec.europa.eu/consumers/archive/safety/rapex/index_en.htm (accessed September 29, 2014).

29 Council of Europe, Committee of Ministers: Resolution ResAP (2003)2 on Tattoos and Permanent Make-Up. Strasbourg, France, Council of Europe, 2003.

30 Council of Europe, Committee of Ministers: Resolution ResAP (2008)1 on Requirements and Criteria for the Safety of Tattoos and Permanent Make-Up (Superseding Resolution ResAP(2003)2 on Tattoos and Permanent Make-Up). Strasbourg, France, Council of Europe, 2008.

31 ISO 11137–1:2006/Amd1:2013. Sterilization of health care products – Radiation – Part 1: Requirements for development, validation and routine control of a sterilization process for medical devices. Geneva, Switzerland, International Organization for Standardization, 2013.

32 European Directorate for the Quality of Medicines, Council of Europe: European Pharmacopoeia, ed 8. Strasbourg, France, Council of Europe, 2014.

Lucia Bonadonna
Istituto Superiore di Sanità
Viale Regina Elena, 299
IT–00161 Rome (Italy)
E-Mail lucia.bonadonna@iss.it

Serup J, Kluger N, Bäumler W (eds): Tattooed Skin and Health.
Curr Probl Dermatol. Basel, Karger, 2015, vol 48, pp 196–200 (DOI: 10.1159/000369227)

The European Landscape of National Regulations of Tattoo Inks and Businesses

Peter Laux · Andreas Luch

German Federal Institute for Risk Assessment (BfR), Department of Chemicals and Product Safety,
Berlin, Germany

Abstract

A rising number of tattooed people in all parts of society and increasing concerns regarding potential health effects triggered the development of specific regulatory measures at the beginning of the 21st century. The first principles considering chemical safety and hygienic aspects were laid down by two resolutions of the Council of Europe, in 2003 and 2008. The applied principle of 'negative lists' of substances that should not be used in tattoo inks has subsequently been transferred to national regulations. However, surveillance data show that in particular, the chemical quality of tattoo inks is still insufficient. The reasons are, amongst others, the lack of analytical methods, the implementation of different thresholds, and the lack of awareness of distributors and producers when it comes to potential health hazards.

As tattooing was originally a practice limited to certain groups in Western society, the development of specific regulatory measures for tattooing started relatively late. Before this millennium, specific regulations were in place only in a few European countries. In Denmark, for example, a law from the year 1966 [1] prohibited tattooing of the head, hands, or neck. In the UK, the 'Tattooing of Minors Act' in 1969 [2] prohibited tattooing of persons under the age of 18 years. In the Netherlands, hepatitis B outbreaks in the 1980s were traced back to unacceptable hygienic conditions in tattoo parlours and led to the first guidelines for the prevention of infections [3]. Minimum ages and hygienic standards were also set in a number of other European countries [4] as a basic instrument for the protection of consumer health. Apart of these basic requirements, the safety of tattoo inks, representing diverse mixtures of substances that may reach the blood and lymph, has so far been the responsibility of the manufacturer or distributor. Because of their main purpose of beautification, tattoo inks are legally considered as products of daily use according to the General Product Safety Directive [5].

However, the rising popularity of tattoos in Europe has increased awareness of governmental bodies towards potential health hazards, such as microbes and potentially toxic substances, that might be present in tattoo inks. As a result, the European Commission has started to assess the safety of tattoos [4], and two resolutions of the Council of Europe on requirements and criteria for the safety of tattoos and permanent make-up were published: that is, ResAP(2003)2 [6] and the revised ResAP(2008)1 [7]. Already in ResAP(2003)2, substances that should not be present in tattoo inks are listed. Besides carcinogenic aromatic amines, these negative lists include a range of harmful pigments and solvents. The resolution further references the European Directives for Cosmetics [8] and Dangerous Substances [9]. Accordingly, substances forbidden or restricted in cosmetic products or classified as carcinogenic, mutagenic, or reprotoxic are not allowed for use in tattoo inks. In addition to these chemical requirements, Resolution ResAP(2003)2 postulates that tattoo inks should not contain preservatives, must be sterile until use, and should be supplied in packaging for single use only. The revised resolution ResAP(2008)1 has superseded ResAP(2003)2 and has introduced maximum allowed concentrations of 13 elements, including cadmium (0.2 ppm), nickel (as low as reasonably achievable), and lead (2 ppm). Polycyclic aromatic hydrocarbons (PAHs) are considered in general, with a limit for benzo[a] pyrene of 5 ppb and a general threshold of 0.5 ppm, without further specification of the kind of PAHs to be measured. Neither for elements nor for PAHs are analytical methods provided, making the application of uniform criteria difficult. According to ResAP(2008)1, tattoo inks have to fulfil the same purity criteria as colours in foodstuffs [10]. Furthermore, *para*-phenylenediamine was added to the 'negative list' of substances. Whereas preservatives were banned for use in tattoo inks according to the first resolution, they became allowed by ResAP(2008)1, but not just

for compensation for insufficient sterility. Both resolutions provide a basis for national regulations; however, they are not legally binding. Furthermore, not all member states have signed up; while ResAP(2003)2 has been worked out by 18 member states, only 16 contributed to ResAP(2008)1. The requirements laid down in these documents were adopted in national regulations in The Netherlands [11], France [12], Slovenia [13], Germany [14], Norway [15], Sweden [16], Spain [17], and Switzerland [18]. In the following, the specifics of the different national regulations, aside from the common requirements given above, are described. In The Netherlands, national legislation based on ResAP(2003)2 was established in 2003 [11]. Additionally, in 2007 an implementation guideline [19] was adopted, setting age limits and prohibiting the tattooing of certain body parts. Market surveillance of tattoo inks in 2013 comprised 701 selectively sampled red, yellow, orange, and green tattoo inks and revealed exceedance of the limits for aromatic amines and elements in 30 and 12%, respectively, of all samples. In France, national legislation on tattoo safety was introduced as part of a law on public health in 2004 [20]. Chemical requirements were adopted according to ResAP(2008)1 in 2013 [12]. Furthermore, the EU Ecolabel criteria applied to textile products were also assigned to tattoo inks [21], thus excluding the use of dyes with harmful properties. Tattoo inks also must not contain carcinogenic azo dyes or aromatic amines, in accordance with an opinion of the Scientific Committee on Cosmetic Products and Non-Food Products that refers to cosmetics [22]. The French vigilance programme [23] on tattoo products has been ongoing since 2008 and involves obligations for professional tattoo artists and medical personnel to give notification of undesirable and serious side effects. For consumers, such a notification of unwanted effects is only voluntary. Furthermore, chemical analysis of 52 tattoo inks in 2012 revealed nonconformity for 7 samples due to elevated levels of o-anisidine, barium, or bacterial contamination. In Switzerland, national regulation of piercing, tattooing, permanent make-up, and related practices came into effect on January 1, 2014, as a part of a decree on items for human contact. Its principles were adapted from ResAP(2003)2 and ResAP(2008)1. Similar to both resolutions' reference to the European Directive for Cosmetics, the Swiss regulation references an equivalent national regulation [24]. However, in contrast to ResAP(2008)1, there are currently no maximum levels defined for antimony and nickel. In Switzerland, surveillance programmes are conducted on a regular basis. In 2013 [25], a total of 60 tattoo inks and permanent make-up samples were investigated, of which 39 (65%) were objectionable, and 33 were banned from further use. The reasons were inaccurate declaration, use of forbidden colourants or preservatives, detection of N-nitrosamines and PAHs, threshold exceedance for preservatives, and the presence of aromatic amines. Among them, two samples contained very high concentrations, or 32 and 84 mg/kg for the total of all (23) PAHs measured. With regard to the 8 carcinogenic PAHs considered in risk characterisation by the European Food Safety Authority, concentrations of 6.6 and 4 mg/kg, respectively, were measured. In Germany, a national regulation based on the principles of ResAP(2008)1 has been effective since May 1, 2009. The requirements are similar to those of ResAP(2008)1, with the exception of CI Solvent Yellow 14 (Sudan I), which is also being excluded from use by the German regulation. A federal surveillance programme on tattoo inks, targeting preservatives and heavy metals, was conducted in 2007 [26]. Out of 782 samples tested for preservatives, positive results were reported in 53 cases. Among the identified compounds were 1,2-benzisothiazolone, benzoic acid, and 2-methyl-4-isothiazolin-3-one. Furthermore, 878 samples were investigated according to the 13 elements mentioned in ResAP(2008)1, and the highest concentrations were found for copper,

iron, chromium, and zinc, with mean concentrations of 4,652, 79.2, 29.5, and 16.3 mg/kg, respectively. A monitoring programme in 2013 investigated 250 coloured and 129 black tattoo inks for its nickel contents. This allergen was found in 54.8 and 21.7%, respectively, of the samples, with maximum concentrations of 65.1 and 60 mg/kg, respectively. In Norway, a regulation assuming the principles of ResAP(2003)2 came into force on January 1, 2009 [15]. As a further regulatory measure, only 26 preservatives with supposedly low sensitisation potential are allowed. These substances have been selected through safety assessment and subsequent elimination of certain substances, such as triclosan, Kathon CG, and formaldehyde, from the 'positive list' of preservatives given in the EU Cosmetics Directive. The list has been suggested by Norway to the Committee of Experts on Cosmetic Products [27] but has not been implemented on the European level yet. A surveillance programme on tattoo inks has been ongoing since 2011. In 2013, 25 out of 35 products tested in total contained prohibited aromatic amines. In Sweden, national legislation on tattoo inks [28] that adopted the principles of ResAP(2008)1 came into force on August 1, 2012. An associated regulation [16] came into effect on February 1, 2013. The Swedish legislation is being enforced by the local municipalities and has predominantly revealed a lack of labelling as well as open questions regarding the legal use of certain pigments. The national regulation in Slovenia is equivalent to ResAP(2008)1 and came into force on January 2, 2010, as part of the regulation of sanitary and health requirements [13]. A survey on 34 tattoo inks in 2010 revealed element concentrations in 12 samples beyond the thresholds given in resolution ResAP(2008)1. Metals exceeding these limits were barium, copper, cadmium, and lead, with maximum concentrations of 900, 3,400, 0.38, and 18 mg/kg, respectively. Nickel was found in all 34 samples at concentrations of up to 3.1 mg/kg. In Spain, tattoo inks are covered by the national regulation of cosmetics

[29]. In 2008, the principles of ResAP(2008)1 were adopted, and tattoo inks have to be approved by the Spanish Agency for Medicines and Health Products on the basis of toxicological and quality data supplied by the distributor [17]. Approved products are included in a registry. In addition to these national requirements, there are regional regulations in the different Spanish provinces regarding hygiene requirements, registration of tattoo studios, and necessary qualification of tattoo artists. In Denmark, there is currently no regulation of tattooing. However, the Danish Ministry of the Environment published a recommendation on the safety of tattoo ink in 2014 [30]. The chemical parameters are similar to those in ResAP(2008)1 but are further modified in certain aspects. Aniline, a primary aromatic amine found in tattoo inks on the Danish market [31], was added to the list of forbidden substances. For the group of PAHs, the single compound benzo[a]pyrene is considered, with a threshold of 0.2 ppm, and an additive threshold of 2 ppm is assigned to benzo[e]pyrene, benz[a]anthracene, chrysene, dibenz[a,h]anthracene, and three isomeric benzofluoranthenes. For lead, a maximum content of 10 ppm is given; other elements are not included. The recommendation contains further practical guidance on how to realise correct labelling, sterility testing, and expiry date setting. In the appendix of the document, guidelines for a safety assessment of tattoo inks, including exemplary calculations of a systemic exposure dosage and the margin of safety, are provided.

Summarising the efforts on national regulations of tattooing in European countries, there has been some progress in a limited number of countries since the first resolution was issued by the Council of Europe in 2003. However, also in these countries, implementation is currently suffering from insufficient analytical methods as well as from limited data on biokinetics and the toxicity of tattoo inks and their ingredients. However, most European countries remain without such a specific regulation at all. In light of the rising popularity of tattooing throughout Europe and the associated risks to human health, this situation actually is unacceptable. Thus, an initiative by both regulators and scientists at the international level appears to be quite urgent in order to overcome current scientific gaps and limited knowledge and to achieve a common protective regulation in all European countries.

References

1 Lov om tatovering. Lovtidende for Kongeriget Danmark 1966, Afdeling A 1966;194:310.
2 Tattooing of Minors Act. Her Majesty's Stationery Office, 1969.
3 Worp J, Boonstra A, Coutinho RA, van den Hoek JA: Tattooing, permanent makeup and piercing in Amsterdam; guidelines, legislation and monitoring. Euro Surveill 2006;11:34–36.
4 Papameletiou D, Schwela D, Zenie A: Workshop on 'Technical/Scientific and Regulatory Issues on the Safety of Tattoos, Body Piercing and Related Practices'. Ispra, European Commission, 2003.
5 Directive 2001/95/EC of the European Parliament and of the Council of 3 December 2001 on general product safety (Text with EEA relevance). Official Journal of the European Communities 2002;L11:4–17.
6 Council of Europe: Resolution ResAP(2003)2 on Tattoos and Permanent Make-Up. Strasbourg, France, Council of Europe, 2003.
7 Council of Europe: Resolution ResAP(2008)1 on Requirements and Criteria for the Safety of Tattoos and Permanent Make-Up (Superseding Resolution ResAP(2003)2 on Tattoos and Permanent Make-Up). Strasbourg, France, Council of Europe, 2008.
8 Council of the European Communities: Council Directive of 27 July 1976 on the Approximation of the Laws of the Member States Relating to Cosmetic Products (76/768/EEC). Brussels, Belgium, European Commission, 1976.
9 Council of the European Communities: Council directive of 27 June 1967 on the approximation of laws, regulations and administrative provisions relating to the classification, packaging and labelling of dangerous substances (67/548/EEC). Official Journal of the European Communities 1967;196:234–255.

10 Commission of the European Communities: Commission Directive 95/45/EC of 26 July 1995 Laying Down Specific Purity Criteria Concerning Colours for Use in Foodstuffs. Official Journal 1995;L226:1–45.

11 Besluit van 14 augustus 2003 tot het stellen van regels betreffende de veiligheid van tatoeagekleurstoffen (Warenwetbesluit tatoeagekleurstoffen). Staatsblad van het Koninkrijk der Nederlanden 2003;342:1–14.

12 Arêté du 6 mars 2013 fixant la liste des substances qui ne peuvent pas entrer dans la composition des produits de tatouage. Journal Officiel de la République Francaise 2013; 0061:4404 (NOR:AFSP1306308A).

13 Rules on minimal sanitary and health requirements for hygiene care and other similar establishments 2009. Official Gazette of the Republic of Slovenia 2009; 104.

14 Verordnung über Mittel zum Tätowieren Einschliesslich Bestimmter Vergleichbarer Stoffe und Zubereitungen aus Stoffen (Tätowiermittel-Verordnung). Bundesministerium der Justiz und fur Verbraucherschutz, 2008.

15 Forskrift for Produksjon, Import og Omsetning mv. av Tatoveringsprodukter og Andre Produkter til Injisering i Huden i Kosmetisk Hensikt. Norsk Lovtidend, 2008, booklet 12.

16 Läkemedelsverkets föreskrifter (LVFS 2012:25) om tatueringsfärger; beslutade den 19 december 2012. Läkemedelsverkets författningssamling LVFS 2012:25.

17 Información Sobre Productos para Maquillaje Permanente (Micropigmentación) y Tatuaje. Agencia Espanola de Medicamentos y Productos Sanitarios, 2008.

18 Verordnung über Gegenstände für den Humankontakt, 817.023.41. Das Eidgenossische Departement des Innern (EDI), 2005.

19 Regeling van de minister van Volksgezondheit. Welzijnen Sport van 9 mei 2007, nr. VGP/PSL 2766859, houdende de aanwijzing van Veiligheidcodes voor het tatoeeren en piercen (Warenwetregeling aanwijzing veiligheidscodes tatoeeren en piercen) Staatscourant 2007;93:26.

20 LOI n° 2004-806 du 9 août 2004 relative à la politique de santé publique (1). Journal Officiel de la République Francaise 2004;185:14277 (NOR: SANX0300055L).

21 Commission Decision of 15 May 2002 establishing the ecological criteria for the award of the community eco-label to textile products and amending Decision 1999/178/EC (2002/371/EC). Official Journal of the European Communities 2002;L133:29–41.

22 Opinion of the Scientific Committee on Cosmetic Products and Non-Food Products Intended for Consumers Concerning the Safety Review of the Use of Certain Azo-Dyes in Cosmetic Products, SCCNFP/0495/01, final2002. SCCNFP, 2002.

23 Décret n° 2008–210 du 3 mars 2008 fixant les règles de fabrication, de conditionnement et d'importation des produits de tatouage, instituant un système national de vigilance et modifiant le code de la santé publique (dispositions réglementaires), NOR: SJSP0766088D2008. Paris, 2008.

24 Verordnung des EDI Über Kosmetische Mittel, in 817.023.31. Das Eidgenossische Departement des Innern (EDI), 2012.

25 Hauri U: Tinten für Permanent Make Up (PMU) und zur Tätowierung/Organische Pigmente, Konservierungsmittel, Verunreinigungen (Nitrosamine, Polyaromatische Kohlenwasserstoffe (PAK), Aromatische Amine). Bereich Gesundheitsschutz, Gesundheitsdepartement des Kantons Basel-Stadt, Kantonales Labor, 2012.

26 Droß A: Schwermetalle und konservierungsstoffe in mitteln zum tätowieren; in Brandt P (ed): Berichte zur Lebensmittelsicherheit 2007: Bundesweiter Überwachungsplan 2007. Basel, Birkhäuser Basel, 2008, pp 76–78.

27 Norwegian Initial List of Preservatives that could be Allowed in Tattooing Products. The Norwegian Delegation of the Council of Europe, 2006.

28 Förordning om Tatueringsfärger, SFS 2012:503. Miljödepartementet, 2012.

29 Real Decreto 1599/1997, de 17 de octubre. Que recoge la regulacion de los Productos cosmeticos (BOE núm. 261, de octubre [RCL 1997, 2572].

30 Recommendation from the Danish Environmental Protection Agency on the Safety of Tattoo Ink. Copenhagen, Miljøstyrelsen, 2014.

31 Jacobsen E, Tønning K, Pedersen E, Bernth N, Serup J, Høgsberg T, Nielsen E: Chemical Substances in Tattoo Ink. Copenhagen, Miljøstyrelsen, 2012.

Peter Laux
German Federal Institute for Risk Assessment (BfR), Department of Chemicals and Product Safety
Max-Dohrn-Strasse 8–10
DE–10589 Berlin (Germany)
E-Mail peter.laux@bfr.bund.de

Serup J, Kluger N, Bäumler W (eds): Tattooed Skin and Health.
Curr Probl Dermatol. Basel, Karger, 2015, vol 48, pp 201–205 (DOI: 10.1159/000369228)

Implementation of European Council Resolution ResAP(2008)1 in Italy. National and Regional Regulation of Tattoo Practices: Diversity and Challenges

Alberto Renzoni[a] · Antonia Pirrera[a] · Francesco Novello[a] ·
Maria Simonetta Diamante[b] · Carmine Guarino[a]

[a]National Centre ONDICO, Istituto Superiore di Sanità, Rome, and [b]Ministry of Economic Development, Rome, Italy

Abstract

In Italy, tattoos and permanent make-up have become increasingly popular in recent years. The number of tattoo parlours has increased from 257 in 2009 to 2,055 in 2014, wich is a eight-fold increase over the last 6 years. Although there is no specific legislation, the Italian Ministry of Health issued a document containing the 'Guidelines for the implementation of procedures for tattooing and piercing in safe conditions'. This document has not been adopted by all Italian regions, principally regarding training course requirements for tattoo professionals, creating a highly fragmented situation that resembles the European scene in miniature. ResAP(2008)1, which is not mandatory in Italy but was made binding by Italian Decree n. 206/2005, has been applied uniformly throughout the country. Thus, as far as the safety of inks is concerned, the surveillance system appears to be working well. However, surveillance has highlighted the presence of non-compliant inks and potentially unsafe preparations for tattoo removal in the market. Updating and rebalancing the situation will be the goal in order to face the challenge of combining well-being with the on-going social demand of looking after and beautifying the body. This would include the growing fashion of tattoos, provided that the products that are used are safe and that tattooing is performed in controlled hygienic conditions that fully guarantee the health of consumers.

Compared with the significant growth of the practice of tattooing in Italy, related legislation has not succeeded in keeping up with its development. This situation is common to many European countries and, in most cases, 'strongly suggested directives' or 'Guidelines' rather than specific regulations have been issued.

The National Centre Organismo Notificato Dispositivi Medici e Cosmetici of the Istituto Superiore di Sanità has, inter alia, the task of making assessments to form the basis of regulatory proposals in areas relevant to public health where there is no specific regulation. The situation regarding tattooing and piercing is a case in point.

At the moment, there are no official data describing the percentage of tattooed individuals in the general population or in specific age groups. Some partial data show that about 20% of adults were tattooed as of 2012 [1] and that the percentage of teenagers (12–18 years of age) with at least one tattoo had increased from 6.6 to 7.5% in the years 2002–2011 [2]. Circumstantial evidence of the growth of tattooing is seen in the number of operating tattoo parlours, which has increased from 257 in 2009 to 2,055 in 2014, which is a eight-fold increase over the last 6 years [3]. Some information regarding awareness, attitudes and the practice of tattooing among the population, although fragmentary, is available in the following scientific publications.

In 2005, a study on a sample of 577 students aged between 14 and 20 years was published to describe the educational initiative involving schools in the Region of Tuscany. This study reported that 4.8% of students had at least one tattoo. A definite increase in frequency of having a tattoo with age was evident among females, but this same frequency could not be detected among males, owing to the low numbers (not significant) in the study. Approximately 95.2% of those questioned were aware of the fact that piercing and tattooing might carry health risks. Of these, 95.2% indicated the possible risk of infections, 21.0% indicated the risk of allergic reactions, and 9.0% indicated the risk of aesthetic damage [4]. It is worth noting that specific regional regulations have been in place in Tuscany since 2004; indeed, Tuscany was the first region to issue specific regional laws. This example leads us to believe that good results regarding the awareness of risks from tattooing and their minimisation can be obtained when the sector is regulated by laws and when a good level of training is required.

In 2010, a study on the prevalence, knowledge and practices of and attitudes towards body art was published. These data, derived from a survey conducted at the University of Palermo, showed that 31.7% of a sample of 1,200 undergraduate university students had at least one tattoo. In general, students from a scientific background showed a higher rate of interest in body art (42.9%) compared with students from the humanities (19.5%). The results of the study supported the conclusion that cultural choice and lifestyle as well as gender (in the humanities and scientific groups, respectively, 31.8 and 47.6% of males had a tattoo, which was significantly more than females, at 14.3 and 26.9%, respectively) were associated with body art. However, there seemed to be no association with physical characteristics such as age, height, or weight. Students in the sample seemed to be clear as to why someone might desire to have a tattoo. On the contrary, the individuals who were questioned had no accurate idea of the consequences of getting a tattoo to their health or body, apart from the general risk of infection [5].

A 2010 study conducted in Northeast Italy evaluated the awareness of health-related risks in a sample of 4,277 secondary school students aged 14–22 years; 6% had a tattoo. Males appeared to be consistently less conscious of the risks of infectious diseases and mandatory hygienic norms when obtaining body art and were less likely to choose a certified parlour to obtain body art or to seek medical advice in the event of related medical complications. In contrast, high school-aged students had a better knowledge of the risks of infectious diseases related to body modifications, were more likely to use certified body art parlours and knew the hygienic norms expected in such salons [6].

In 2012, a study was published to verify the practices and knowledge of the risks related to body art among university freshmen in Bari and Naples, both cities in Southern Italy. Of a sample of 3,868 people selected from 26 degree courses, 597 (19.8%) were tattooed. The mean age when the first tattoo was obtained was 17 years. Of the respondents, 84.4% claimed to know the infectious risks associated with body art practices, but only 4.1% correctly identified the infectious diseases that could be transmitted through these procedures. While 59.2% of the sample declared that non-infectious diseases could occur after a tattoo or a piercing, only 5.4% of them correctly identified allergies, cysts, bleeding and scars. Of the sample, 23.4% reported complications [7].

The Italian Ministry of Health first addressed the problem of tattooing in 1998, when it issued document no. 2.9/156 'Guidelines for the implementation of procedures for tattooing and piercing in safe conditions' [8] and the subsequent interpretive letter no. 2.8/633 of the same year [9]. These documents focused on the risk of infection caused by blood-borne pathogens, of skin infections, of toxic effects due to substances used for pigmentation of the dermis as well as of the measures that should be applied, in particular, the basic rules for hygiene and environmental control. The Ministry requirements for a professional tattooist are as follows: at least 18 years of age and in possession of a certificate of participation in a training course for tattoo artists. In 1998, health hazards related to tattoo practice had limited impact at the national level and were consequently underestimated. Therefore, the public health departments of the Italian regions were allowed to adopt the guidelines with modifications and the consequent promulgation of regional directives and/or other legislative measures. Most of the regions simply enforced the Ministry guidelines, a few issued more stringent rules, and others had no regulations at all (see table 1). From the table, it is evident that the regulatory fragmentation is also reflected in the length of the required training courses; the qualifications of tattoo artists are extremely varied at the regional level, and the courses range from 14 h to 600 h. Some regions require 10 years of compulsory schooling as a threshold level of education. The great variability of the duration of the training courses poses serious issues. Differences in the authorisation processes for establishing a tattooing business mean that there is a lack of equivalence and that the level of health

Table 1. Status of tattoo regulation in the Italian regions

Regions	Regional regulation	Training courses for tattoo artists/hours (minimum)
Abruzzo	no	–
Basilicata	no	–
Calabria	yes	90 (planned)
Campania	yes	50
Emilia-Romagna	yes	14
Friuli-Venezia Giulia	awaiting approval	–
Lazio	yes	90
Liguria	yes	30
Lombardia	yes	90
Marche	awaiting approval	–
Molise	no	–
Piemonte	yes	awaiting approval
Puglia	yes	90
Sardegna	yes	60
Sicilia	yes	90
Toscana	yes	600
Trentino	yes	60
Alto Adige	yes	30
Umbria	yes	90 + public register
Valle d'Aosta	no	–
Veneto	yes	90

protection varies across the different regions. Clearly, the recognition status of a tattoo artist varies from one region to another, and there is the additional problem of the recognition of qualifications of tattoo artists from foreign countries. Consistent criteria are essential for the definition of a uniform professional profile for tattooists that will ensure a minimum technical level of skill to protect consumers and to allow comparison and competition on equal terms for market access.

The responsibility for issuing authorisation to establish a tattooing enterprise and for the routine monitoring of licensed tattoo parlours rests with Aziende Sanitarie Locali (Local Health Units). These units operate within the National Health Service; however, even in this case, there is considerable variation in the licensing requirements and monitoring frequency. In this context, on a small scale, Italy reflects the EU situation.

The 'Resolution ResAP(2008)1 on requirements and criteria for the safety of tattoos and permanent make-up', hereafter referred to as ResAP, is not mandatory in Italy. Nevertheless, the Italian Decree n. 206/2005 [10], based on the 'EU General Product Safety Directive (GPSD) 2001/95/CE', confers a binding nature on ResAP; indeed, art. 105 of the Decree states that '...in the absence of law, product safety is assessed on the basis of voluntary national standards transposing European standards ..., European Commission recommendations..., or referral to codes of good practices relating to safety in the sector concerned, to the latest technology, to the level of safety which consumers may reasonably expect'. Accordingly, tattoo inks must comply with ResAP before being marketed; otherwise, the national authority can ban their importation/sale. The national authority can also order the seizure of unsafe tattoo products. A substantial consequence is the immediate notification to all EU Countries through the RAPEX system. So, in Italy, ResAP is applied uniformly throughout the country and, as far as the safety of inks is concerned, the surveillance system, which is coordinated by the Ministry of Health, together with the Regional Agencies for the Protection of the Environment, Local Health Units, Carabinieri Healthcare Command (Carabinieri NAS). Office of Maritime, Air and Border Health (Uffici di Sanità Marittima, Aerea e di Frontiera) and Istituto Superiore di Sanità, appears to be working well. Based on the results of analyses of inks that were undertaken after either RAPEX warnings or individual complaints or as part of routine controls following sampling campaigns, approximately 40% of samples that were investigated were found to be non-compliant with ResAP requirements. Such campaigns revealed the presence in the market of fake inks of unknown composition that mimicked brands of inks that com-

plied with ResAP requirements; the results of this surveillance are published on the website of the Ministry of Health. This raises the problem of traceability and product control, an issue that should be addressed at the EU level.

Other issues waiting to be addressed are the harmonisation of methods for analysing inks and the safety of products for tattoo removal. The compliance of inks to the ResAP is assessed by methods that may differ in the preparation and/or subsequent analysis. Official Italian laboratories, which perform the control analysis upon request by the Ministry of Health, adopt more restrictive methods because they are inspired by the precautionary principle. Methods used in other EU states provide different results. The risk related to the substances used for tattoo removal represents another emerging problem. Whereas ResAP has addressed the safety of the substances contained in tattoo ink, there has been no provision for the substances used for their removal. A variety of special preparations are commercially available. These preparations are applied on or beneath the skin and are not listed as cosmetics, medical devices or drugs. Evidence is piling up about the adverse effects of such substances and, once again, they need to be regulated.

An area of tattoo practice worthy of study and regulation is that performed for medical purposes, e.g. reconstruction of the nipple-areola complex after mastectomy, camouflage of scars, and endoscopic tattoos for gastrointestinal investigations. These medical tattoos require special procedures that must comply with the fundamental rules of sterility and are very similar to those used for surgical operations. Some medical tattoos are included in the list of medical devices of the Italian National Classification of Medical Devices, according to Directive 93/42/EEC of June 14, 1993.

Awaiting European legislation, the next step will be the proposal for an update of the 1998 'Guidelines' of the Ministry of Health to include relevant scientific and technological evolutions and to standardise the training of tattooists. Some final, but not less important, objectives include the following:

- The creation of an Italian network for the reporting of complications and adverse events related to tattoos (database included), with the collaboration of first aid locations and health care facilities as well as of general practitioners and dermatologists.
- Obtaining more reliable data to know the exact size of the tattooed population, in general and by age groups as well as sex, including gathering further detailed information on the knowledge and awareness of and on the attitudes towards the risks of tattooing.
- Institution of a national register of certified tattoo artists on the basis of standardised training courses all over the country, which would supersede the fragmentary regional requirements, would impose a well-defined profile for tattooists and would ensure a technical level of skill by the tattooists to protect consumers.

- Institution of a register of ink and tattoo equipment manufacturers to overcome the problem of traceability.

The final goal of the Italian Health Authority aligns perfectly with the statements made at the meeting of the European Commission SANCO B3, Consumer Safety Network, Subgroup Tattoos of June 23rd, 2014: '…creation of a European system of registration or recognition of tattooists, a tattoo vigilance system where undesirable effects could be registered and be available to all Member States and information campaigns to increase awareness of consumers of the risks of receiving tattoos, in particular by unqualified tattooists'. In conclusion, one of the challenges that awaits us deals with a lifestyles in which well-being is coupled with a growing social demand for looking after and beautifying the body. This also includes the growing fashion of tattoos, provided that the products that are used are safe and that the tattooing is performed in controlled, hygienic conditions that fully guarantee the health of the consumers.

References

1 SWG Trieste: Sondaggio online dal titolo: I tatuaggi. 2012. www.agcom.it (accessed August 3, 2012).
2 EURISPES: Indagine Conoscitiva sulla Condizione dell'Infanzia e dell'Adolescenza in Italia 2011.
3 Unioncamere-Infocamere: Registro delle Imprese 2014.
4 Boncompagni G, Lazzeri G, Martiello MA, Incandela L, Santori R, Spinelli GM, Senatore R, Gentili G, Giacchi M, Pozzi T: Related risks of tattooing and body piercing: prevalence study in a convenience sample. J Prev Med Hyg 2005;46:153–158.

5 Sidoti E, Paolini G, Tringali G: Prevalence, knowledge, attitudes and practices towards body art in university students: body art as an indicator of risk taking behaviours? Ital J Public Health 2010;7:386–394.
6 Cegolon L, Miatto E, Bortolotto M, Benetton M, Mazzoleni F, Mastrangelo G, VAHP Working Group: Body piercing and tattoo: awareness of health related risks among 4,277 Italian secondary school adolescents. BMC Public Health 2010;10:73–81.

7 Gallè F, Quaranta A, Napoli C, Di Onofrio V, Alfano V, Montagna MT, Liguori G: Body art and health risks: young adults' knowledge in two regions of southern Italy. Ann Ig 2012;24:535–542.
8 Ministero della Sanità: Linee Guida del Ministero della Sanità per l'Esecuzione di Procedure di Tatuaggio e Piercing in Condizioni di Sicurezza. Circolare 5 Febbraio 1998 n. 2.9/156.
9 Ministero della Sanità: Chiarimenti Forniti dal Consiglio Superiore della Sanità. Circolare 16 Luglio 1998 n. 2.8/633.
10 Decreto Legislativo del 6 Settembre 2005 no. 206 'Codice del Consumo'.

Dr. Antonia Pirrera
ONDICO, Istituto Superiore di Sanità
Viale Regina Elena, 299
IT–00161 Rome (Italy)
E-Mail antonia.pirrera@iss.it

Serup J, Kluger N, Bäumler W (eds): Tattooed Skin and Health.
Curr Probl Dermatol. Basel, Karger, 2015, vol 48, pp 206–209 (DOI: 10.1159/000369229)

EU Actions to Ensure the Safety of Tattoos and the Protection of Consumers

Ana María Blass Rico*

European Commission, Justice and Consumers Directorate General Unit Product and Service Safety,
Brussels, Belgium

Abstract

The number of tattooed persons has been continuously increasing in the last few years, particularly in the younger population. At the same time, the possibility of purchasing tattoo inks online is easier than ever worldwide. Consumers are not always sufficiently aware of the possible health problems associated with this 'cool fashion' if hygiene conditions are not respected and/or if the injected mixtures contain dangerous chemicals. Concerns about the possible health risks associated with such practices arise from the absence of a clear legislative framework, the lack of proper risk assessment of the chemicals used, and non-harmonised or missing hygiene and purity requirements, among other factors. There is a general consensus among all active stakeholders that EU harmonised rules would help to ensure a consistent high level of protection of consumers across the EU.

© 2015 S. Karger AG, Basel

Background

In 2000, the Scientific Committee on Cosmetic Products and Non-Food Products delivered an opinion regarding the safety of tattoos. The committee recommended that a systematic effort be undertaken to amass the needed chemical and toxicological information so that a proper risk assessment could be conducted. In this light, the European Commission (EC) decided to undertake action to establish a common knowledge basis on the safety of tattoos and body piercing. The Directorate General for Health and Consumers (DG SANCO) asked the Joint Research Centre (JRC) to carry out this activity as part of the EIS-ChemRisks project, which aimed to collect process and assess information on consumer exposure to chemicals in consumer products and articles and associated health risks. The work resulted in a report summarising the final conclusions and recommendations for regulatory action on the safety of tattoos, body piercing, and related practices in the EU [1].

In the meantime, considering that tattoos and permanent make-up (PMU) were not covered either by national legislation or by EU legislation, the Council of Europe published a resolution on

* The views expressed in this article are those of the author and cannot be considered as an official position of the European Commission.

requirements and criteria for the safety of tattoos and PMU in 2003, which was superseded by a new resolution in 2008, or ResAP(2008)1 [2]. The resolution provides a recommendation on chemical and microbiological quality and on safety assessment, including a negative list of substances that should not be present in tattoos and PMU as well as the maximum allowed concentrations of a number of impurities. The recommendation provides criteria for the safety assessment of the chemicals used and encourages establishing a positive list of chemicals proven safe for this use under certain conditions.

The market surveillance authorities of several Member States have taken action (e.g. withdrawal from the market, import rejection) against tattoo inks that pose serious risks to the health and safety of consumers and have reported these inks to the EC through the Rapid Alert System for non-food dangerous products (RAPEX) [3]. From 2010 to 2014, around 100 RAPEX notifications concerned dangerous tattoo inks, mostly due to the presence of carcinogenic and/or sensitising substances (e.g. polycyclic aromatic hydrocarbons; benzene-a-pyrene; azodyes; aromatic amines; or heavy metals such as nickel, cadmium, lead, and arsenic). ResAP(2008)1 is the benchmark for the RAPEX notifications.

It is the responsibility of the business operator to fulfil the EU legislation requirement that only safe products are put on the market. In the case of products for tattooing, this involves not only those operators supplying the tattoo ink but also the artist who is supplying the tattoo ink to the public in the course of providing the tattooing service.

Some Member States have adopted national measures that are based on ResAP(2008)1, prohibiting the presence of tattoo inks containing certain chemicals on the market, whilst in other measures, the general safety requirements laid down in Directive 2001/95/EC, or the General Product Safety Directive (GPSD) [4], applies. Therefore, the approaches adopted by Member States to deal with the same risk differ. As a result, there could be problems with the free circulation of products in the EU, and furthermore, EU consumers are not equally protected. However, all EU consumers should be assured that tattoo inks are safe, irrespective of the EU country where they get the tattoo. The adoption of an EU measure is a way to ensure a consistent high level of protection of the health and safety of consumers and the proper functioning of the internal market.

With the purpose of exchanging information on the current regulatory approaches and common practices and on safety issues related to tattoos all around the world, DG SANCO organised an international virtual symposium on tattoos in April 2014. The exchange took place within the context of the International Consumer Product Safety Caucus and the Organisation for Economic Co-operation and Development. There were participants from the US, Canada, Australia, Peru, Norway and EU Member States, as well as the Organisation for Economic Co-operation and Development and the JRC of the EC at the virtual symposium. Live presentations from the EC, DG SANCO, and the US Food and Drug Administration were followed by oral contributions from various jurisdictions on their current regulatory approaches, data on inks' ingredients, market data, and statistics on undesirable effects.

In the EU, the EC invited Member States to designate national experts and identify possible stakeholders from the tattooing industry, scientists, practitioners, and others to participate in an expert working sub-group of the Consumer Safety Network. On June 23, 2014, DG SANCO organised the first meeting of the expert group on tattoos, with participants from 13 Member States (and Norway), stakeholders (tattoo ink producers, dermatologists, tattoo associations), the Council of Europe, the European Association for the Co-ordination of Consumer Representation in Standardisation (the European consumer voice in standardisation), and the JRC.

EU Member States having national legislation based on ResAP(2008)1 explained their experience and their suggestions for improvement. The stakeholders also expressed their views, and ink producers, consumer associations, and tattoo artist associations were in favour of a legislative measure based on ResAP(2008)1 and asked for stricter rules.

Tattoo Inks Must Be Safe

The GPSD applies to tattoo inks, irrespective of whether they are purchased for self-application or by a professional tattooist and inserted under the skin of a consumer by this service provider.

The GPSD empowers the EC to adopt so-called emergency measures valid for 1 year (renewable) to address serious risks to the health and safety of consumers emanating from certain products. This is applicable when Member States differ significantly on the approach to deal with the risk, when the risk cannot be dealt with as quickly as necessary under other EU legislation applicable to the products concerned, and when the risk can be eliminated effectively only by EU measures in order to ensure a consistent high level of protection of consumers and the proper functioning of the internal market.

Based on the results of the consultation of different stakeholders and the support of Member State experts that have asked the European Commission to take actions towards EU harmonised rules for tattoos, it seems that an 'emergency' measure allowed in certain circumstances by the existing legislation governing general product safety would be generally welcomed.

The measure could incorporate parts of the recommendations in ResAP(2008)1, with some updates with regards to the negative list of chemicals. There is, however, some legal basis for limitations to what can be done through this measure. It should be noted that any such 'emergency' measure should be followed in due course by a permanent measure under existing legislative powers, either as an amendment to existing legislation or as a self-standing text.

Furthermore, the Commission is at the time of writing still assessing whether all the necessary conditions for an urgent and temporary 'emergency' EU level measure are met. This process includes gathering data about number of tattooed people in the EU, health issues associated to tattoos as well as assessment of other socioeconomic aspects that could affect stakeholders, according to the different measures that could be adopted to protect consumers from the potential hazards of tattoos.

Next Steps

With the aim of comprehensively addressing all safety issues related to tattoos and their removal, DG SANCO (as from 1 January 2015 DG JUST and CONSUMERS) has asked for the collaboration of the JRC to continue with the work of the working group of experts on tattoos as an 18-month project.

Some additional potential participants have been identified, like additional tattoo associations, experts from additional Member States and third countries (Switzerland), and the European Network of Official Cosmetics Control laboratories. Open consultations and discussions are also foreseen and will be an important part of the study.

The main goal of this project is to provide scientific and technical support to prepare future legislative actions if deemed necessary.

The JRC, with the support of the experts, will gather data on the percentage of tattooed persons in the population, the ink market, ink ingredients, health effects, toxicological aspects, removal processes, the fate of the chemicals within the human body in the long term, and regulatory review (national legislations on tattoos in and outside the EU) and will assess and update ResAP(2008)1 with regards to the list of restricted chemicals and limits as well as analytical methods, labelling requirements, safety assessment, and hygiene/sterility requirements. Finally, the group will also look at risk perception and communication aspects, data gaps, and research needs and lessons learnt. The project should provide conclusions on the elements to be addressed by the EU action on tattoos.

References

1 Papameletiou D, Schwela D, Zenié A, et al: Recommendations for Regulatory Action in the EU on the Safety of Tattoos, Body Piercing and of Related Practices in the EU. Ispra (VA), Italy, European Commission, Joint Research Centre (JRC), Institute for Health and Consumer Protection (IHCP), Physical and Chemical Exposure (PCE) Unit, 2003.

2 Council of Europe: Resolution ResAP (2008)1 on requirements and criteria for the safety of tattoos and permanent make-up (superseding Resolution ResAP (2003)2 on tattoos and permanent make-up). Strasbourg, France, Council of Europe, 2008.

3 European Commission: RAPEX: The rapid alert system for non-food dangerous products managed by the European Commission. http://ec.europa.eu/rapex (accessed January 1, 2015).

4 Directive 2001/95/EC of the European Parliament and of the Council of 3 December 2001 on general product safety. Official Journal of the European Communities 2002;L11:4–17.

Ana María Blass Rico
European Commission, Justice and Consumers Directorate General, Unit Product and Service Safety
Rue Belliard 232
BE–1049 Brussels (Belgium)
E-Mail Ana-Maria.Blass-Rico@ec.europa.eu

Serup J, Kluger N, Bäumler W (eds): Tattooed Skin and Health.
Curr Probl Dermatol. Basel, Karger, 2015, vol 48, pp 210–217 (DOI: 10.1159/000369230)

Surveillance of Tattoo-Related Adverse Events by the EU RAPEX System and by National Monitoring

Cécile Verdier

Non-Clinical Assessor, Industrial Biology Engineer and Master Degree in Toxicology, Marines, France

Abstract

A resolution of the Council of Europe in 2008 (ResAP (2008)1) helped to define requirements and criteria for the safety of tattoos and permanent make-up in order to increase the level of consumer health protection for these products. Tattoo product usage is not without risk. These products are injected into the skin and may represent a risk to human health due to possible microbiological contamination and/or contamination by the presence of hazardous substances in the products. ResAP (2008) laid the foundation for the safety of tattoo products in Europe. This has generated awareness by European Member States and has encouraged them to adapt this resolution in their own law or to use it as a model to define their own regulation on tattoos. In order, to communicate on the hazard associated with these products between Member States and the European Commission, the European RAPEX system was created; this system will be further explained in this article. Finally, some Member States have created a specific vigilance system related to the adverse effects of tattoos. In this respect, a European national example will be presented.

© 2015 S. Karger AG, Basel

Surveillance of Tattoo-Related Adverse Events by the EU RAPEX System

The resolution of the Council of Europe in 2008 (ResAP (2008)1) [1] set up the basis for the safety of tattoo products.

This resolution has recommended that the Member States take into account the principles described in the resolution in their national laws and regulations on tattoos and permanent make-up. More specifically, this resolution states which information should be put on the labeling, discusses the safety assessment of tattoo products, and states which substances should not be found. Moreover, vigilance of these products is not specifically addressed.

Nevertheless, despite the lack of European regulations on tattoos to date, a European system for monitoring adverse effects associated with tattoo products does exist. It is presented following this section.

Introduction

Tattoo products are not covered by any specific regulation or directive. Therefore, the directive 2001/95/EC of the European Parliament and of the Council of 3 December 2001 on general product safety [2] applies to these products by default. This European legislation ensures high and uniform protection of the health and safety of consumers. Products placed on the internal market are subject to general safety requirements. The European Union has also set up a rapid alert system (RAPEX) for products presenting a serious risk to consumers.

According to the decision of 16 December 2009 [3], laying down guidelines for the management of RAPEX, in section 2.1.1, tattoo products are covered by RAPEX.

Context and Purpose of Notification of RAPEX

In the decision of 16 December 2009 [3], it is stated that RAPEX, which was established by Article 12 of the directive on general product safety [2], applies to measures designed to prevent, limit, or control the sale and use of consumer products presenting a serious risk to the health and safety of consumers. Members States are required to participate in the RAPEX system and to inform the European Commission whenever the four criteria below are met:

– the product is a consumer product;
– the concerned product is the subject of measures to prevent, limit, or control its marketing and use;
– the concerned product presents a serious risk to the health and safety of consumers;
– the serious risk has cross-border implications.

When Member States identify products that present a serious risk to health and safety, they pursue rapid intervention measures to protect consumers. In this case, Member States must immediately inform the Commission through the RAPEX system. The purpose of this system is to quickly circulate information about risk and measures between Member States and the European Commission.

Requirements for Notification of RAPEX

There are 2 types of RAPEX notifications:
– 'Article 12 notification', which responds to the above-mentioned criteria;
– 'Article 12 notification requiring emergency action', which indicates that the product poses a life-threatening risk and/or that there have been fatal accidents and in other cases where a RAPEX notification requires emergency action by all Member States.

There is also the possibility of receiving 'notifications for information' when some items are missing in order to complete the notification form correctly. A confirmation of measures may also be required when the notification was sent before measures were adopted. These notifications are subject to different deadlines.

According to the directive 2001/95/CE [2], Member States must provide all available details. In particular, the notification must contain at least
– information enabling the product to be identified;
– a description of the risk involved, including a summary of the results of any tests/analyses

and of their conclusions that are relevant to assessing the level of risk;
– the nature and the duration of the measures or action taken or decided on, if applicable;
– information on the supply chains and distribution of the product, and particularly on destination countries.

The decision 2010/15/UE [3] provides an example of Section IV of the notification form of RAPEX.

Notification Form

In Section IV and section 3.2.2, the decision 2010/15 [3] shows the standard notification form to be filled out by Member States. Notifications should be as complete as possible; all sections must be completed. An opportunity to update the notification form is allowed as soon as the information becomes available. The record is then reviewed by the European Commission before being published. The main fields to be filled out on the notification form are described below.

Field 1: General Information

The type of notification is requested: 'Article 12 notification requiring emergency action', 'Article 12 notification', 'Notification for information', or 'Article 11 notification'. The number, date, and country and the person in charge of notification are also requested.

Field 2: Product Identification

Many pieces of information are requested: the product category, name, brand, model and/or type number, barcode, batch or serial number, and custom code; a description of the product and its packaging, with pictures of the product, packaging, and labels; and the total number of open items for notification.

Field 3: Regulations and Standards Applicable

Information on the safety requirements applicable to the notified product is requested, including legal provisions (directive, decision, and regula-

tion), standards, means of attestation of conformity, and indication of whether the product is counterfeit or not.

Field 4: Traceability

Information establishing the product's origin is requested: the contact details of the manufacturer or its representative, of the exporter(s), of the importer(s), of the distributor(s), and of the retailer(s). Information regarding the product's destination countries is also requested.

Field 5: Risk Description

A risk category description is required. A summary of test results, legal provisions, and standards (with clauses) against which the product was tested and with which it did not comply must be provided. A risk assessment, conclusions, and information on known incidents and accidents are also required.

Field 6: Measures

Information on the measures taken, the category (withdrawal from the market, recall from consumers), the scope and date of entry into force, and the duration of the measures must be provided.

Field 7: Confidentiality

Indication of whether the entire notification or part of it and/or its attachment(s) are covered by confidentiality must be provided. A request for confidentiality must always be accompanied by a justification clearly stating the reasons for such a request.

Member States are encouraged to obtain and provide information on the supply chains of the notified product in non-EU countries that cooperate closely with the EU on product safety.

Examples of Notification/Review of Notifications from 2005 to 2014

RAPEX notifications are available on the website of the European Commission at the following address: http://ec.europa.eu/consumers/safety/

rapex/alerts/main/index.cfm?event=main.list Notifications&selectedTabIdx=1.

To illustrate the work of Members States at the European level, it is interesting to consider tattoo ink notifications. The following is a review of all notifications on tattoo inks presenting a serious risk to human health from 2005 to September 30th, 2014. The research based on the European database was performed using the word 'tattoo' in the field 'product'. The results regarding Rapex notifications review from 2005 to end of September 2014 are presented in table 1.

The main notifying countries are Germany and Italy. The main origin countries of tattoo inks presenting a serious risk to human health are the USA and China. Nevertheless, it is noted that in several cases, the origin country is unknown.

The main types of risk reported concern the presence of heavy metals, aromatic amines released by azo dyes, or polycyclic aromatic hydrocarbon. Few notifications indicate microbiological contaminations. The standard claimed in most of the notifications is the resolution of the Council of Europe in 2008 [1]. The measures taken by Member States are either compulsory measures, such as import rejection at the border, a ban of the product from the market, withdrawal of the product from the market, or recall of the product from end users, or voluntary measures, such as withdrawal of the product from the market or destruction of the product.

Surveillance of Tattoo-Related Adverse Events by a National System: the French Example

An example of the French vigilance system for tattoo products is explained below.

Introduction

Up to 2004, there was no French regulation on tattoo products. France adopted a regulation on tat-

toos on August 9th, 2004, by the publication of Law n°2004–806. This law, and particularly article 149 [4], relates to public health policy regarding tattoo products other than medical devices in the regulatory framework for public health. Tattoos were then added to the field missions of the competent authority of the French National Agency for Medicines and Health Products Safety (ANSM).

Main Principles of the Regulation of Tattoo Products in France

We can distinguish technical and administrative requirements.

French regulations establish technical requirements for tattoo products:
- a definition: tattoo products are any substance or preparation intended for coloring by cutaneous effraction to create a mark on the external parts of the human body, except for products that are medical devices;
- tattoo products do not require any authorization to be put on the market;
- a tattoo product can be put on the market if it meets certain regulatory requirements, and particularly the absence of harm to the health of the consumer, meaning that manufacturers are responsible for the safety of the product and that tattoo products should not affect human health;
- tattoo products must comply with the definition;
- the composition of tattoo products must comply with the lists of substances;
- tattoo products must meet the labeling requirements.

French regulations also establish administrative requirements:
- reporting by the responsible person to the competent authority is required;
- technical documentation must be kept available to the control authorities;

Table 1. RAPEX notifications review from 2005 to the end of September 2014

Year	Number of notifications	Notifying country and number of notifications per country	Country of origin of tattoo products and number of times the country is cited
2014 (until September 30th, 2014)	17	Germany: 12 Italy: 5	USA: 10 China: 4 Germany: 1 Japan: 1 Italy: 1
2013	32	Germany: 22 Italy: 3 The Netherlands: 3 Slovenia: 2 France: 1 Austria: 1	USA: 17 China: 4 Unknown: 3 Brazil: 2 Japan: 2 Italy: 2 Germany: 1 France: 1
2012	36	Italy: 27 Germany: 9	USA: 30 Germany: 2 Spain: 1 China: 1 Unknown: 1 Italy: 1
2011	13	Germany: 6 Denmark: 5 Italy: 2	USA: 10 Unknown: 3
2010	7	Italy: 7	USA: 4 Unknown: 3
2009	1	The Netherlands: 1	USA: 1
2008	1	Germany: 1	USA: 1
2007	5	The Netherlands: 4 Germany: 1	UK: 3 USA: 1 Italy: 1
2006	0	–	–
2005	0	–	–
Total	112	Germany: 51 Italy: 44 The Netherlands: 8 Slovenia: 2 France: 1 Austria: 1	USA: 74 Unknown: 10 China: 9 Germany: 4 Japan: 3 Italy: 5 UK: 3 Brazil: 2 Spain: 1 France: 1

- the manufacture of tattoo products must be conducted in accordance with Good Manufacturing Practices;
- safety assessment of the human health effects of tattoo products must be performed in compliance with Good Laboratory Practice.

To ensure safety of tattoo products, the French competent authority (ANSM) organizes a vigilance system to monitor the risk of side effects from the use of tattoo products. Vigilance is directed toward all products once they are on the market.

Introduction to the National Vigilance System

Vigilance of tattoo products always involves monitoring of the adverse effects resulting from their use. It is directed toward all tattoo products once they are available on the market.

This vigilance includes

- reporting of all adverse events and collecting information about them;
- registration, evaluation, and use of the information related to those effects for the purpose of prevention;
- performance of all studies on the safety of use of tattoo products;
- implementation and monitoring of corrective actions if necessary.

Definitions

French regulations provide the following definitions:

Undesirable Effect: This adverse effect is a harmful and unintended reaction that occurs during the normal use of a tattoo product in humans or results from its misuse.

Serious Undesirable Effect: This effect is defined as an undesirable effect that results in hospitalization, temporary or permanent functional incapacity, a disability, an immediate vital risk, death, an anomaly, or a birth defect.

Misuse: This is incorrect use of a product during routine use, with special precautions mentioned in 7° of article R.513–10–5.

Scope of Notification of Undesirable Effects

In the French regulation [5], many actors can be identified: the responsible person, the health professional, the person making tattoos, and the consumer.

Responsible persons must notify the competent authority, without delay, of all serious undesirable effects. Moreover, the responsible persons must notify the competent authority about other undesirable effects. In the latter case, there is no concept of time. A lack of reporting of serious undesirable effects as soon as responsible persons have knowledge and by any means is punishable by 2 years' imprisonment and a penalty of EUR 30,000.

Health professionals and persons making tattoos must notify the competent authority, without delay, of all serious undesirable effects. Moreover, health professionals and persons making tattoos must notify the competent authority of other undesirable effects, with no concept of time. In his notification, the health professional specifies if the undesirable effect results from misuse and describes the conditions under which the tattoo has been applied. A lack of reporting of serious undesirable effects as soon as health professionals or persons making tattoos have knowledge and by any means is punishable by 2 years' imprisonment and a penalty of EUR 30,000.

Consumers can report undesirable effects, indicating any misuse and describing the conditions under which the tattoo was applied.

Manufacturers or their representatives and the persons on whose behalf tattoo products are manufactured are notably required to report all undesirable effects contrary to the requirement of safety of tattoo products to the General Directorate for Competition Policy, Consumer Affairs, and Fraud Control (DGCCRF).

ANSM has developed a notification form for an undesirable effect occurring after the realization of a tattoo. On this form, it is stipulated that tattoo products with an undesirable effect must be kept for at least 3 months. This notification form can be downloaded from the ANSM website and then sent to the vigilance department of ANSM.

This notification form includes several fields to fill out:

Field 1: Notifier
All person involved in the reporting system for vigilance of tattoo products are indicated: responsible persons, health professionals (physicians, pharmacists), tattooists, tattooed persons, and other. It is advisable to write the full name, telephone number, and e-mail address of the person designated above. The date of issue of the notification form is requested.

Field 2: Tattooed Person
It is requested that the date of birth of the tattooed person, the person's gender, and whether there is a current pregnancy be specified.

Field 3: Product(s)
The following information on tattoo products is requested: the name of the product(s), the batch number, and the color index of the colorants inside the tattoo product(s). The address and local contact details of suppliers, distributors, and/or manufacturers must also be provided.

Field 4: Tattoo Realization
Completion of the fields regarding the address and local contact details of the tattooist is requested. The notifier should indicate if the notification concerns a monochrome tattoo or a polychrome tattoo. The colors constituting the tattoo and the date of the realization of the tattoo must be clarified. The body area where the tattoo was performed is worth mentioning. If associated products are used, such as anaesthetic, antiseptic, etc. they may be included. At last, the date of occurrence of the adverse effect is requested.

Field 5: Consequences of Adverse Effect
Many fields are available: consulting a physician; consulting a pharmacist; social inconvenience (specify); work stoppage; urgent medical intervention; hospitalization; sequelae, disability, or incapacity; and other (specify).

Field 6: Special Exposure to Product
Specification of professional use or misuse and if there are old tattoos is requested.

Field 7: Kinds of Undesirable Effects
Clarification of whether the effect of the events took place at or away from the area of the realization of the tattoo is requested.

Field 8: Description and Time of Occurrence of the Adverse Effect
In the notification form, an open field is left available to the notifier, to describe the adverse effect and the occurence time of the effect.

Field 9: Medical History of the Person Concerned by the Adverse Reaction
Information on whether the person has allergies and/or skin diseases or other diseases is requested.

The development of the undesirable effect is investigated, such as if there was a spontaneous resolution of the effect and whether local and/or a general treatment was carried out.

Information on whether further investigations were carried out is requested, such as microbiological sampling, blood assessment, a biopsy, or an allergy survey. Finally, which final diagnosis was made and whether there is a causal link between the effects observed and the realization of the tattoo must be indicated.

Treatment of an Undesirable Effect by the French Competent Authority

The vigilance of tattoo products is led by the French competent authority, or ANSM, which defines the approach and leads and coordinates the action of different stakeholders, including

- notification of the undesirable effect and collection of information about it;
- registration, evaluation, and use of this information for the purpose of prevention, with the information analyzed while taking into account the available data on the sales and use practices of tattoo products;
- realization of all studies and all work on safety regarding tattoo products;
- realization and monitoring of corrective actions;
- possibly also research and analysis of data contained in the file of the finished product.

Example of a Survey of Tattoo Products on the Market

In terms of market surveillance, ANSM works in strong coordination with DGCCRF to monitor the implementation of the text. Given the collaboration agreement between the two French competent authorities, ANSM and DGCCRF, in France, tattoo inks were subject to a survey from 2012 to 2013. In total, 35 tattoo inks were examined by ANSM. Sterility tests were performed on 26, and research on aromatic amines was carried out on 28 samples. The DGCCRF laboratory focused on finding heavy metals. Three products were found to be nonsterile, and the presentation and/or labeling of 11 products were considered noncompliant with regulations [6].

References

1 Council of Europe: Resolution ResAP (2008)1 on Requirements and Criteria for the Safety of Tattoos and Permanent Make-Up (Superseding Resolution ResAP(2003)2 on Tattoos and Permanent Make-Up). Strasbourg, France, Council of Europe, 2008.
2 Directive 2001/95/EC of the European Parliament and the Council of 3 December 2001 on general product safety. Official Journal of the European Communities 2002;L 11: 4–17.

3 Commission Decision of 16 December 2009 laying down guidelines for the management of the Community Rapid Information System 'RAPEX' established under Article 12 and of the notification procedure established under Article 11 of Directive 2001/95/EC (the General Product Safety Directive), decision 2010/15/EU. Official Journal of the European Union 2010;53:1–64.

4 Loi n°2004–806 du 9 août 2004 relative à la politique de santé publique, NOR: SANX0300055L, article 149.
5 Loi n°2014–201 du 24 février 2014 portant diverses dispositions d'adaptation au droit de l'Union européenne dans le domaine de la santé, NOR: AFSX1315898L, article L.513–10–2 to L.513–10–10, L.5437–2 to L.5437–5.
6 ANSM: Rapport d'Activité 2013. Saint-Denis, ANSM, 2014.

Cécile Verdier
29 rue vieille de Chars
FR–95640 Marines (France)
E-Mail cecile.verdier@gmail.com

Serup J, Kluger N, Bäumler W (eds): Tattooed Skin and Health.
Curr Probl Dermatol. Basel, Karger, 2015, vol 48, pp 218–222 (DOI: 10.1159/000369945)

The Amsterdam Model for Control of Tattoo Parlours and Businesses

Thijs Veenstra

National Institute for Public Health and the Environment, Amsterdam, The Netherlands

Abstract

In the early 1980s, an outbreak of hepatitis B in Amsterdam stood at the start of the development of the first hygiene guidelines for tattooists in The Netherlands. Ever since, infection control in tattoo practice has continued to prove its importance as tattoo-related outbreaks of infectious diseases have continued to be reported in Europe. Furthermore, the act of tattooing includes breaking the skin barrier but is performed by professionals who are not medically trained. The Ministry of Health has now implemented uniform regulations that apply to professionals who perform tattooing and apply permanent make-up. These regulations include hygiene guidelines that were developed by the National Institute for Public Health and the Environment in cooperation with representatives of the tattooing associations. The guidelines contain a list of requirements, including for the studio interior, the cleanness of the studio, the safe use of permitted equipment and products, sterilization methods, and the information provided to the customer. A permit may be granted after an inspection by the local health service, during which the act of tattooing has to be performed. It is now estimated that over 95% of all tattoos in The Netherlands were obtained at one of the almost 900 licensed studios. Reports of complications are generally low in number. We suggest that uniform European hygiene guidelines would further contribute to the safety of tattooing.

© 2015 S. Karger AG, Basel

The Amsterdam Model

Infection control in tattoo studios is important. Over the past three decades, preliminary regulation in Amsterdam has grown into an effective national policy. Currently, tattoo practice in The Netherlands is subject to national hygiene guidelines that are created by tattooist organizations and infection-control professionals.

Hygiene in the Early 1980s

In the early 1980s, an outbreak of hepatitis B among eight American soldiers stood at the start of regulated practice in The Netherlands. The outbreak alerted the public health service of Amsterdam to bad hygienic conditions in a vast and growing number of tattoo shops in the city when investigation of this outbreak revealed a tattoo studio with extremely unhygienic conditions [1]. The findings included reusing needles, testing needles on the tattooist's skin, and cleaning the client's skin with water that was previously used to rinse another person's tattoo. A survey among tattoo studios indicated that similar conditions were found in several other tattoo studios. Aware of the urgent need for regulation of tattooing practice, the public health service set up a preliminary guideline for tattoo parlours. In cooperation with a known local tattoo artist, ten 'golden rules' for infection prevention in tattoo studios were formulated [2].

After these ten golden rules were established, the local government applied local regulations to tattoo practice. This made it possible to enforce the regulations when a health risk was identified. Health inspectors were authorized to access the premises of registered studios at all times and to issue a warning when unacceptable conditions were identified. In The Netherlands, the city of Amsterdam gained a reputation for keeping a close eye on hygienic practices in tattoo studios.

Aim for Regulated Hygienic Practice

The act of tattooing is actually very similar to nursing or medical activities that should only be carried out by trained professionals. With tattooing, the natural skin barrier is broken, making the skin vulnerable to invasion by micro-organisms via needles, ink, or contact with contaminated materials or fluids before the skin has healed. Of course, using safe ink, with an absence of micro-

biological contamination when leaving the manufacturer, is an important standard. There is, however, a variety of activities prior to the actual act of tattooing that may lead to the contamination of ink. These activities may be as simple as opening the bottle and touching the nozzle or as complicated as bacterial growth in bottles of diluted ink that have been used for too long. The process of tattooing consists of a chain of activities that are vulnerable to errors [3]. A sterile working field can be compromised by a lack of hand hygiene or ineffective disinfection of, for instance, the tattoo machine, after which bacteria may be introduced onto the skin by contact with the skin during tattooing. Furthermore, unprofessional use of a steam sterilizer will lead to the use of unsterile materials as safe materials.

Unlike training for health care workers, there is no universal professional education for tattoo artists that covers all aspects needed for safe practice. This does not mean that every artist poses a health risk when tattooing without hygiene guidelines, but it leaves room for serious errors, as we have seen in the last few years, when errors in practice led to infections in clients [4]. In The Netherlands, initiatives by tattooist organizations to introduce universal professional education have still not led to a sufficient training program. The increasing number of consumers who choose to get a tattoo has also led to a rise in the number of persons at risk for tattoo-related infections. Consumers have little knowledge of infection control in tattooing practice and rely on the artist's professional skills [5]. This means that there is a need for a system that ensures the safety of tattoo artists' clients by regulating the practice of tattooists and the use of safe products.

Hygiene Guidelines

More elaborate guidelines were established in The Netherlands in 1987 [Bronnen van Joy]. Several organizations contributed to these guidelines, including organizations for tattooists, infection-control specialists from the public health service, dermatologists, and health inspectors. Since then, the guidelines have been subject to revision every 4 years, which makes it possible to update the guidelines with new insights as well as with information about new activities in tattooing practice that need specific safety measures. The current guidelines [6] date from 2014 and are divided into several chapters. The main chapter relates directly to the act of placing a tattoo. This includes general measures such as sufficient hand hygiene and personal protective equipment, e.g. gloves that meet international standards. The chapter provides principles for safe practice with regard to cleaning instruments, inks, and needles; using sterile packaging before and during tattooing; safely disposing of contaminated materials and sharps; and providing instructions for safe aftercare. The second chapter covers the cleaning, disinfection, and sterilization of surfaces and materials, which are categorized based on whether they penetrate or have contact with the skin and whether they can be contaminated by blood or ink from a used needle. This chapter provides principles for carrying out these activities in a professional way. A special chapter is dedicated to building, equipping, and furnishing the area. An orderly, non-cramped working space with well-cleanable surfaces is the main required condition. Tattooing must be carried out separately from other activities and from waiting clients. A hand-washing facility must be within close range and has to be located in the same room. The last chapter contains information to be provided to the client about correct aftercare and about seeking the right medical assistance in the case of a complication.

National Legislation

In 2007, national legislation was established by the Dutch Ministry of Health, Welfare, and Sports. It contained regulations for tattooing ac-

tivities as well as for permanent make-up and piercing and was based on the Amsterdam model. In addition to hygiene guidelines, age limits were set for clients getting a tattoo. In the national program, an owner of a studio must obtain a license for using tattooing materials. The license has to be renewed every 3 years. In order to obtain a license, the holder must request an inspection by the public health service, during which all aspects of the guidelines are assessed. Furthermore, the artist has to demonstrate the act of tattooing as well as preparations to show his/her ability to work according to the hygienic principles. When not all aspects are in accordance with the guidelines, a re-inspection is issued before the shop may operate. During the 3-year period of the license, authorities may visit a studio unannounced to ensure that the guidelines are still being followed. Failing to comply with the hygiene guidelines may lead to an official warning, and failing to improve practice may result in the license being withdrawn. Performing commercial tattooing activities without a license is now illegal and may lead to a EUR 1,500 penalty.

In addition to the legislation, the government assigned the National Centre for Public Health and the Environment to establishing a public website for consumers that provides information about getting a tattoo safely [7]. The website mainly consists of a database containing all currently licensed studios. Furthermore, it provides information about tattooing and health, assessing hygiene in a studio, proper aftercare, how to act when a complication occurs, and where to submit complaints.

Effects

Since 2007, the number of licensed tattoo shops in The Netherlands has increased almost three-fold (fig. 1). It is difficult to measure the exact effect of hygienic practice and legislation, as

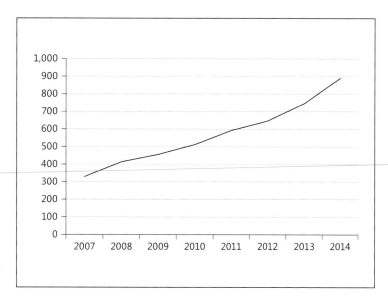

Fig. 1. Number of licensed tattoo studios in The Netherlands.

complications are not registered. Unfortunately, serious complications such as hepatitis B infection are often difficult to relate to a specific cause. In 2009, the authorities in The Netherlands ordered a survey of 292 persons who had recently gotten a tattoo [8]. Based on the survey, it was estimated that 95% of the tattoos had been obtained at a licensed studio. Only 2% reported a complicated healing process. It is remarkable that five out of the seven people who reported complications after getting a tattoo had gotten their tattoo at an unlicensed studio. Unfortunately, the study lacked baseline data. A study in 2009 showed no increased prevalence of hepatitis B and C among tattoo artists in Amsterdam [9]. However, this study was not intended to measure the effects of the regulation on the number of hepatitis B and C infections.

Resistance to the legislation exists among a number of Dutch tattoo artists. Their main counterargument is the fact that illegal activities (kitchen-table scratchers) are still reported. Some artists claim that staff from foreign countries are unfamiliar with the Dutch guidelines and have difficulties in complying. Furthermore, tattoo artists as well as consumers argue that the fact that the license solely covers safety and does not cover the quality provided by the tattoo artist is confusing to some.

A Uniform Model

The Amsterdam model is an example of an effective way to regulate the practice of tattooing. Still, a licensing system has both benefits and limitations, and there are other types of legislation that can be considered for implementation to ensure that tattooists provide safe practice. The importance of universally implementing hygiene guidelines has been acknowledged, as the act of tattooing is not limited by national borders. Many artists operate in more than one country, and many consumers get their tattoo abroad. The current diversity in legislation and guidelines does not support compliance, as artists need to adapt to different instructions when operating abroad. Universal European guidelines would contribute to compliance with hygiene guidelines.

References

1 Worp J, Boonstra A, Coutinho R-A, van den Hoek J-A-R: Tattooing, permanent make-up and piercing in Amsterdam; guidelines, legislation and monitoring. Euro Surveill 2006;11:34–36.

2 Worp J, Boonstra A: Evaluation Report of Tattoo and Piercing Studios in Amsterdam (in Dutch). Public Health Service of Amsterdam, 1999.

3 LeBlanc P-M, Hollinger K-A, Klontz K-C: Tattoo ink-related infections – awareness, diagnosis, reporting, and prevention. New Engl J Med 2012;367: 985–987.

4 Conaglen P-D, Laurenson I-F, Sergeant A, Thorn S-N, Rayner A, Stevenson J: Systematic review of tattoo-associated skin infection with rapidly growing mycobacteria and public health investigation of a cluster in Scotland, 2010. Euro Surveill 2013;18:20553.

5 Quaranta A, Napoli C, Fasano F, Montagna C, Caggiano G, Montagna M-T: Body piercing and tattoos: a survey on young adults' knowledge of the risks and practices in body art. BMC Public Health 2011;11:774.

6 Veenstra T: Tattoo Hygiene Guidelines. The Netherlands, National Institute for Public Health and the Environment, 2014.

7 Veilig tatoeëren en piercen. http://www.veiligtatoeeeren.nl/ (accessed November 15, 2014).

8 Zweers J, Grimmius T: Report, Evaluation of Legislation Tattoo and Piercing (in Dutch). Research voor Beleid, 2011.

9 Urbanus A-T, van den Hoek A, Boonstra A, van Houdt R, de Bruijn L-J, Heijman T, Coutinho R-A, Prins M: People with multiple tattoos and/or piercings are not at increased risk for HBV or HCV in The Netherlands. PLoS One 2011;6:e24736.

Thijs Veenstra, MSc
National Institute for Public Health and the Environment
PO Box 2200
NL–1000 CE Amsterdam (The Netherlands)
E-Mail tveenstra@ggd.amsterdam.nl

Serup J, Kluger N, Bäumler W (eds): Tattooed Skin and Health.
Curr Probl Dermatol. Basel, Karger, 2015, vol 48, pp 223–227 (DOI: 10.1159/000369840)

Hygiene Standards for Tattooists

Andy Schmidt

2nd Chairman DOT e.V., Willich-Neersen, Germany

Abstract

The following excerpt is taken from the hygiene guidelines written by Deutsche Organisierte Tätowierer (DOT e.V. Germany; German Association of Professional Tattoo Artists) and United European Tattoo Artists e.V. (UETA). It has been published with the intention of creating a standard that is understandable and accomplishable in practice, focusing on a minimum standard level that guarantees the highest possible safety for tattooists and customers at the same time. The DOT and UETA consistently strive to participate in the research of tattoo hygiene and tattoo colours because important insider information can be provided by professional tattoo artists with many years of work experience.

The following hygiene guidelines have been developed by the Deutsche Organisierte Tätowierer (DOT; German Association of Professional Tattoo Artists) and United European Tattoo Artists e.V. (UETA) especially for tattoo studios. The main intention was to create a standard that is easily understandable and easily applicable in practice, focusing on a minimum standard level that guarantees 100% safety for tattooists and customers at the same time. Presented here is the version from 2008. Based on this version, we

are currently developing a Comité Européen de Normalisation (European Committee for Standardisation) norm for Europe assisted by the Deutsches Institut für Normung (German Institute for Standardisation); therefore, there may be possible alterations in the cooperation with further European partners.

Since its creation in 1995, the DOT has continuously tried to improve the image of the art of tattooing. To a large extent, this has included the creation of hygienic standards and also cooperation with the relevant authorities. Many local health authorities in Germany adhere to our standards. Further, the DOT has participated in the Arbeitsgemeinschaft industrieller Forschungsvereinigungen (Consortium of Industrial Research, Collective Research Networking). Within this cooperation, hygiene has been evaluated in tattoo studios in Germany, Belgium and Austria, and the first tests on tattoo colours have been carried out.

The DOT is a founding member of the European Society of Tattoo and Pigment Research. The DOT consistently strives to participate in the research of tattoo colours specifically. However, tattooing should not be dealt with only under medicine or cosmetics, it needs to be considered under a special status. Unfortunately, there is little data to review. Research is important but requires funding that neither the DOT nor the manufacturers of tattoo colours can supply.

Excerpt from the 'Hygiene Standards for Tattooists'

As of May 2008. All rights reserved by the DOT and UETA.

Health Risks and Infections during Tattooing
The process of tattooing poses a theoretical risk of infection with viruses transmittable through the blood, although this risk has not been verified with scientific data. Even a mathematical implication of the data at hand is inconclusive. According to the literature, the prevalence of tattooing in the German population is 10%; hence, approximately 8 million persons are tattooed in Germany. Many have more than 1 tattoo and have large tattoos that require several sessions to complete. If we multiply these 8 million tattoos by a factor of 2.5, we are talking about 20 million tattoo sessions in Germany. If only 1% of these sessions resulted in infectious complications, a total of 200,000 infections would have occurred. Assuming those 20 million tattoo sessions took place during the last 10 years and assuming a 1% infection rate, in Germany alone, 20,000 infections would have been contracted annually through tattooing. Even at a 0.1% infection rate, there would still be 2,000 cases per year.

Vocational Training
Individuals who apply tattoos must have basic knowledge in the following areas:
- general and specific microbiology, germinal sources and ways of transmission, causative organisms of skin and wound infections, and viruses transmitted by the blood, especially hepatitis B virus (HBV), hepatitis C virus (HCV) and human immunodeficiency virus (HIV)
- general hygiene (germinal sources and ways of transmission and possibilities and methods of preventing transmission
- specific hygiene (cleaning, disinfection and sterilisation, the treatment of instruments relevant to the transmission of pathogenic germs, hand disinfection, skin disinfection, surface disinfection, protection against re-contamination, the handling of sterile materials, water requirements, the handling of disposables, and waste disposal)
- personal protection (disposable medical gloves, protective gear, the washing and disinfection of hands and clothing, and the prevention of environmental contamination)
- procedures that support the fast healing of wounds sustained through tattooing

Work Area
The work area has to be easily cleanable, well ventilated and adequately lit. Flooring and work surfaces must be smooth and water repellent and/or easy to wipe and disinfect (e.g. tiles, polyvinyl chloride, and linoleum). A washstand should be close to the work area but placed in such a location that the contamination of the work area through splashing or aerosols may not take place.

The following equipment is needed:
- a hand disinfectant dispenser
- a liquid soap dispenser
- paper towels
- a waste disposal container

A smooth and easy-to-clean work space for setting down instruments is required. The work space should be covered with disposables (e.g. foil and paper towels). All furniture and fixtures (tattoo chair/arm rest) must have smooth and easy-to-clean and easily disinfectable surfaces. If necessary, liquid-repelling or impermeable disposable covers have to be used to cover chairs and gurneys.

If disposable materials are not used exclusively, equipment must be available to prepare and treat instruments and objects (cleaning, disinfection, and sterilisation) on site.

Sterilisation and Autoclaving
Sterilisation is safer because it leaves materials cleaner and lowers contamination levels. Through prior cleaning and disinfection, the initial germ count should be reduced to a low level. Manufacturer's specifications concerning concentration and disinfection and sterilisation times must be followed to inactivate or kill microorganisms on or inside of the processed materials to eliminate their infectivities if the materials possess a common grade of contamination. Dry heat is sufficient for sterilising grips and needle holders.

Used Needle Disposal
Standard commercial needle disposal containers for used needles must be available. The container has to stay securely shut, and once full, it must be disposed of.

Tattoo Machines
Tattoo machines and clip cords have to be freshly bagged for each customer. Commercial plastic bags, such as freezer bags and plastic wrap, are adequate. After tattooing, bags must be removed, and instruments must be cleaned and disinfected with an appropriate agent. Instruments must be disconnected from their power sources.

Materials and Instruments Needed
- for operator safety, disposable medical gloves (non-sterile) must be available in adequate quantities
- an appropriate alcohol-based hand disinfectant has to be in stock if possible as well as an attached dispenser or a pump bottle
- for skin disinfection prior to tattooing, an alcohol-based disinfectant must be used. (Note: this is considered the use of an approved drug,

therefore, make sure to strictly follow the manufacturer's instructions)
- disposable cleaning cloths/tissues for cleaning the work space (work table, tattoo chair, and arm rest). Disposable paper towels can be used.
- an alcohol-based surface disinfectant for the disinfection of small instruments
- a surface disinfectant for flooring and appropriate towels
- disposable tattoo needles
- if necessary, disposable needle jigs and grips

If disposable needles, needle jigs and grips are used exclusively, additional resources for the treatment of the instruments are not required.
- disposable bowls for inks (separate ones for each customer)
- an ultrasonic cleaner to clean the needle jigs and grips
- a disinfectant for instruments that is effective against HBV, HCV and HIV
- a disinfectant pan
- running water to rinse instruments (of drinking-water quality)
- if necessary, a steriliser
- appropriate packaging material for sterilised needle jigs
- a closed storage system (lockable drawers and cabinets) to prevent the contamination of sterilised materials
- quality control to ensure for the efficiency of the sterilisation procedures

Colours
Ink bottles must be stored closed and protected from dust to prevent microorganisms from contaminating the contents. Colours have to comply with current tattoo guidelines.

The following information must be included on the ink bottle label:
- 'for tattoo purpose' or 'tattoo ink' or 'tattoo colour'
- lot number
- manufacturer information

- expiration date
- storage life after opening bottle
- list of ingredients

Disinfection Procedures

Hands
Hand disinfection is one of the most important measures to prevent infections. The washing of hands should be reduced to a minimum. In cases of an increased risk of infection or contamination, especially while handling customer's excretions or objects contaminated with blood or sputum, the wearing of disposable medical gloves to protect the hands is mandatory. Contaminated hands may be washed with water and soap only after proper disinfection. Hand disinfection is mandatory in the following situations:
- after contact with blood, secretions or excretions
- before physical contact with customers or before touching the skin area to be tattooed
- after contact with contaminated surfaces or objects
- after taking off disposable gloves

Skin
Objective: To attain an adequate reduction of germs on the respective skin area prior to the procedure. The shaving of large areas of skin to be tattooed has to be done directly before beginning the tattoo session, and a suitable disinfectant has to be sprayed on with an exposure time of at least 15 seconds. Only original containers with the manufacturer's labels may be used. Do not decant.

Preparation of Hygiene-Relevant Equipment

Using the same colours for different customers and using reprocessed needles are the main risks in tattooing. Therefore, using new, disposable ink cups and new, disposable needles for each cus-

tomer are the most important and effective hygienic measures.

Because needle jigs may be contaminated with blood, they may also be contaminated with viruses transmitted through the blood, and because under certain circumstances, jigs may be in direct contact with the skin, another major risk of transferring relevant microorganisms is related to the use of reusable needle jigs. Additional increased safety can be achieved by using disposable needle jigs.

If disposable needle jigs are used exclusively, preparation and sterilisation procedures are redundant (see preliminary note on sterilisation).

Contamination of the tattoo machine during or because of its use cannot be ruled out. Therefore, a theoretical possibility of cross-contamination exists. The disinfection of tattoo machines is limited, and sterilisation is not possible at all.

Preparation of Needle Jigs and Grips
Risk Assessment
- no direct contact with blood, contamination with blood and ink are possible and likely
- effective cleaning and quality control of cleaning efficiency is possible
- only dismountable needle jigs and grips should be used, with components that do not have significant air pockets to impact sterilisation
- treatments must follow proper and controlled procedures

Measures
- cleaning, disinfection and sterilisation after each usage
- locked storage in appropriate packaging (lockable cases, drawers, and cabinets)
- removal only immediately prior to use
- if necessary, assembly prior to use
- the placement of materials and instruments on disposable paper towels or foil

Preparation for Treatment
After Usage: Temporary storage on disposable paper towels, disassembly into its parts only while

wearing non-sterile disposable gloves, and the placement of components into an appropriate container (to disinfect or dispose of them).

Cleaning

Thorough cleaning is a precondition for the effectiveness of later disinfection and sterilisation processes. Adherent blood and ink residues may significantly impact disinfection and sterilisation.

Non-disinfected components, especially sharp and pointed objects, bear the risk of injury and the infection of personnel. Protective disposable gloves must be worn while handling contaminated objects.

Because of hard-to-remove pigment particles, particularly when they are mixed with blood, it is recommended to subject such contaminated objects to an ultrasonic cleaning procedure. Ultrasonic cleaning procedures should only be applied to the components. The ultrasonic bath must be filled with disinfectant solution, which allows for the effective inactivation of HBV/HCV/HIV.

Furthermore, the instrument disinfectant agent must be suitable for ultrasonic cleaning. The change of the disinfectant agent must take place according to the manufacturer's instructions daily or earlier depending on the level of contamination (and for longer periods only with a certificate provided by the manufacturer).

Inspection for Residues

A thorough visual inspection with sufficient lighting and, if necessary, the use of a magnifying glass ensures that objects are free of residue (clean). Particular attention must be paid to hollow spaces, edges and corners. If needed, hollow spaces should be checked against the light. If necessary, targeted cleaning and drying procedures should be repeated, followed by inspection.

These were abstracts of the paper 'Hygiene standards for tattooists'.

The entire paper can be seen on: http://www.ueta.org/service/guidelines/.

Hygiene standards established by:
- Heribert Nentwig, (former) Chairman UETA e.V., (former) Hygiene Supervisor DOT.e.V. c/o Tattoo-Center Koblenz, Triererstrasse 38, DE–56072 Koblenz (Germany)
- Andy Schmidt, 2nd Chairman DOT e.V., Hauptstrasse 60, DE–47877 Willich-Neersen (Germany)

Hygiene standards verified and revised by:
- Prof. Dr. med. Burkard Wille, Arzt für Hygiene und Umweltmedizin und Arzt für Mikrobiologie und Infektionsepidemiologie, iki Institut für Krankenhaushygiene Gbr., Siemensstrasse 18, DE–35394 Giessen (Germany), Tel.: +49 641 9790 50

Physician for Hygiene and Environmental Medicine and Physician for Micro-Biology and Infectious Epidemiology:
- Prof. Dr. med. Burkard Wille, Siemensstrasse 18, DE–35394 Giessen (Germany) Tel.: +49 641 9790 50

General contact DOT e.V. *(Deutsche Organisierte Tätowierer = German Association of professional tattoo artists)*
- www.dot-ev.de, 2nd Chairman Andy Schmidt, Hauptstr. 60, DE–47877 Willich-Neersen (Germany) Tel.: +49 21 56 52 40

General contact UETA e.V. *(United European Tattoo Artists)*
- www.ueta.org, Chairman Maik Frey, Sirnauer Strasse 23, DE–73728 Esslingen (Germany) Tel. +49 711 5357277

Andy Schmidt
2nd Chairman DOT e.V.
Hauptstrasse 60
DE–47877 Willich-Neersen (Germany)
E-Mail andysbodyelectric@yahoo.de

Serup J, Kluger N, Bäumler W (eds): Tattooed Skin and Health.
Curr Probl Dermatol. Basel, Karger, 2015, vol 48, pp 228–235 (DOI: 10.1159/000369178)

Hygiene Standards in the Tattoo Parlour and Practices for Prevention of Infection

Jens Bergström[a] · Max Bodlund[b]

[a] Tattoo Artist, Head Chairman of SRT, Founder of Tattoo and Piercing Education Scandinavia, Åkersberga,
[b] Tattoo Artist, Editor of the SRT book, Board member of SRT, Helsingborg, Sweden

Abstract

The tattoo studio and the procedures and operations of practicing tattooing may help to reduce the risk of infections associated with tattooing or, if improper, increase the risk. Thus, as a preventive measure, the tattoo studio should be optimized. All procedures should be carefully chosen to eliminate microbial contamination from the environment (from needles, machines, and other utilities) and also from persons. This chapter provides a detailed generic description of the organization of a safe tattoo procedure, i.e. guidance for professional tattooists on how to set up or reorganize their studio with the aim of the highest standard possible, which may satisfy customers' needs and make the procedure safe for the end consumer as well as the practitioner. These practices are necessary to meet upcoming official requirements in the future.   © 2015 S. Karger AG, Basel

Regardless of what anyone thinks about body modification, there are few negative aspects or even great risks associated with either a tattoo or a piercing. This modification is part of a magical ritual practiced for thousands of years. No one can explain why, but it's just as natural for many indigenous people as sleeping, eating, or providing food for the day: a part of life. This practice has become similarly so in the West. Body modification is a way of life and an art form that has been of great importance for many people, and it is a natural way for us to express ourselves. The risks are not in the procedure itself, but in our behaviors. It is when we do not take the few risks that are involved seriously that tattooing can have unintended consequences.

Studio Routines and General Shop Flow

A tattoo studio is dependent on its flow and the planned venue, which are based on what you will use it for (fig. 1). You have an obligation as a practitioner to ensure that the premises meet the requirements of the decision-making authorities.

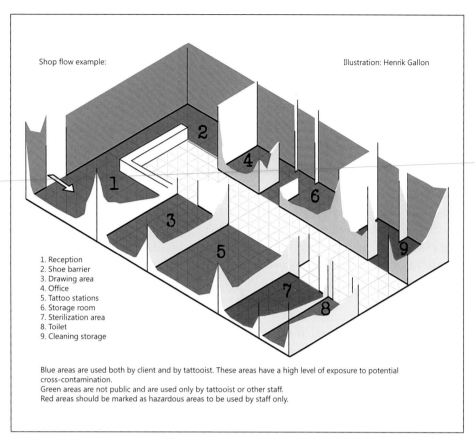

Shop flow example:

1. Reception
2. Shoe barrier
3. Drawing area
4. Office
5. Tattoo stations
6. Storage room
7. Sterilization area
8. Toilet
9. Cleaning storage

Blue areas are used both by client and by tattooist. These areas have a high level of exposure to potential cross-contamination.
Green areas are not public and are used only by tattooist or other staff.
Red areas should be marked as hazardous areas to be used by staff only.

Fig. 1. Shop flow.

A tattoo artist is also considered to be required to be well versed in all aspects of his or her craft, even if it does not include any requirements for the esthetic knowledge that the practitioner should have or not have. The look and the methods differ in various parts of the world, and primitive methods are still used. This also applies to the degree of knowledge on hygiene, and in many cultures, tattoos are still performed under very dirty conditions. However, these cultures cannot be blamed for the problems that we, in the West, experience; the eventual problems caused by remote cultures dedicated to body modification can be seen as socially negligible.

When we break the skin barrier, we commit ourselves to taking responsibility for some simple factors. We have, by penetrating the skin, made it possible for outside circumstances to damage the internal organs. The skin is the body's largest living organ, designed to a big degree to protect what is inside the body. We and whom we are working with while damaging the skin barrier must therefore make it our responsibility to ensure that the injury heals as quickly as possible and that the effect of the procedure is as small as possible. This is ensured through good practice, appropriate flow of the area, and a well-thought-out plan for after care; it doesn't have to be more complicated than that.

When it comes to the areas of the shop, it is good to have a clear idea of what each room is for and how it is used. The workstation must be planned so that it provides as little risk as possible and so that it is safe to work from. Creating a workable flow in the lounge, workroom, sterile room, and common areas is the easiest way to ensure a good and safe procedure.

There should also be a written standard for the shop for other duties on the premises used for the procedure. Cleanliness is of utmost importance to reduce the risk of cross-contamination, and all surfaces are of the same weight. Having knowledge of the management of materials and keeping the surfaces clean are critical to ensure the safety of the environment that you are working in.

It is also evident through the research done, e.g. that of the European Society of Tattoo and Pigment Research, that much of the problems that occur are actually caused by the customer in connection with healing. To prevent unwanted infections, a health declaration before the procedure is recommended when the customer's general condition may form the basis for many common problems. It is also important to have understandable after-care advice to give after treatment, when the most common incident is infection associated with healing. A good practice is to give this advice in written form.

Procedure

Use purpose-designed disposable gloves when handling contaminated items as well as during the actual tattoo session.

Good hand hygiene is extremely important. By washing our hands with soap and water, only the visible dirt comes off. Disinfection of the hands is more effective in reducing microorganisms and may therefore be appropriate to perform often, especially at jobs where the risk of infection is greater during daily treatment routines (tattooing). Hand sanitizer does not have to

be preceded by washing hands that are not visibly dirty. However, visibly dirty hands must first be cleaned with soap and water and then with hand sanitizer.

- Never touch the contaminated goods or the newly tattooed skin without gloves.
- Never touch anything that does not have to do with the session with contaminated gloves.

Of the utmost importance is that all that will be touched during the session must be wrapped in plastic so that the dirty (contaminated) plastic can be removed when the work is done. Some examples of what must be wrapped in plastic are tattoo machines, the bottle of water for washing the skin during the process, the power supply, and even the customer's chair (fig. 2, 3). There are more examples, but those we will mention in detail later in the text. After the session, all contaminated plastic should be thrown away, and the workspace, the customer's chair, and all equipment used should be thoroughly disinfected.

During the working process, the tattoo artist must always take off his or her gloves if he or she needs to touch something that is not protected with disposable plastic. For example, if the phone rings or if he or she needs to go to the bathroom, the contaminated gloves must first be thrown away before anything else is done. If this rule is broken for some reason, the mistakenly contaminated surface must immediately be disinfected.

Only sterilized goods should be used on each and every new customer. During the session, only disposable needles should be used on the customer. Disposable goods should be used as much as possible, unless it is inconsistent with environmental considerations.

Make sure that everyone working in the studio on a daily basis understands the risks and consequences of cross-contamination. Everybody working in a tattoo shop is a risk factor, so it's crucial that any person working in the shop environment has the required education regard-

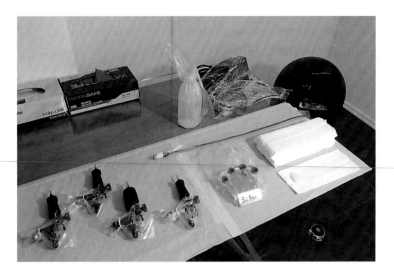

Fig. 2. Set up.

ing blood pathogens and cross-contamination (fig. 4).

A special standard regarding the hygiene procedure for the client is preferable. The client is NOT necessarily aware of the hazards of cross-contamination, so a document explaining the risks for the client in the shop can be helpful.

If there are any errors in the pre-procedure, start over. Never take a chance regarding the client's or your own safety.

How to Choose Materials When Designing the Workspace

The work area should be well thought out, as should material choices, as these will facilitate the daily hygiene work. The workspace should not be right next to the space where you clean the machines and tubes after the procedure. It should have its own place: not necessarily a separate room but separated from anything that can affect the hygiene work negatively.

- The table that is used as a surface to put the tattoo machines on while performing the tattoo must be of a material that is easy to

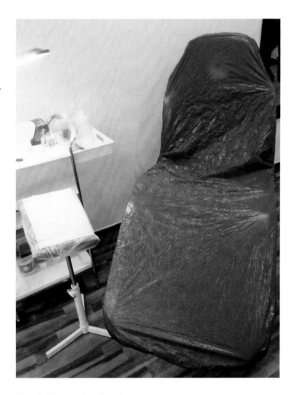

Fig. 3. Protection barrier.

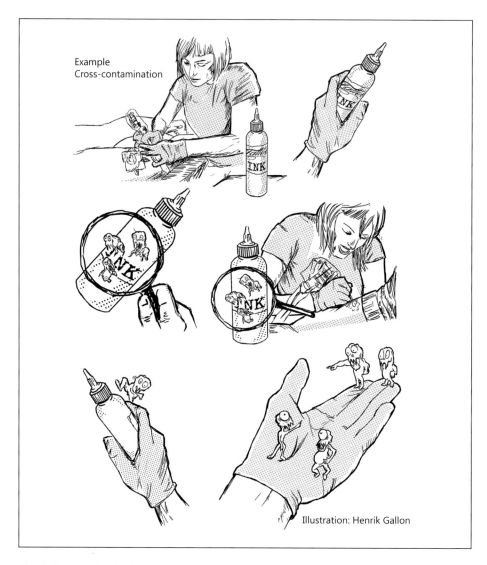

Example
Cross-contamination

Illustration: Henrik Gallon

Fig. 4. Cross-contamination.

wipe clean, such as glass or stainless steel. Wood should be avoided because it can be difficult to disinfect due to the fact that the wood grain can hide bacteria in the deeper structures.

- The customer's chair and bunk and the tattooist's chair must be easy to wrap and have a surface texture that, just like the tabletop, must be easy to wipe clean. These should be easy to disinfect, and not plain soft fabric-covered chairs or any other material that is impossible to disinfect if necessary.

- All storage of either single-use, sterile, or ultraclean equipment should be in a dry, dust-free environment. This applies to all of the inks and fluids that are used during the procedure. Cabinets with doors are preferable for material storage (fig. 5).

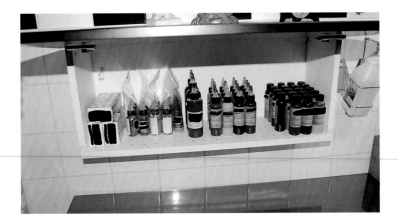

Fig. 5. Material storage.

- The studio should have good ventilation.
- It is good to have a shoe limit so that the customer minimizes the risk of bringing dirt from the outside into the working area.
- The studio should have a well-separated area for cleaning and sterilizing the machines and goods. An area where you won't need to open a door to get there is preferable.

Preparation of the Work Area and the Machines

All preparation work is done with well-washed hands (soap and water) that are then cleaned with hand sanitizer. In addition, disposable gloves are used when it comes to the plastic wrapping procedure.

Work Preparation

The tattoo artist should first, before anything else, clean the table and chairs (all of the surfaces used during the session) by disinfecting them. Do not forget the clip cord and machinery.

Step two is to wrap everything with plastic that risks being touched during the work. What you need to understand here is that if you don't do this, sooner or later, cross-contamination will be inevitable and will lead to bacteria spreading. Thus, the basic rule is that anything that may be touched during the session must have a protective barrier of the disposable kind that should be thrown away after each and every finished tattoo (fig. 2).

Some Specific Steps that Cannot Be Neglected

- The front of the electric transformer should be well covered with disposable plastic wrap. All water bottles or the equivalent should also be covered with plastic bags, leaving only the top of the plastic bag open for the bottle. We recommend that the tattoo artist use dropper bottles rather than spray bottles.
- The tabletop should be protected with plastic or a protective sheet made of paper and plastic. It is enough to cover the area used the most during the session.
- The part of the clip cord that is touched when changing machines or when you unplug the machines at the end of the session should be covered with a plastic bag. Remember that the cord can touch with the tattoo during the session, so the plastic bag designed for the cord should be at least 70–80 cm long.

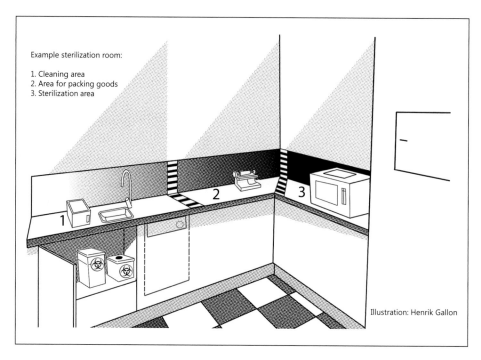

Example sterilization room:

1. Cleaning area
2. Area for packing goods
3. Sterilization area

Illustration: Henrik Gallon

Fig. 6. Sterile room.

- Use only disposable ink caps. The ink cap holder should also be covered with a plastic bag.
- Each tattoo machine must also be covered with a well-suited plastic bag. This is vital due to the fact that the machine is hard to clean because of its nooks and crannies. It is also impossible not to touch the machine when you replace it with another machine, so the protective barrier is as important as everything else that we emphasize here.
- Vaseline is to be taken out of the jar with a disposable tongue depressor or the tattooist's hand, of course protected with a disposable glove.
- Only disposable plastic cups should be used to wash out or dilute the ink during the session and should be thrown away after each and every customer. The tattooist should never refill an ink cap during the procedure; use a new one

if a refill is needed to avoid cross-contamination of the bottle.
- Only disposable razors should be used for preparation of the skin's surface.
- The chair or the bunk that the customer sits or lies on must also be covered properly. The parts of the tattooist's chair that will be touched during the session must also be covered (e.g. the height-adjusting lever).

Machine Preparation

Start by cleaning the machines. Very important is that the machines are washed and cleaned with disinfectant after the session with the previous customer and before the set up for the new customer.

The new set up with needles, grips, and tubes must be placed in an area made only for this purpose. It would be appropriate to do so on a sheet of glass that can be cleaned with disinfectant regularly. This specific area cannot be near the sink where the dismantling of equipment is done or near the sink where you clean and sterilize the contaminated grips and tubes.

Needles, grips, and tubes are to be stored in sterile bags or put into the autoclave just before use.

When the needle, grip, and tube are to be mounted on a tattoo machine, only disposable gloves should be used. Rubber bands and the 'nipple' (to hold the end of the needle in place) must be disposable; otherwise, they can be contaminated if used more than once. The last thing before using the machines: put a suitable plastic bag over each machine. A must!

Regarding sterilization equipment in the shop, it is of major importance that the practitioner is well aware that the equipment needs to be maintained and serviced. The responsible parties also need to know the difference between different types of autoclaves and procedures. The regulations for this equipment look different throughout Europe, but harmonization of the rules is desirable. In-house sterilization is the best way to control and maintain sterile conditions, but this also calls for a great deal of responsibility for the practitioner, who needs to have a strict plan for how the routines should be followed and how to minimize the risk of cross-contamination (fig. 6).

Recommended Reading

1 The National Board of Health and Welfare. http://www.socialstyrelsen.se/english (accessed January 15, 2015).

2 Swedish Work Environment Authority. http://www.av.se/inenglish (accessed January 15, 2015).

3 Swedish Medical Products Agency. http://www.lakemedelsverket.se/english/ (accessed January 15, 2015).

4 Public Health Agency of Sweden. http://www.folkhalsomyndigheten.se/ (accessed January 15, 2015).

Jens Bergström
Tattoo Artist
Bivägen 1
SE-184 38 Åkersberga (Sweden)
E-Mail info@tattooeducation.se

Serup J, Kluger N, Bäumler W (eds): Tattooed Skin and Health.
Curr Probl Dermatol. Basel, Karger, 2015, vol 48, pp 236–247 (DOI: 10.1159/000370017)

Seamless Prevention of Adverse Events from Tattooing: Integrated Strategy Emphasising the Customer-Tattooist Interaction

Jørgen Serup

Bispebjerg University Hospital, Department of Dermatology, the 'Tattoo Clinic', Copenhagen, Denmark

Abstract

The boom in tattooing has been paralleled by more frequent adverse events, which may be localised in the skin or systemic and manifested clinically or latent. Infections, allergic reactions from red-coloured tattoos and papulonodular reactions from black tattoos dominate. Mild complaints are very common, with 1/5 of all tattooed individuals having acquired sensitivity to sunlight in the tattooed skin. The potential risk of cancer due to potential carcinogens in some tattoo inks has hitherto *not* manifested in clinical reports, despite the millions of people who have been tattooed over many decades. A risk of death from tattooing remains associated with severe infection, i.e. sepsis. Preventive strategies may rely on focused preventions, and sterility and preservation of ink is essential, rational and knowledge-based. The chemical and particle contents of ink nanoparticles cannot be unrestricted; however, focused control of ink is facing many uncertainties, including analytical problems, lack of identification of allergens in ink and discrepancies between the content of potential carcinogens and manifestation of cancer in the clinic. The concept of seamless prevention is introduced as a pragmatic strategy that emphasises the customer-tattooist interaction, which is the 'engine' of tattoo safety. This strategy amalgamates the range of narrow-scope preventive instruments and shall ensure that any relevant instrument is used actively and without deficiency or drop out, thus resulting in a complete orchestration of a multi-targeted strategy. High-priority elements of this strategy shall facilitate a qualified 'go' or 'no go' decision by the customer before the tattoo is made and should involve informed consent, qualification of the tattooist and the parlour, including supplies of inks etc., and attention to hygienic security. Records and documentation of tattoo cases with complications and the culprit inks as well as the establishment of national or European-based surveillance systems that are properly equipped to deliver efficient clarification and handling of adverse events and hazards of tattooing and inks, which needs attention and timely action to prevent additional cases and epidemic outbreaks, are part of this seamless strategy, along with optimised medical therapy and research.

© 2015 S. Karger AG, Basel

Introduction

Tattooing is, with some 100 million Europeans being tattooed, the largest on-going experiment involving the injection of chemicals and microparticles into the skin and body of man. Tattooing is an old art and is felt to belong to the roots of the people; thus, it is culturally difficult to approach this issue with authoritative restrictions. It is already solidly established in societies and has an established culture of its own. People may feel that they are within their democratic and human rights to exert ownership of their own skin and decide to run the risk that comes with the satisfaction of putting their personal signature on their skin.

However, from a toxicological and medical point of view, the practice of tattooing is an obvious risk to health. The scattered regulation of tattooing and inks in countries is out of proportion with the world-wide heavy regulation of pharmaceuticals, in which the new registration and international launch of just one new drug with just one pure chemical requires an investment on the order of a billion dollars.

Nevertheless, it shall be recognised that tattooing, despite its widespread use all over the world and the number and occurrences of tattoos, has caused remarkably few identified medical complications and alerts. However, the development of the global tattoo business is dynamic and involves the constant introduction of new practices, tattoo ink ingredients, contaminants and products, as well as the risk of adverse events and hazards that present an ever-lasting threat to health.

This chapter launches the concept of the 'seamless prevention' of tattoo adverse events, as worked out in more detail in a recent report of the Council on Health and Disease Prevention, which is incorporated with the Danish Medical Association [1]. This concept is pragmatic and attempts to face facts and reality for the fulfilment of its aims, while understanding the necessity of the acceptance and partnership with stakeholders in order to become implemented and truly improve the situation.

Tattoo Risks, Aims and Targets of Prevention

Tattoo complaints and complications and their diagnosis and spectrum are described in a separate chapter of this book and in a number of reports and reviews in the medical literature [2–7].

In brief, the observed adverse events, which are candidate objects of prevention, are described below.

The Known Risks of Tattooing
Medical complications and interactions
- Bacterial infections manifested as acute infections after tattooing and during the course of healing of the tattoo. These may be local or systemic and ultimately progress to sepsis.
- Traumatic and other local skin events due to improper tattoo technique and amateurism, with acute, subchronic or chronic consequences.
- Chronic infections introduced with the tattoo, especially viral hepatitis B and C and HIV infections.
- Chronic allergies originated from the ink, especially those occurring in tattoos with red or shades of red, which are supposed to be somehow associated with azo-pigments but are also occasionally seen in green and blue tattoos.
- Chronic papulo-nodular reactions in black tattoos that are supposed to be associated with pigment overload and agglomeration inside the skin that happens spontaneously over time.
- Special chronic reaction patterns that are, to examplify, associated with the lymphatic system and pain syndromes that are associated with the sensory nervous system.

- Interactions with skin diseases and skin conditions, generally and specifically, and interactions with general diseases and weaknesses of the body.

Mild complaints
- Intermittent or constant itch and swelling, with discomfort and photosensitivity; the latter is observed in 1/5 of tattooed individuals [8, 9].

Regret of tattoos, psycho-social consequences and tattoo removal by lasers
- Regret of a tattoo is frequent.
- Regret of a tattoo and psychic and social complications, which may be severe, limit life and block opportunities.
- Removal of a tattoo using laser or other methods resulting in scar formation, abnormal melanin pigmentation, allergic reaction or other complications. Many tattoos cannot be removed efficiently with an aesthetically acceptable result and without scarring using lasers.

Life-threatening and exceptional hazards
- Bacterial infection with sepsis, multiple organ failure and death, by incident.
- Anaphylactic allergic reactions, with the allergen released during laser treatment, or latex protein allergy induced by the tattooist's gloves, which is exceptional.
- Syncopes during tattooing due to a new or pre-existing medical disease or condition, i.e. cardiac problems and arrest.

The Potential Risks of Tattooing
- Manifestations of *carcinogenic, mutagenic and reproduction-toxic (CMR) ingredients* of inks and manifestations of the toxic or allergic effects of metals. Risks remain potential since clinical reports and epidemiological data have not confirmed such risks to be clinically significant with the use of present tattoo inks.
- Manifestations related to pigments which, as *nanoparticles and microparticles*, might exert

hitherto unknown effects in the body; however, these are presently not a subject of specific study or reporting.

The list of isolated risks and scenarios of risk related to tattooing uncovers a broad range of mechanisms, unwanted effects and safety end points, which prevention shall ideally address. The list is exhaustive, and prevention as a whole goes far beyond the narrow regulation of tattoo inks and hygiene. The more common adverse events shall be the primary aims of prevention. Sepsis is uncommon but remains the primary reason for death, unless treatment is efficient. Severe infection has for more than a century been the main cause of severe disability, amputations and deaths from tattooing [10].

State of the Knowledge and Need for Research as a Back-Up for Preventive Measures

The incidence and prevalence of tattoo complications have not been studied systematically, and prevention has to rely on clinical and epidemiological evidence that has accumulated over the years and is reported in the medical literature by professionals of different backgrounds who may be confronted with such events. A search of the National Library database for medical reports (as of 15 November 2014, PubMed) resulted in the hits that are shown in table 1.

The literature includes many individual case reports and may provide limited evidence; however, the figures support the impression that allergic reactions and infections are prominent and that red and black tattoos, which are the more popular colours, generate more frequent reports. Tattoo problems are clearly underreported [11]. Since its start in 2008, the 'Tattoo Clinic' of Bispebjerg University Hospital has collected some 400 cases of tattoo complications from the Copenhagen major region. The EU Rapid Alert System for non-food (RAPEX) products has very few reports

Table 1. Incidence and prevalence of tattoo complications illustrated from the National Library database, index words and hits

Tattoo	1,533
Tattoo reactions	158
Tattoo complication	48
Tattoo allergy	133
Tattoo red	134
Tattoo blue	67
Tattoo green	46
Tattoo yellow	22
Tattoo black	166
Tattoo infection	186
Tattoo sepsis	5
Tattoo laser	289
Tattoo laser removal	188
Tattoo cancer*	244
Tattoo lymph node	51
Skin cancer	146,473

* Includes black tattoos used for medical purposes, i.e. marking of the radiation field in breast cancer.

of problematic tattoo inks and cannot contribute significant information on the clinical adverse reactions associated with tattooing because it is not a clinical database.

The reports of cancer from tattoos are consistent with the recent review of the world medical literature as searched by Kluger and Koljonen [12]. These authors checked the reports and traced only 50 valid cases of cancers (including keratoacanthoma, a dubious 'cancer' that is benign in clinical development but shares features with squamous cell carcinoma by histology) arising in tattoos. They concluded that these cancers likely originated by coincidence, since cancers may easily arise in the epidermis, independent of tattoo pigment. This conclusion is in agreement with two studies of 25-year follow ups of patients with psoriasis and atopic dermatitis who were repeatedly treated with tar on large areas of their skin over several weeks, sometimes combined with ultraviolet-B light (i.e. the Goeckerman regimen) [13, 14]. Follow up showed no increase in

skin cancer. The skin organ, in contrast to airway epithelium and lung tissue, appears to be remarkably resistant to the development of cancer from tar, which is rich in polycyclic aromatic hydrocarbons (PAHs). This contrasts data from the chemical screening of tattoo inks, which found PAHs and primary aromatic amines (PAAs) in the inks, but apparently these do not cause clinical cancer in tattooed skin [15]. Today, tar treatment is accepted and used as an efficient treatment of psoriasis and eczema in dermatology, used as 2nd- or 3rd-line treatment because of its unpleasant smell and staining.

The preventative measures for skin cancer due to tattooing and ink ingredients, which are based on register data on potential carcinogenicity, is not applicable in this situation since such cancers in the tattooed skin, regional lymph nodes and other organs apparently do not occur under real-life conditions. What is not present, of course, cannot be reduced through prevention.

It shall, nevertheless, be noted that the adverse effects of CMR substances in tattoo inks that manifest in any organ can not be academically excluded, particularly reproduction-toxic effects, when a single dose of a mutagen at a critical stage of cell division might potentially cause harm.

It shall also be noted that tattoo inks cannot acceptably have unlimited amounts of CMR substances; therefore, there is an urgent need for some regulatory limitation, if not based on conclusive research then, as a minimum, shaped as a 'soft' regulation.

With respect to allergic reactions to tattoos, especially to tattoos using red and shades of red, it was demonstrated in a large study involving allergy-patch testing of ninety patients that patients who had allergic reactions did not react to a chemical or allergen from the specific culprit tattoo ink stock bottle and thus had not reacted to the free PAAs in the products [16]. Allergic tattoo reactions typically occur after weeks, months or years and are thought to occur due to a hapten that has formed in the tattooed skin by local metabolism.

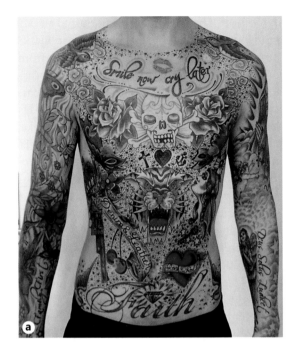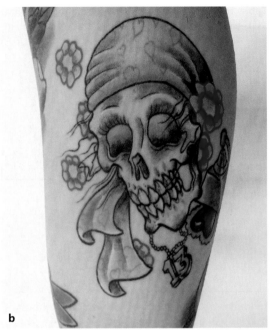

Fig. 1. a Extensively tattooed young man. The tattoo shown in the photo covers 27% of the person's skin, i.e. about 0.5 m^2 or 5,000 cm^2, according to 'the rule of nine'. However, the extensive skin fields inside the frame of the tattoo are not completely tattooed, and about 10 different colours were used at varying intensity to create shades. The dose of each colour per cm^2 is much lower than the outline of the tattoo and is very difficult to estimate unless sophisticated computer technology is used to assess the area. The toxicological risk is assumed to be colour-specific. Thus, the simple measurement of the size of a tattoo is imprecise when measuring the area-wise exposure to tattoo ink of a defined colour. **b** The same problem illustrated for a tattoo on the shoulder of a young woman.

The hapten, epitope and substrate raw material in tattoo ink are presently unidentified and thus cannot be analysed, delineated or eliminated from inks. The substrate of allergic reaction to azochemical is not simply a PAA or paraphenylene diamine, as shown in studies on allergic reactions to textile dyes.

Prevention based on the elimination of dangerous ingredients of tattoo inks suffers from a lack of fundamental knowledge, especially on dosage and biokinetics. The local dose of ink in the skin and the absorption, distribution, metabolism and excretion of soluble and insoluble agents, i.e. ingredients and pigment particles, is not understood (fig. 1a, b). Soluble and insoluble ingredients that may slowly release chemicals over years are likely to have very different kinetic profiles and thus very different exposure scenarios. This field is massively under-researched. The translation of register data on PAHs and PAAs and cancer risk in humans is not correlated. Cancer from tattoos appears to not be a problem. The sensitisation potential of isolated PAAs in inks, as mentioned, has not been confirmed, although red ink containing azo chemicals appears to be associated with clinical tattoo allergy. However, the raw material ingredient in ink and the haptens that stimulate allergic reactions are unknown.

The limited knowledge of the aetiology, mechanism and manifestations of tattoo complications calls for pragmatic strategies for the realistic prevention of tattoo complications.

In contrast to the risks of chemical ingredients and pigment particles, the potential risks of infectious complications are well understood with respect to clinical manifestations, the spectrum of causative microorganisms and the routes of infection. These ingredients can be modified as part of a preventative effort. This rationale is behind infection control well established and universally accepted [17, 18]. Some part of the microbial risk is attributed to contaminated tattoo ink products, which may include about 10% of new inks [19, 20]. This threat to tattooed individuals obviously needs to be addressed through development of hygiene policies and guidance for the tattoo parlours.

In conclusion, an overwhelming problem for preventive strategies is that the translation of the potential risk of the chemical and particle contents of tattoo inks, based on register data, into clinical risk to humans is presently poorly understood, premature, limited in predictive value and backed up by little research and validation. This lack of knowledge even includes essential knowledge, such as the nomination of valid standard methods for the chemical analyses of risk elements, which is a key prerequisite for the establishment of meaningful threshold levels of chemical risk elements that are allowed or forbidden in commercial tattoo inks.

Society, Culture and Tattooing in the Perspective of Prevention

Tattooing is in a boom that has been promoted by media and celebrities. During the last decades, tattooing has propagated from the lower social classes and has become diffusely absorbed by all social segments. Tattooing has become gender neutral and widespread, and populations other than youngsters and gangsters are now tattooed [21]. With tattoo prevalence in the range of 10–20% of adults and about 30% of youngsters, prevention is facing a difficult task and a physical barrier due to the size and power of the tattooed population. This development has been paralleled with the opening of a huge number of professional tattoo parlours and even more amateur tattooists, who uncritically buy cheap machines and inks (fig. 2). Furthermore, in modern society, communication using images, which is a modern language that is competing with traditional textual communication, has become mainstream, resulting in massive cultural pressure on individuals in the direction of being tattooed and having personal images and signatures on the skin. On the other hand, the efficient modern society has posed massive pressure and conformity standards on citizens' private lives, limiting their individualism and freedom. Preventive measures limiting the risk of tattooing shall operate in this environment of contrast and incongruence and is bound to have a weak position from the start simply due to the magnitude and popularity of the tattoo business. Any preventive measure must have rationale and concordance with the situation in society to become efficient. Unpopular, authoritative regulation may require extensive control and policing functions to come into operation, which risks the vanishing of the regulations and their ending as a failure, making the construction of such regulations a 'suicide mission'. Tattooing has maintained a rebellious spirit and, even today, is non-obedient in nature and is a signal of setting orders and tight standards aside and saying 'I am my own'.

The Customer-Tattooist Interaction

The customer-tattooist interaction and mutual confidence described in other chapters of this book appears powerful and important in a preventive perspective. The customer starts with curiosity about tattooing and, under the influence of the surrounding society and his personal environment, friends and close relatives, he or she may decide to contact a tattooist. The tattooist may modify or propose the desired tattoo and in-

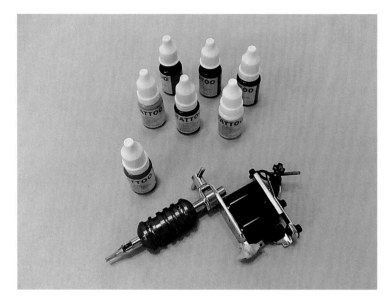

Fig. 2. Low-cost beginner tattooist's kit that is popular among amateurs, supplied with a few disposable needles. The cost of the kit is about EUR 75. The inks named 'Tattoo' are, according to the label, produced in Taiwan, but there is no information on the ingredients or identity of the manufacturer; the origin and legal responsibility cannot be traced.

struct the customer, or not, on the risks of tattooing. This is mostly well-accepted, since the customer wishes that his private and permanent signature on his own skin be unique and a mark for life. In that situation, the customer may need to explain the details of his life to the tattooist. This interaction resembles patient-doctor or client-lawyer interactions, and this is a situation when the tattooist may influence a customer's decision on the type of tattoo, its size, location on the body, motive, choice of colour, etc. in a direction that poses more or less risk to the customer, ideally in a spirit of ethical tattooing and high professional standards. The customer-tattooist interaction is the engine of physical tattooing, customer satisfaction and the associated health risk. The tattooist can, as many other professionals, be requested to perform his role up to the requirements given by the society and guidelines from associations of professional tattooists that define professional standards. The job of the tattooist involves the practical execution of the decision to get a tattoo, and for that part, the physical requisites, such as a clean parlour, hygienic instruments and the utilities that should be used. The tattooist should also

be educated and experienced. Of course, the ink should be of high quality so that its quality can be ensured and it poses minimum risk; any risk from the ink should be predicted and guaranteed by the manufacturer and distributor. The customer-tattooist interaction also includes advice on aftercare and support in case healing does not occur smoothly. This interaction is of major importance in a preventive perspective because it is individual and because the very act of being tattooed at any time enters a zone of physical risk.

The Supply Industry

The supply industry comprises manufacturers of tattoo machines, tattoo needles, tattoo ink stock products and other supplies. The supply industry sells their products internationally via local or regional suppliers and via the internet. Any layperson can buy the products. The market is competitive, and the prices of the machines, needles and ink are generally low. American as well as European industries appear to be the leading suppliers of machines and inks. In Europe, tattoo inks are only produced in some countries, especially the UK, Germany and Italy, and the majority of European countries have no national production. Inexpensive machines and inks from Asia are important players in the market that help to keep prices low. The market has no obvious room for an increase in the price of supplies. The market is thus price sensitive and appears to have little room for higher price justified by claims of improved safety.

Focused Preventative Strategies

A focused strategy of prevention targets a selected issue or a sequence of events of major importance in a risk panorama and may act as a key that can lock a door to a disease outcome (by negative listing) or open a door to a safe outcome (by positive listing). Regulation based on specific requirements regarding the chemical composition of tattoo inks, as specified by ResAp(2008)1 of the Council of Europe, represents a focused strategy that operates by negative listing [22]. To address the real problem, i.e. clinical complications arising from tattooing, the strategy must be essentially rational and thus knowledge based, deemed suited to help the real problem, and be possible to implement, not only sporadically but also coherently in a larger territory, since the tattoo business is international. A critical point is its acceptance by stakeholders and the market. From the start, focused regulation of the negative listing type is positioned weakly when held against the size and nature of tattooing and the tattoo business. If not acceptable, the regulation runs major risk of being neglected and ultimately creating an even more chaotic situation in the market. ResAP(2008)1, originally introduced as a resolution in 2003, regulates the amounts of PAHs, PAAs, metals and microbes in inks, with sterility of inks being a fundamental requirement. The resolution did not manage to become generally accepted in Europe. In countries where

the resolution was implemented, follow up showed that inks with PAHs, PAAs and metals had become less frequently found on the shelves of tattoo parlours upon monitored visits and examinations. In addition, the percentage of inks that were contaminated with bacteria decreased. However, per definition unsafe inks were far from eliminated, and there is no indication or evidence that the registered minor change of ink status was accompanied by any reduction in complications from tattooing. No European country (except, very recently, France) has installed a surveillance system to monitor clinical adverse events from tattooing.

ResAP(2008)1 operates only by the negative listing of chemicals and thus faces firm obstacles to being accepted and implemented. Therefore, stakeholders will need advice on alternative routes. A positive listing of acceptable ingredients in tattoo inks is an obvious and critical need if focused regulation of chemical composition of inks shall ever be successful.

As mentioned above, the rationale behind the focused regulation of microbial contamination of tattoo inks is clear, and since tattoo infections are relatively common and can potentially cause death, this is both a logical and obvious need that can be argued, insisted on and finally accepted. The regulation of microbial contamination of inks may benefit from being separated from the regulation of the chemical content of inks, and from focusing specifically on the sterility and preservation of products. The elimination of microbes in inks and the improvement of hygiene in parlours are synergistic and independent of chemical content.

Integrated/Seamless Prevention Strategy in Tattooing

In the seamless prevention strategy, a holistic view is taken that recognises the actions of the tattoo customer over time and attempts to influ-

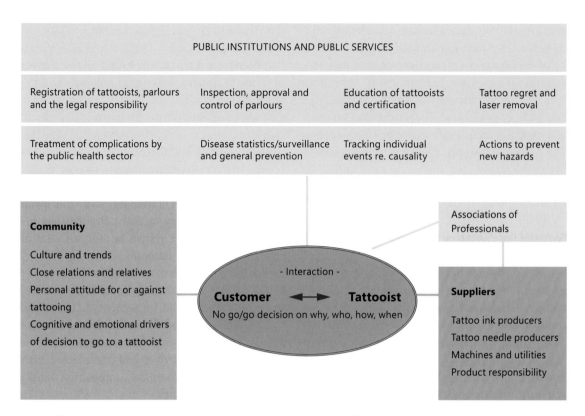

Fig. 3. The seamless prevention model shown as a schematic drawing. The customer-tattooist interaction is essential and the 'engine'. The customer is influenced by society and personal relationships, and the tattooist is influenced by suppliers and professional associations. The suppliers include manufacturers of needles, machines, inks and other utensils. The activity is performed within a legal framework with regulations, guidance, detailed control and surveillance. The responsible society provides medical service and health statistics, and the society shall have both a general strategy and instruments for handling adverse events, which may need timely action to prevent new cases and outbreaks. The strategy has an observational component and, in some aspects, a defensive or pro-active profile. However, in principle, this strategy may function and be efficient with or without the establishment of efficient control of the chemical ingredients of the inks.

ence any element of that action at any time when the process can be qualified, thus reducing the risk taken by the tattooed individual. This concept is inspired by seamless or integrated care, which has been successfully implemented in the health sector [23]. The concept of seamless prevention in tattooing is illustrated in figure 3. The multi-target, preventive construction shall be active in every important cell, and there shall be no transitional friction or inconsistency and no defects in the range of executed preventive exercises as the customer moves from curiosity about tattooing, which is influenced by society, to interaction with the tattooist and finally to the long-term situation, which is when complications shall be limited and, if present, treated properly, diagnosed, registered and tracked backwards to learn and prevent similar occurrences from happening in the future.

As described previously in this chapter, the crucial points, or the 'engines', are the customer's decision to become tattooed and the act of tattooing, i.e. the customer-tattooist interaction. Making this interaction as qualified and safety-oriented as possible is a core object of the seamless strategy.

The customer is influenced by the surrounding society and culture, with the present trendy promotion of tattooing and little public attention to safety issues. *Public information and campaigns shall be instituted and make use of the most important media.* The customer ultimately relies on close friends and relatives and his personal desires; however, both society and culture influence his decision.

The tattooist and customer interact at a level that may become intimate. If properly informed, in writing through an *authorised brochure* and verbally by the tattooist, about the limitations and risks of having a tattoo, the customer may decide *not* to be tattooed, which is the perfect form of prevention. However, the customer may of course decide to have the tattoo done after having the pros and cons being explained to him. Before giving his *informed consent*, there shall be an opportunity for a *qualified 'go' or 'no go'*.

To do a good job, tattooists should practice *ethical conduct,* be *qualified through formal education,* and *follow the laws and regulations.* The *tattooist and the tattoo parlour should be registered by a competent authority, which shall regularly inspect the facility to ensure that it is clean and suited for tattooing. The authority shall also ensure that the process of tattooing in the parlour, from A–Z, is up to the defined standards, including the proper use of the machines, needles and tattoo inks.* The *parlour shall have and follow an authorised hygiene standard* that describes situations and sources that can expose the customer to risk of infection. The parlour shall also have a policy to prevent the tattooist himself from being infected by a customer through blood-borne viral agents. The parlour shall have a procedure for buying, maintaining and storing supplies and, if applicable, list the expiration date of the products. There shall be a defined procedure for pre-treatment and after-care that includes written information to the customer about the latter. *The tattooist shall perform systematic filing of all relevant data, including precise data on the ink used, for the purpose of keeping a track record in the case of complications from tattooing for a particular customer.* The *tattooist shall on the day the tattoo is performed routinely supply the customer with a written record about the tattoo and the specific ink used, to be kept by the customer at home in his private files.*

The suppliers of inks, tattoo needles and other utilities shall ensure that inks, needles and utilities are produced under *good manufacturing standards and meet the highest achievable safety for a product for human use. This cannot be achieved unless there is a legal basis and standards. Needles and inks must be effectively sterile, with the method and date of sterilisation documented.* Inks shall be delivered in unbroken and undamaged containers that are constructed to minimise contamination during use. The labelling of content, manufacturer, production date etc. shall follow requirements given by the relevant competent authority. The expiration date of inks is presently no more that a guess and some print on the product and is not documented in any way. In contrast, in the pharmaceutical industry, the expiration date and shelf life of a product is carefully measured and documented to become useful and reliable.

As mentioned above, competent authorities have a number of jobs related to the system and the daily business of tattoo parlours. Their role is to ensure that an appropriate system is established, implemented and followed.

Authorities have another important role, namely *establishing a surveillance system for reporting clinical adverse events due to tattooing, especially medical events requiring treatment by medical health providers, clinics and hospitals. Such a system, to which customers, tattooists, clinics and hospitals may report, is needed to trace inks that pose a risk and other hazards,* which need to be identified and handled without delay to minimise subsequent events and timely and efficiently eliminate the cause of problems. Such a system should be national and ideally involve European countries reporting on a European platform. A surveillance system is a major need since the chemical and particle safety of tattoo inks remain uncertain.

Adverse Events from Tattooing and Their Medical Treatment and Service

The tattoo boom is paralleled by adverse medical events that require medical diagnosis and treatment and are in line with any other significant disease that causes health problems. Sufferers are presently diffused among different specialties, such as general practice, dermatology, internal medicine, infectious medicine, general surgery, plastic surgery, laser surgery etc., and consequently may be seen as isolated cases. It is necessary to improve the diagnosis and treatment of complications from tattoos and register these complications case-by-case to generate experience, research and education that matches the present and future situation of the hundreds of millions of Europeans being tattooed and the hundred of thousands having complaints or complications specific for tattoos. Health care systems need to establish dedicated and qualified service to sufferers of tattoo complications, who are diseased and documented as burdened and disabled to the same degree as other patients who are offered public care [24]. Societies also need a knowledge reference in order to efficiently monitor the tattoo field.

References

1 Council on Health and Disease Prevention, Denmark. Tattooing, Health, Risks and Culture. Report under publication, 2015.
2 De Cuyper C, Perez-Cotapos M-L: Dermatologic Complications with Body Art. Tattooos, Piercings and Permanent Make-Up. Berlin/Heidelberg, Springer Verlag, 2010.
3 Kazandjieva J, Tsankov N: Tattoos: dermatological complications. Clin Dermatol 2007;25:375–382.
4 Kaatz M, Elsner P, Bauer A: Body-modifying concepts and dermatologic problems. Clin Dermatol 2008;26:35–44.
5 Kluger N: Cutaneous complications related to permanent decorative tattooing. Expert Rev Clin Immunonol 2010;6: 363–371.
6 Desai NA, Smith ML: Body art in adolescents: paint, piercings and perils. Adolesc Med 2011;22:97–118.
7 Wenzel SM, Rittman I, Landthaler M, Bäumler W: Adverse reactions after tattooing: review of the literature and comparison to results of a survey. Dermatology 2013;226:138–147.

8 Høgsberg T, Carlsen KH, Serup J: High prevalence of minor symptoms in tattooos among a young population tattooed with carbon black and organic pigments. J Eur Acad Dermatol Venereol 2013;27:846–852.
9 Hutton Carlsen K, Serup J: Photosensitivity and photodynamic events in balck, red and blue tattooos are common. A 'Beach Study'. J Eur Acad Dermatol Venereol 2013, DOI: 10.1111/jdv.12093.
10 Berchon E: Histoire Médicale du Tatouage. Paris, J-B Baillié et Fils, 1869.
11 Klügl I, Hiller K-A, Landthaler M, Bäumler W: Incidence of health problems associated with tattooed skin: a nation-wide survey in German-speaking countries. Dermatology 2010;221:43–50.
12 Kluger N, Koljonen V: Tattoos, inks and cancer. Lancet Oncol 2012;13:e161–e168.
13 Pittelkow MR, Perry HO, Muller SA, Maughan WZ, O'Brian PC: Skin cancer in patients with psoriasis trteated with coal tar: a 25-year follow-up study. Arch Dermatol 1981;117:465–468.

14 Maughan WZ, Muller SA, Perry HO, Pittelkow MR, O'Brian PC: Incidence of skin cancers in patients with atopic dermatitis treated with coal tar: a 25-years follow-up study. J Am Acad Dermatol 1980;3:612–615.
15 The Danish Ministry of the Environment. Chemical substances in tattoo inks. Reports 215/216, 2012. ISBS 978–87–92779–86–1. www.mst.dk.
16 Serup J, Hutton Carlsen K: Patch test study of 90 patients with tattoo reactions: negative outcome of allergy patch to baseline batteries and culprit inks suggests allergen(s) are generated in the skin through haptinization. Contact Dermatitis 2014;71:255–263.
17 Long GE, Rickman LS: Infectious complications of tattoos. Clin Infect Dis 1994;18:610–619.
18 Kluger N: Complications infectieuses cutanées assciées au tatouage permanent. Méd Mal Infect 2011;41:115–122.
19 Høgsberg T, Saunte DM, Frimodt-Møller N, Serup J: Microbial status and product labelling of 58 original tattoo inks. J Eur Acad Dermatol Venereol 2013;27:73–80.

20 Baumgartner A, Gautsch S: Hygienic-microbiological quality of tattoo- and permanent make-up colours. J Verbrauch Lebensm 2011;6:319–325.

21 Laumann AE: History and epidemiology of tattoos and piercings, legislation in the United States; in: de Cuyoer C, Perez-Cotapos M-L (eds): Dermatologic Complications with Body Art. Berlin-Heidelberg, Springer Verlag, 2010, pp 1–11.

22 Council of Europe. Resolution ResAP(2008)1 on Requirements and Criteria for the Safety of Tattoos and Permanent Make-Up. Strasbourg, Council of Europe, 2008.

23 Thaldorf C, Liberman A: Integration of health care organizations: using the power strategies of horizontal and vertical integration in public and private health systems. Health Care Manag 2007;2:116–127.

24 Hutton Carlsen K, Serup J: Patients with tattoo reactions have reduced quality of life and suffer from itch: dermatology Life Quality Index and Itch Severity Score measurements. Skin Res Technol 2015, DOI: 10.1111/srt 12164.

Prof. Jørgen Serup, MD
Department of Dermatology D41, Bispebjerg University Hospital
Bispebjerg Bakke 23
DK–2400 Copenhagen NV (Denmark)
E-Mail Joergen.vedelskov.serup@regionh.dk

Serup J, Kluger N, Bäumler W (eds): Tattooed Skin and Health.
Curr Probl Dermatol. Basel, Karger, 2015, vol 48, pp 248–252 (DOI: 10.1159/000369231)

Regulation of Tattoo Ink Production and the Tattoo Business in the US

I.M. Haugh[a] · S.L. Laumann[b] · Anne E. Laumann[a]

[a]Dermatology Department, Feinberg School of Medicine, Northwestern University, Chicago, Ill.,
[b]Chicago, Ill., USA

Abstract

The production of tattoo ink and pigments in the US is unregulated. There are no guidelines or standards issued by national agencies. However, the practice of tattooing is regulated at the state and local levels but varies widely. Adverse events are addressed when a problem is reported. © 2015 S. Karger AG, Basel

One out of five adults (21%) in the US today has a tattoo. This amounts to over 50 million people, and the number is increasing. The fact that the art of tattooing is associated with health risks is undeniable and openly acknowledged by the US Food and Drug Administration (FDA) [1]. Therefore, due to the large number of people at risk for adverse reactions from tattooing procedures and the deposition of pigment into the body, meaningful regulation of tattoo ink production and the tattoo industry in the US is crucial.

The structure of the legal system in the US differs from that in Europe. The country's Constitution grants specific powers to the national or 'federal' government. The 10th Amendment to the US Constitution states that 'powers not delegated to the United States by the Constitution, nor prohibited by it to the States, are reserved to the States, respectively, or to the people'. Therefore, the individual states have the power to regulate everything else. As laws governing the tattoo artistry are not outlined in the US Constitution, rules relating to this field are controlled independently by each of the 50 states. The result is that different rules apply in different states, with the extent of regulation varying widely. Some jurisdictions have stringent laws in place, whereas others have very minimal requirements (table 1). Within the states, at the local level, agencies such as a city or county board of health have the power to enact and enforce laws.

Sandra Laumann, BA, JD studied Political Science at the University of Michigan and completed her education as a lawyer at Fordham University School of Law.
Isabel Haugh, MB BAO BCh, Dermatology Research Fellow, Northwestern University, Ann & Robert H. Lurie Children's Hospital of Chicago, Chicago, Ill., USA.

Table 1. A comparison of selected tattoo regulations between the 50 states

State	Educational standards for artists for infection control	Disclosure of potential risks to consumers	Standards for sterile technique	Tattoo artists required to wear gloves	Hepatitis B vaccine offered to tattoo artists	Artist health screening, including for hepatitis B, required	Artists required to report adverse events
Alabama	Y	Y	Y	Y	Y	N	Y
Alaska	Y	Y	N	N	N	N	N
Arizona	N	N	N	N	N	N	N
Arkansas	Y	N	Y	Y	N	Y	Y
California	Y	Y	Y	Y	Y	N	N
Colorado	Y	Y	Y	Y	Y	N	N
Connecticut	Y	N	N	N	N	N	N
Delaware	Y	Y	Y	Y	Y	N	N
Florida	Y	N	Y	Y	N	N	N
Georgia	N	N	Y	Y	Y	N	N
Hawaii	Y	N	Y	N	N	N	N
Idaho	N	N	N	N	N	N	N
Illinois	Y	Y	Y	Y	N	N	Y
Indiana	Y	N	Y	Y	Y	N	N
Iowa	Y	N	Y	Y	N	N	N
Kansas	Y	Y	Y	Y	N	N	N
Kentucky	N	Y	Y	Y	N	N	N
Louisiana	Y	Y	Y	Y	Y	N	N
Maine	Y	N	Y	Y	N	N	Y
Maryland	N	N	Y	Y	Y	N	N
Massachusetts	Y	Y	Y	Y	Y	N	Y
Michigan	Y	N	Y	Y	Y	N	N
Minnesota	Y	N	Y	Y	N	N	Y
Mississippi	Y	Y	Y	Y	N	N	N
Missouri	Y	Y	Y	Y	N	N	N
Montana	Y	Y	Y	Y	Y	N	N
Nebraska	Y	N	Y	Y	N	N	N
Nevada	Y	N	N	Y	N	N	Y
New Hampshire	Y	N	Y	N	N	N	N
New Jersey	Y	Y	Y	Y	Y	N	Y
New Mexico	Y	N	N	N	Y	N	N
New York	Y	N	N	N	N	N	N
North Carolina	N	N	Y	Y	N	N	N
North Dakota	Y	Y	Y	Y	Y	Y	Y
Ohio	N	Y	Y	Y	N	N	N
Oklahoma	Y	Y	Y	Y	Y	Y	Y
Oregon	Y	N	N	N	N	N	N
Pennsylvania	Y	Y	Y	Y	Y	Y	N
Rhode Island	Y	N	Y	Y	Y	N	N
South Carolina	Y	Y	Y	Y	Y	N	Y
South Dakota	N	N	Y	Y	N	N	Y
Tennessee	Y	N	Y	Y	Y	N	N
Texas	Y	N	Y	Y	N	N	Y
Utah	N	N	N	N	N	N	N
Vermont	Y	N	N	N	N	N	N
Virginia	N	N	Y	N	N	N	N

Table 1. Continued

State	Educational standards for artists for infection control	Disclosure of potential risks to consumers	Standards for sterile technique	Tattoo artists required to wear gloves	Hepatitis B vaccine offered to tattoo artists	Artist health screening, including for hepatitis B, required	Artists required to report adverse events
Washington	Y	N	Y	Y	N	N	N
West Virginia	N	Y	Y	Y	N	N	N
Wisconsin	N	Y	Y	Y	N	Y	N
Wyoming	N	N	N	N	N	N	N

Y = Yes; N = no.
Data obtained from http://www.cdc.gov/niosh/topics/body_art/stateRegs.html, accessed September 30, 2014.

Engaging in tattoo artistry is not a risk-free process for either the tattoo artist or the tattooee. Gaps in the regulatory system create the potential for widespread harm. Pathogen contamination of tattoo materials to be injected into the skin can occur during ink production as well as during the tattooing process. During the tattooing process, bacteria can be introduced through a nonsterile needle, the tattoo artist not wearing gloves, or the tattoo artist or the tattooee carrying and passing on a blood-borne disease through failure to use proper aseptic techniques. The composite parts of the pigments may include carcinogens and allergens. The deposition of these into the body is another source of risk. An area of particular concern with any needle-using activity is the transmission of human immunodeficiency virus and hepatitis, as these infections can have devastating potential sequelae. In order to ensure safety, each step requires oversight.

Another agency regulating and overseeing disease control within the US is the Occupational Safety and Health Administration, a federal agency within the US Department of Labor. This federal department outlines safety and health standards for employees in contact with toxic and hazardous substances. These include standards for handling contaminated materials, planning exposure control, washing hands, disposing of sharps,

wearing gloves, and offering hepatitis B vaccination for employees. Within these regulations, hepatitis B vaccination is not compulsory, and employers need only make hepatitis B vaccinations available to employees who have had an occupational exposure such as a needle stick injury. However, some workplaces are exempt from these regulations. These include independent contractors and other self-employed individuals, and therefore, it is likely that many tattoo facilities are excluded from these rules. Local governments and municipalities have the power to enact and enforce such regulations but are not obliged to do so.

The FDA has the power to regulate the production of the ink and pigments used in intradermal tattoos, yet it has chosen not to due to 'competing health priorities and a lack of evidence of safety problems specifically associated with these pigments' (FDA website: Tattoos and Permanent Makeup: Fact Sheet). Tattoo inks have been classified as cosmetics and are not regulated before going to market. This is in contrast to other 'colors', such as colors in food and drugs for ingestion and colors in cosmetics for external placement on the skin, which the FDA does regulate. As the pigments used in tattoo inks are color additives, they could be subject to premarket approval under the Federal Food, Drug, and Cosmetic Act. The FDA's goal is to encourage consumers as well as tattoo and permanent make-up artists to take precautions and to urge potentially infected clients to seek medical care. Adverse event reporting is important in order for the FDA to be able to investigate and take action. The FDA posts warnings to consumers about adverse events and recalls. These are publicly available to enable both consumers and tattoo artists to take steps in order to help to decrease the likelihood of further problems.

Instead of carrying out premarket approval of tattoo inks, the FDA reacts to adverse events to prevent further consumer injury or illness. The FDA investigates incidents that are reported and takes action as appropriate [1]. An example of the FDA responding to such an event occurred following an outbreak of *Mycobacterium chelonae* skin infections in Monroe County, New York, in 2011, which led to a voluntary recall of the contaminated ink. There were also cases in Washington, Iowa, and Colorado that were unrelated to the New York cases. The contaminated ink in those cases was identified, and there were voluntary recalls involving multiple ink manufacturers. This emergency response was a joint effort between the FDA and the Centers for Disease Control and Prevention. As with the FDA, the Centers for Disease Control and Prevention are reactive, not proactive, and only act in response to outbreaks of infections related to tattooing. No agency is taking precautionary measures to prevent the occurrence of such crises.

Interestingly, the FDA has carved out a medical exception to its solely reactive role in the tattoo business. Tattooing devices, which were developed for tattooing radiotherapy targets on the skin of radiation oncology patients, have been approved by the FDA. They are described as tools to 'to permanently mark the central axis or field borders of any radiation fields used to treat a patient'. These were approved under the 'medicinal device category' as FDA class 1 exempt devices, and therefore, one could argue that the ink within was also approved. In fact, the tattoo pigment used within these devices may be regular ink sold for use in fountain pens. This FDA safety 'guarantee' is reassuring to both physicians and patients. It appears as though these devices or a similar device could be developed or approved for cosmetic use. Today, many pigments used in tattoo inks are industrial-grade colors suitable for printers' ink or automobile paint. The FDA could theoretically develop an administrative code to create standards and criteria for tattoo ink in order to prevent distribution of contaminated inks or inks containing known allergenic components.

The risk of immediate introduction of infection with tattooing is undeniable. Another area of concern is the long-term safety of intradermal pigment. The implications of this have not been thoroughly investigated. Recently, tattoo inks that contain azo and polycyclic pigments are becoming more widely used. Not one of these products has been adequately studied to determine whether it is safe for use in humans. At the FDA's Arkansas-based National Center for Toxicological Research, investigations are being performed into the chemical composition of some tattoo inks and their metabolism in the human body, in addition to other studies to clarify their safety [2]. Tattoo pigments can drain from the skin and move deeper into the body through the lymphatic system, a collection of fluid-carrying vessels in the body that filter out disease-causing organisms. The long-term effects of this have not yet been established.

In conclusion, the production of tattoo ink and pigments in the US is an unregulated industry. There are no guidelines or standards issued by federal agencies. Furthermore, there is no screening of tattoo pigments prior to placement on the market for permanent introduction into the body. Adverse events such as infections are addressed only once a problem is reported.

For the physical act of tattooing, regulation is controlled at the state and local levels. The degree to which this is regulated differs widely by location. Regulations sufficient to safeguard the health and safety of consumers in tattoo parlors are dependent on the local jurisdictions across the US. Interestingly, probably due to a cultural moral preference, regulations regarding the age at which a minor may get a tattoo, who must give consent and be present at such a time, and what records must be kept do exist in a meaningful form in virtually every state.

At the federal level, the FDA is prepared to react quickly when there is a crisis. Recently, the FDA discovered and forced a recall of a do-it-yourself tattoo kit being sold online in which the ink was contaminated with multiple bacteria, thus stopping a potentially large-scale outbreak of infection in the US. However, tattoo inks, pigments, and do-it-yourself at-home tattoo kits are still readily available online, and due to the fact that the FDA has to rely on reporting of adverse incidents by consumers in order to act, the timely reporting of such incidents to this agency is the only way that consumers can be protected and protect others. Despite the lack of regulation and the large numbers of Americans who get tattoos annually in this growing industry, the fact is that getting a tattoo remains reasonably safe, with a very low reported occurrence of adverse events.

References

1 Braverman S: One in Five Adults Now Has a Tattoo. New York, Harris Interactive, 2012. http://www.harrisinteractive.com/NewsRoom/HarrisPolls/tabid/447/mid/1508/articleId/970/ctl/ReadCustom%20Default/Default.aspx (accessed September 30, 2014).

2 Tattoo & Permanent Makeup: Fact Sheet. Silver Spring, MD, US Food and Drug Administration, 2012. http://www.fda.gov/Cosmetics/ProductsIngredients/Products/ucm108530.htm (accessed September 27, 2014).

Anne E. Laumann, MBChB, MRCP (UK)
Professor of Dermatology, Division Chief of Medical Dermatology
Director of the Collagen Vascular Disorders Clinic, Feinberg School of Medicine, Northwestern University
676 N. St. Clair Suite 1600
Chicago, IL 60611 (USA)
E-Mail a-laumann@northwestern.edu

Author Index

Subject Index